THE SUPERFAMILY WITH VON WILLEBRAND FACTOR VA DOMAINS

Alfonso Colombatti, M.D.

Roberto Doliana, Ph.D.

Centro di Riferimento Oncologico
Istituto Nazionale Tumori Centroeuropeo
Aviano, Italy
Departmento di Scienze
eTechnologie Biomediche, Universitá di Voline
Voline, Italy

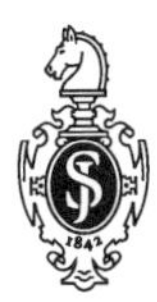

Springer
New York Berlin Heidelberg London Paris
Tokyo Hong Kong Barcelona Budapest

R.G. LANDES COMPANY
AUSTIN

MOLECULAR BIOLOGY INTELLIGENCE UNIT
THE SUPERFAMILY WITH VON WILLEBRAND FACTOR VA DOMAINS

R.G. LANDES COMPANY
Austin, Texas, U.S.A.

Please address all inquiries to the Publishers:
R.G. Landes Company, 909 Pine Street, Georgetown, Texas, U.S.A. 78626
Phone: 512/ 863 7762; FAX: 512/ 863 0081

International distributor (except North America):

Springer-Verlag GmbH & Co. KG
Tiergartenstrasse 17, D-69121 Heidelberg, Germany

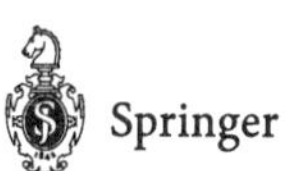
Springer

International ISBN: 3-540-61448-6

Library of Congress Cataloging-in-Publication Data
Colombatti, Alfonso.
    The superfamily with von Willebrand factor VA domains / Alfonso
Colombatti. Robert Doliana.
       p. cm. — (Molecular biology intelligence unit)
    Includes bibliographical references and index.
    ISBN 0-57059-387-6 (RGL : alk. paper). — ISBN 3-540-61448-6 (SV : alk. paper)
    1. von Willebrand factor — Structure.   I. Doliana, Roberto. II. Title. III. Series.
    [DNLM: 1. von Willebrand factor — physiology. 2. Molecular
Structure. WH 310 C718s 1996]
QP93.7.V65C65 1996
612.1'2—dc20
DNLM/DLC
for Library of Congress   96-28891
                                               CIP r96

Publisher's Note

R.G. Landes Company publishes six book series: *Medical Intelligence Unit, Molecular Biology Intelligence Unit, Neuroscience Intelligence Unit, Tissue Engineering Intelligence Unit, Biotechnology Intelligence Unit* and *Environmental Intelligence Unit.* The authors of our books are acknowledged leaders in their fields and the topics are unique. Almost without exception, no other similar books exist on these topics.

Our goal is to publish books in important and rapidly changing areas of bioscience and environment for sophisticated researchers and clinicians. To achieve this goal, we have accelerated our publishing program to conform to the fast pace in which information grows in bioscience. Most of our books are published within 90 to 120 days of receipt of the manuscript. We would like to thank our readers for their continuing interest and welcome any comments or suggestions they may have for future books.

Shyamali Ghosh
Publications Director
R.G. Landes Company

CONTENTS

PREFACE

The exponential growth of sequence databases has revealed that an increasing number of proteins, which exert diversified functions, contain homologous modules with primary sequences that can present even very low similarity but possess similar tertiary structures. The superfamily of proteins with von Willebrand factor type A modules (VWFA) consists of 27 members present in a wide range of species including man, pig, cow, dog, chicken, parasites, *Xenopus* and *C. elegans* with 50 different VWFA modules. Several recent findings have spurred the interest in VWFA modules: the suggestion based on multiple alignment secondary structure predictions that the structure of a VWFA module is similar to the three-dimensional doubly-wound α/β open twisted sheet structure of p21[ras]; the determination of the high resolution crystal structure of other VWFA modules; and finally, the identification of a new cation binding motif (metal ion dependent adhesion site = MIDAS) within the VWFA module. Furthermore, the molecular cloning, expression and mutagenesis investigations are yielding important new insights into the structure-function relationships of several numbers of the VWFA superfamily. This is going to contribute soon also to the understanding of mechanisms of action of the less studied members of the superfamily.

The first chapter in this book introduces the terminology and focuses on the primary sequences and structural organization of the VWFA modules. The remaining chapters detail the role of the different protein classes which harbor VWFA modules including: (1) von Willebrand factor, its fundamental role in haemostasis and thrombosis and the consequences of its alterations in von Willebrand disease (chapter 2); (2) $\beta 1$ integrins and their relationships with extracellular matrix molecules, laminins and collagens in particular (chapter 3); (3) $\beta 2$ integrins and their function in cell/cell adhesion phenomena, in immune responses, in leukocyte homing as well as their interaction with soluble ligands (chapter 4); (4) proteins involved in the complement activation cascade (chapter 5); (5) several extracellular matrix constituents and their molecular networks (chapter 6); and (6) other proteins including the integrin of intraepithelial lymphocyte ($\alpha E\beta 7$), the L-type voltage gated Ca^{2+}-channel, the inter-α-inhibitor family of protease inhibitors and proteins of parasites such as *Plasmodium falciparum*.

We have attempted to present a comprehensive picture of the VWFA superfamily with the primary scope to foster the interdisciplinary connections prompted by the widespread presence of the members of the superfamily in different biological systems.

We would like to thank our colleagues in the laboratory who managed the daily work while we were spending a great deal of our time writing chapters for this book. I (AC) thank my wife Emilia and our five children for their patience and continuous support during my long weekends spent at home polishing this book.

Alfonso Colombatti
Roberto Doliana
April 1996

ACKNOWLEDGMENTS

The work of the authors is supported by grants from the Associazione Italiana per la Ricerca sul Cancro, the Consiglio Nazionale delle Ricerche-Progetto Finalizzato ACRO and Ministero della Sanità-Ricerca Finalizzata 1994-1995.

CHAPTER 1

INTRODUCTION

It is becoming apparent that, as the number of known protein sequences grows, many extracellular as well as intracellular proteins are built from relatively few (probably less than 100 for extracellular proteins) different kind of modular units, repeatedly used as 'building blocks' in functionally distinct proteins. In the course of evolution, these structural units have been used over and over again and the successive divergence confer to them different sequence characteristics and hence also different functional tasks.

Similar stretches of amino acid sequences, found in one or more proteins, have been variously called "Structural Units", "Repeats", "Modules", "Motifs" or "Domains". In particular, the term "Domain" describes a spatially distinct unit, not necessarily contiguous in sequence, having characteristic structural features and capable of folding up independently of neighboring sequences.[1] In contrast, "Modules" are contiguous in sequence, and are repeatedly used as building blocks in functionally diverse proteins. The two terms are very often, but not always, interchangeable. The "Module" definition is then used when referring to the particular kind of domain that is clearly associated with exon shuffling and duplication. The term "Superfamily" defines a set of related sequences belonging to two or more families and whose different proteins may or may not share sequence similarity with all members of the family in the set.[2] The module we will describe herein is constituted by a consensus sequence, about 200 amino acid residues long, first identified in the von Willebrand factor (vWF) hemostatic protein as a triplicated unit called "A" module.[3] Similar modules recognized in other proteins have usually been denoted vWF type A-like domains by scholars of the ECM field, and "I" domain by scholars of the integrin field (as they appeared to be "Inserted" segments in some integrin α chains). Although this consensus sequence fits into definitions of both "module" and "domain", we will refer mainly to VWFA as a "module" throughout this book.

A recent international workshop on extracellular protein modules has outlined a standardized nomenclature for about 50 distinct modules identified in extracellular proteins.[1] The common abbreviations adopt 3-5 characters, while a two-letter designation is suggested for use in cartoons and figures. Following this nomenclature, we will refer to the vWF type A-like module as VWFA in the text, and as VA in the figures.

The Superfamily with von Willebrand Factor VA Domains, edited by
Alfonso Colombatti and Roberto Doliana. © 1996 R.G. Landes Company.

SPREADING OF MODULES IN EXTRACELLULAR PROTEINS

The insertion or deletion of building blocks in many multimodular proteins can be traced over too short phylogenetic timescales to involve gene duplication and gene fusion alone. The most probable evolutionary mechanism employed in building mosaic proteins, i.e., proteins containing a set of different structural units, is exon shuffling, which is the promotion of nonhomologous rearrangements between genes.[4] By this mechanism complex genetic information can be built up by joining previously independent exons, thus giving rise to more complex proteins and to novel functions. The exon shuffling theory assumes that modules are encoded by exons flanked by introns that, acting as a buffer during shuffling events, preventing gene destruction. Moreover, the large size of introns implies that random rearrangements can bring exons into new combinations with much higher frequency than would be possible for rearrangement in a continuous coding sequence. Depending upon the position in which the first codon of an exon is interrupted by an intronic sequence, three different intron phase types are possible and are denoted 0, I and II. To avoid frame shift during mRNA translation, phase compatibility between the "donor" and "receiver" genes is necessary. If the phase of the inserted intron were different from the phase of the accepting intron, the downstream exons would be translated in a different frame and this would mean disruption of the protein structure. Almost all the module gene structures, including those encoding VWFA modules, are at phase I-I. The reason for the predominance of phase I-I exons is not understood yet, but it could result from a random selection among primordial sequences.[5] A low degree of homology in exon-intron structures and between intron sequences is frequently detected among repeated modules. While this finding is in contrast with the exon shuffling theory, the well known mechanism of intron mobility and the high rate of mutation in intronic sequences may explain this apparent discrepancy. In fact, it is rather common that even genes coding for the same protein in evolutionarily close species, present a quite high variability in the number, length and sequences of the intronic regions.

LOCALIZATION OF MODULES

Approximately 50 distinct modules have been identified thus far that are shuffled about in various extracellular proteins. A distinction between extra/and intracellular protein modules is justified as their localization is usually not interchangeable. If extra/and intracellular modules are mixed in the same protein they are well separated in terms of cellular compartments. For example, fibronectin type III (FN3) modules, and Immunoglobulin (Ig)-like modules are found in the extracellular portion of many tyrosine kinase receptors where they can interact with specific ligands, while in the cytoplasmatic portion of the same proteins are confined the classical intracellular modules SH2 and SH3. There are some exceptions to the rule: the FN3 and Ig-like modules are found in the intracellular muscle protein Titin.[6-7] The latter is also found in other intracellular proteins such as projectin.[8] Also phylogenetic restrictions have turned out to be less rigid than originally believed: the Ig[9] and the ankyrin modules[10] have been found in both eukaryotes and prokaryotes without a specific cellular location, whereas FN3 modules sporadically have moved to prokaryotes for a phenomenon of horizontal transmission.[11] All the VWFA modules identified to date are localized in the extracellular compartment, both in ECM proteins and in the extracellular part of transmembrane proteins.

ASSIGNMENT OF A SEQUENCE TO A FAMILY OF MODULES

Assignment of an amino acid sequence to a family of modules is hampered by the fact that module shuffling is frequently accompanied by a change in its function and the relaxation of functional constraints usually leads to significant sequence divergence. Many modules lack homogeneous homology along the primary sequence, but may exhibit instead an alternance between well conserved and often similarly short stretches of amino acids, and stretches of different length with very low or no detectable homology. The latter description is certainly the case for FN3 and VWFA modules. In other instances a module is characterized by a specific cysteine pattern where disulfide bridges help stabilize the folded structure; the overall homology for this kind of modules is usually very low, sometimes below 30%. The EGF module is a good example: six cysteines similarly spaced in all the known EGF modules forming disulfide bonds are found along the sequence while some glycins and aromatic residues are present in fixed positions to permit β-strand arrangment.[12] In accordance with a wide functional diversity demonstrated for the EGF modules, no homologous functional residues are detectable, and the connecting segments between cysteines are very flexible in length as well in amino acid composition. Nevertheless, the few conserved amino acids are able to confer a similar tertiary structure to all the EGF modules analysed by NMR: the dominant feature of the structure is a β-sheet platform with three disulfide bonds radiating up from one face to various other loops and turns.[13] The fact that sequences having very low homology undergo folding in similar tertiary structures is not surprising considering that amino acid sequences are eroded during evolution at a much faster rate than their three-dimensional structures. Thus, two modules derived from a common ancestor may share similarity only at the tertiary structural level. In contrast, two topologically similar sequences might be the result of a convergent evolution of noncorrelated primary sequences toward a similar three-dimensional folding having a stable core structure. The functional specifity of the modules with similar tertiary structure but different primary sequence is given by different surface "patches" of amino acids able to interact with rather distinct ligand molecules. It has been shown for example that CYTR, the N-terminal domain of the cytokine receptor superfamily, has a three-dimensional structure very similar to that of the widespread, and apparently non-correlated, FN3 module.[14] Moreover a G domain from factor IX has the same fold as an EGF module.[15] Also the VWFA domain has a three-dimensional "twin": using multiple alignment-based secondary structure prediction and protein fold recognition algorithms, Edward and Perkins found a striking three-dimensional similarity between the known structure of the GTP binding fold of human $p21^{ras}$ and the predicted structure of the VWFA module.[16] This prediction has been later confirmed by the high resolution crystal analysis of the recombinant VWFA module of the β2 integrin Mac-1,[17] whose structure differs from that of $p21^{ras}$ only in the orientation of two β-strands. The almost perfect match between the three-dimensional structure calculated comparing the primary sequences of 75 VWFA modules, and the crystal structure of the VWFA module of Mac-1, suggests that the large majority of or even all modules of this family might fold up in a very similar way, conserving the same number, alternance and relative spatial disposition of their secondary motifs.

PROTEINS CONTAINING VWFA MODULES

To date 27 polypeptides are known to contain one or more VWFA modules contributing to the structure of 25 proteins. The total number of different VWFA modules is 50, but as some of them have been sequenced in more species, overall the sequences of 99 VWFA modules are presently stored in the database. The proteins included in the VWFA superfamily may be grouped in different classes depending upon their localization and/or function.

Extracellular Matrix Proteins

The vast majority of VWFA modules are expressed in this class of proteins with close to half of the known VWFA modules encompassing the nonfibrillar type VI collagen.[18-31] This collagen is the only member of the superfamily constituted by different chains each carrying VWFA modules, and the only one in which VWFA modules are singularly involved in alternative splicing phenomena.[21,23] Type VI collagen is expressed in many connective tissues including cartilage and it is one of the major components of the extracellular matrix (ECM). This collagen presents a complex multimodular structure reflecting a variety of interactions with ECM components and cells in diverse biological phenomena such as ECM assembly, cell adhesion and cell migration during embryogenesis. Another non-fibrillar collagen, type VII, the major if not the exclusive component of the anchoring fibrils, attachment structures at the dermal-epidermal basement membrane zone, bears 2 VWFA modules.[32-35] The FACIT (Fibril Associated Collagens with Interrupted Triple helix) types XII[36-39] and XIV[40-42] collagens contain 2-4 and 2 modules, respectively. These collagens do not form fibrils by themselves, but appear to be intimately associated with the surface of interstitial collagen fibrils, perhaps mediating their interactions with other matrix molecules. The only ECM noncollagenous protein carrying VWFA modules is Cartilage Matrix Protein (CMP),[43-45] a very unique protein as it is formed only by two VWFA modules separated by a single EGF module. CMP is a major component of cartilage matrix interacting with collagen fibrils[46] and proteoglycans.[47] It has been suggested that CMP may be involved in type II collagen fibrillogenesis and in the organization of the cartilage matrix.[48]

Plasma Proteins

The prototype of the VWFA superfamily, von Willebrand Factor, contains three VWFA modules.[49-54] This multimeric glycoprotein mediates platelet adhesion to exposed subendothelium and stabilizes clotting factor VIII.[55] In the plasma compartment two key elements of the classical and alternative activation pathways of complement, factor B[56-60] and C2,[61,62] each carrying one module are also included. Finally, one VWFA module is part of the four noninhibitory subunits components H1,

H2, H3 and H4 of the inter-α-inhibitor (IαI) family,[63-68] a representative group of the superfamily of Kunitz type proteinase inhibitors in mammals.

Plasma Membrane Proteins

Seven of the 15 known integrin α subunits contain a VWFA module (called usually "I" domain). The α1β1 (VLA-1)[69-71] and α2β1 (VLA-2)[72-75] belong to the class of cell surface receptors for ECM molecules, whereas LFA-1 (CD11a/CD18, αLβ2),[76] Mac-1 (CD11b/CD18, αMβ2),[77-79] p150,95 (CD 11c/CD18, αXβ2)[80,81] and the recently isolated αDβ2[82] belong to the leukocyte β2 family of receptors that function as general adhesion proteins in immune interactions, contribute to leukocyte adhesion to endothelial cells and mediate cell activation and signaling. The last α chain containing a VWFA domain is αE,[83] that associates with β7 subunit and is primarily expressed on intraepithelial lymphocytes. Other plasma membrane proteins containing VWFA modules are: the α2δ subunit of L-type voltage-dependent dihydropyridine-sensitive calcium channel;[84] the protozoan parasite-derived proteins *Plasmodium falciparum* malarial thrombospondin-related anonymous protein (TRAP)[85] and the similar protein of the *Plasmodium yoelii* (PySSP2)[86] that might both offer a chance for parasites to mimic host functions; the *Eimeria tenella* microneme protein Etp100[87] and the corresponding protein isolated in *Eimeria maxima*,[88] herewith called Emp100 by analogy with Etp100; and finally the *C. elegans*-derived hyphothetical protein (337.6), with a putative membrane spanning region (partial sequence reported in ref. 17).

GENOMIC STRUCTURE

The genomic structure of several members of the VWFA superfamily has been elucidated and a distinct pattern of organization of the exons encoding the characteristic modules in the different proteins has emerged. The position of the exon/intron boundaries and the phase class of the intervening sequences vary considerably among different genes. Even in the case of

CMP, where the two repeats show 55% sequence similarity at the protein level, the splice junctions do not occur at corresponding positions.

As shown in Fig. 1.1, VWFA modules are encoded within 1-5 exons. Notable exceptions exist in the vWF gene, in which the modules A1 and A2 are encoded within a single exon also encoding part of VWFD module, and in Etp100, in which the sequence coding for a VWFA module is part of a large exon also coding for unrelated parts of the protein. In spite of these differences in gene organization, the translation products are quite similar: all the homologous repeats are approximately 200 amino acids long and, conforming to the shuffling theory, the splice sites at the beginning and at the end of the coding sequences are conserved at the same phase class (ph I-I), with the exception of one module of the α2 chain of type VI collagen, that has an I-0 phase class (module D3, according to the nomenclature reported in ref 25) and of the H1 gene of the IaI family that has a 0-0 phase class. That all

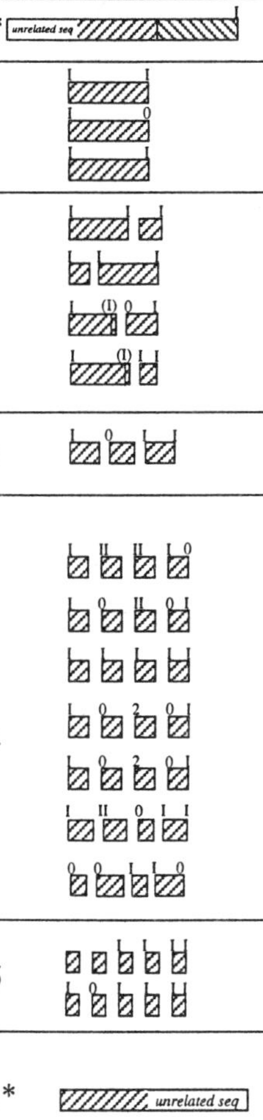

N. of exons/module	protein	module(s)	species	ref.
1/2*	vWF	A1+A2	h	54
1	α1(VI)	C1	c	25,
	α2(VI)	N1, C1	h, c	29,25
	α3(VI)	N10,N9,N8,N7,N6,N5,N4,N3,N2	h, c	28,21
2	α3(VI)	N1	h	28
	α2(VI)	C2	h, c	29,25
	CMP	CMP-1	h, c	45,44
	CMP	CMP-2	h, c	44
3	a1(VII)	VII-2	h	33
4	α1(VI)	C1	c	25
	α1(VI)	C2	c	25
	vWF	A3	h	54
	p150,95	I	h	81
	Mac-1	I	h	79
	a1(VII)	VII-1	h	33
	ITI-H1		h	68
5	factor B		h, m	56,62
	C2		m	62
1*	ETP 100		e	87

Fig. 1.1. Comparison of the structure of the exons encoding VWFA modules. The number and the approximate relative size of the exons are shown. The location of splice boundaries is indicated by vertical lines. The phase class of intervening sequences appears in Roman numerals above the exons, if known.

the known genes containing VWFA modules express at least one or several entire VWFA modules, is highly suggestive of the existence of a primordial structural domain encoded within one single exon. In spite of the insertion in some modules of one or more introns interrupting the original exon, genes expressing incomplete VWFA modules have never been isolated, indicating that the VWFA module needs to be expressed in its entirety to maintain a stable three-dimensional structure. A notable exception is a splicing form of C2 mRNA in kidney that is lacking exons 6, 7 and 18. Exons 6 and 7 code for the first half of the VWFA module. However, it is not yet known whether this form is translated in a functional protein. For some of the proteins, a phylogenetic tree has been proposed on the basis of the amino acid sequence homology and gene structures.

TYPE VI COLLAGEN

A module of about 600 bp, flanked by introns of phase class I, might have encoded the precursor of each of the globular domains A1, A2 and A3 (also called N1, C1 and C2 in the human molecule). This module later joined with a gene coding for a collagenic segment to form a primordial version of a type VI collagen gene. The striking conservation of the exon/intron pattern of the α1 (VI) and the α2 (VI) genes[25] together with the synthetic location on the long arm of chromosome 21 in the human genome,[24] strongly suggest that the two genes evolved by gene duplication. The α3 (VI) chain is much more complex, containing 9 additional VWFA modules at the N-terminus, one FN3 module and a Kunitz-like module in the C-terminus. In order to explain the formation of the α3 gene, Stokes et al[28] have proposed that a first duplication of the type VI primordial gene originated the prototype for the α3 (VI) gene and the prototype for the α1/α2 (VI) gene, and the latter more recently duplicated to form the distinct α1 (VI) and α2 (VI) genes. The VWFA modules at the N-terminus of the α3 (VI) gene, duplicated once before the acquisition of one intron (still present in both human and chicken

genes). Finally, the newly formed VWFA module duplicated sequentially originating the present gene in which there are 9 N-terminus VWFA modules coded by one exon each, called N2-N10 in the human gene and A2 -A9 in the chicken gene, that share higher sequence identity within themselves than to subdomains N1, C1 and C2 (A1', A2' and A3' in the chicken, respectively).

CARTILAGE MATRIX PROTEIN

This protein is formed by two VWFA modules, CMP1 and CMP2, separated by an EGF-like module. Each of the two homologous VWFA modules is encoded by two exons.[44,45] The present structure of the VWFA modules at the genomic level could derive either from a duplication of a primitive small exon or from an insertion of an intron in a primitive single exon. Different observations support the latter mechanism. Firstly, the introns flanking the two exonic sequences coding for the CMP1 module are at different phase class and therefore an hypotetical duplication of a primitive small exon would have destroyed the reading frame. Secondly, the segments of the VWFA modules coded by exons 1 and 2 (CMP1) and 4 and 5 (CMP2) do not show any internal detectable homology, as would be expected in the case of a duplication phenomenon. Thirdly, the locations of the splice sites of the exons coding for CMP1 and CMP2 do not correspond, as would have been expected in the case of an independent phenomenon of intron insertion. The probable evolution of the CMP gene therefore should have involved a first duplication of an uninterrupted exon coding for a VWFA module followed by an independent insertion of one intronic sequence in each of the two exons.

α CHAINS ASSOCIATED WITH THE β2 SUBUNIT

The genomic organization of the single VWFA module present in the α chains of p150,95[81] and Mac-1[79] is very similar and quite complex, as there are four exons coding for 43, 48, 50 and 51 residues, respectively, separated by introns at different phase classes. However, in spite of this complexity, the introns flanking both 5' and 3' ends are conserved at phase class I, supporting the notion that also in this case the prototype VWFA module could have been inserted as a single exon that was interrupted by several introns later in evolution. As the splice junctions are sites in which an enhanced sequence variability of amino acids present at the protein surface is usually observed,[89] it is possible that the multiple intron insertions in the exons coding for the VWFA modules of Mac-1 and p150,95 shuffled in one of the primitive integrin genes contributed to confer the specific functions and binding specificities of this class of molecules.

PRIMARY STRUCTURE OF VWFA MODULES

A comprehensive list of the known VWFA modules has been reported by Perkins et al[90] who aligned the amino acid sequences of 75 VWFA modules. An updated (99 sequences) comparison based on that alignment including the following 22 VWFA modules amino acid sequences is shown in Fig. 1.2. The new entries are: (1) the previously called CMP-like domain present at the N-terminal of type VII collagen (VII-2); (2) the I module present in the αE chain; (3) the module "N10" belonging to the α3 chain of the human type VI collagen; (4) the VWFA modules present in the H3 and H4 subunits of human IαI, and the similar modules of the murine H1, H2 and H3 subunits; (5) the A1 and A2 modules of canine vWF (Gene Bank accession number L16903, Mancuso DJ); (6) the I module of the human α1β1 and those of the murine, pig and bovine α2β1; (7) the VWFA module of the *Plasmodium yoelii* sporozoites PySSP2,[86] and those of Etp100

and Emp100,[87-88] isolated from *Eimeria tenella* and *Eimeria maxima*, respectively; (8) one VWFA module sequenced from the type XII collagen of an urodele, corresponding to that numbered "III" in chicken;[39] (9) the VWFA modules contained in complement factor B of mouse,[62] lamprey[58] and *xenopus*[59,60] (in which two variants of factor B, called A and B have been identified); (10) the VWFA present in mouse complement factor C2;[62] and (11) the module present in the chicken α subunit of the α1β1 integrin.[71]

When considering only the VWFA modules whose genomic organization is known, the length varies between 190 and 215 amino acids, with an average length of 205 amino acid residues. The degree of conservation is rather low: only 38% of the residues are conserved or conservatively replaced in at least half of the 99 sequences, 18% in at least 70% and only 8 residues (7.5%) are almost invariable in the 99 aligned sequences. Six of the latter are hydrophobic (I,L,M,V,Y,P), and may be important for the structure of the inner protein core of the VWFA module. The remaining two are hydrophilic amino acids, a D/E and a S separated in the sequence by only one variable residue, and these have been found to play a key role for the function of VWFA modules (see below).

As it is emerging from other families of modules, the cysteine patterns in the VWFA modules is extremely variable: the cysteines residues are in a conserved position in only 20% of the 99 VWFA sequences and are almost all located at the module boundaries. Also the number of the cysteines is highly variable, ranging from none (in 16 of the 43 modules of the α3 chain of type VI collagen), to 9 (in the domain C2 of the same chain). The

Fig.1.2. (Next page) Alignment of VWFA module sequences. Criteria used are as in Perkins et al.[16] Each sequence, with the residues in the single letter code, is subdivided into 3 sections for readability (subseq a,b,c) Sequences that are defined by known intron exon boundaries are indicated to the left of the sequence. Groups of similar residues are defined: Tiny, G,A,S; aliphatic, I,L,V,M; aromatic, H,F,Y,W; positive, R,H,K; negative, D,E; hydroxyl, S,T; amide, N,Q. An asterisk above the sequences marks residue conservation of at least 50%; two asterisks mark those over 70% conservation. Residues that belong to these groups are shaded. The location of the α helices and β strands according to the crystal of Mac-1[17] and according to the prediction from Edward and Perkins[16] are shown beneath the sequence (arrowed ranges βA to α7). Arrowheads indicate the residues of the MIDAS motif. Abbreviation are: HUM, human; POR, porcine; BOV, bovine; MOU, mouse; RAB, rabbit; CHI, chick; XEN, xenopus; URO, urodele.

```
                                     1                           30    31           46    47               65
                  70% conservation                    ********* *        *   *  *  ** *      *        *****
                  50% conservation                    ********* ***      *   * ** ** *        *       *******
                                                       ▼  ▼  ▼

HUM vWF-1   (ex)               CSRLLDLVFLLDGSSRLSEA    EFEVLKAFVVDMMERL    RISQKWVRVAVVEYHDGSH
POR vWF-1                      CSKLLDLVFLLDGSDKLSEA    DFEALKVFVVGMMEHL    HISQKHIRVAVVEYHDGSH
BOV vWF-1                      CSKLLDLVFLLDGSDKLSEA    DFEALKAFVVGMMERL    HISQKRIRVAVVEYHDGSH
CAN vWF-1                      CSRLLDLVFLLDGSSKLSED    EFEVLKVFVVGMMEHL    HISQKRIRVAVVEYHDGSH
HUM vWF-2   (ex)   TVGPGLLGVSTLGPKRNSMVLDVAFVLEGSDKIGEA    DFNRSKEFMEEVIQRM    DVGQDSIHVTVLQYSYMVT
POR vWF-2          TVAPELPGVSTLEPKKR MVLDVVFVLEGSDKVGEA    NFNRSTEFVEEVIRRM    DVGRDSVHVTVLQYSYVVA
BOV vWF-2          TVGPQLLGPSLPGPKRSSVVLDVAFLLEGSDEVGEA    NFNRSAEFVEEVIRRM    DVGQDGIHVTVL
CAN vWF-2          TVGSELLGVSSPGPKRNSMVLDVVFVLEGSDKIGEA    NFNKSREFMEEVIQRM    DVGQDRIHVTVLQYSYMVT
HUM vWF-3   (ex)               DCSQPLDVILLLDGSSSFPAS    YFDEMKSFAKAFISKA    NIGPRLTQVSVLQYGSITT
HUM FACTOR B (ex)      PGEQQKRKIVLDPSGSMNIYLVLDGSDSIGAS    NFTGAKKCLVNLIEKV    ASYGVKPRYGLVTYATYPK
MOU FACTOR B (ex)      PGEQQKRKIVLDPSGSMNIYLVLDGSDSIGSS    NFTGAKRCLTNLIEKV    ASYGVRPRYGLLTYATVPK
XEN FACTOR Ba              RSVRILKDGLMNIFIVLDTSKSVGQN    RFDEAKSASILFIEKM    SNYDIKPRYCIISYASKAI
XEN FACTOR Bb              RSVQILKDGLMNIFIVLDTSKSVGEE    KFEEAKEASKLFIEKM    ADYDIKPRYCIISYASVAI
LAM FACTOR B                SINLTSLYDTHIYLVIDASYSVGKE    DFDTGLNFVKDLINRI    GMYVRNIRYSIVMYATNPS
HUM FACTOR C2          TKSLGRKIQIQRSGHLNLYLLLDCSQSVSEN    DFLIFKESASLMVDRI    FSFEINVSVAIITFASEPK
MOU FACTOR C2 (ex)     TKSLGRKIIIQRSGHLNLYLLLDASQSVTEK    DFDIFKKSAELMVERI    FSFEVNVTVAIITFASQPK
HUM IaI H1 (ex)    DLLVANNHFAHFFAPQNLTNMNKNVVFVIDISGSMRGQ    KVKQTKEALLKILGDM    QPGDYFDLVLFGTRVQ
MOU IaI H1         DLLVANNYFTHFFAPKNLTNMSKNLVFVIDISGSMEGQ    KVRQTKEALLKILEDM    RPVDNFDLVLVQSWKG
HUM IaI H2         ELEVFNGYFVHFFAPDNLDPIPKNILFVIDVSGSMWGV    KMKQTVEAMKTILDDL    RAEDHFSVIDFNQNIR
MOU IaI H2         NVQIVNGYFVHFFAPQGLPVVPKNIVFVIDVSGSMSGR    KIQQTREALLKILDDV    KEDDYLNFILFSTDVT
HUM IaI H3         NVQIVNGYFVHFFAPQGLPVVPKNVAFVIDISGSMAGR    KLEQTKEALLRILEDM    QEEDYLNFILFSGDVS
MOU IaI H3         NVQIVNGYFVHFFAPQGLPVVPKNIVFVIDVSGSMSGR    KIQQTREALLKILDDV    KEDDYLNFILFSTDVT
HUM IaI H4         SIQIENGYFVHYFAPEGLTTMPKNVVFVIDKSGSMSGR    KIQQTREALIKILDDL    SPRDQFNLIVFPSTEAT

HUM LFA-1 (aL)                 CIKGNVDLVFLFDGSMSLQPD    EFQKILDFMKDVMKKL    SNTSYQFAAVQFSTSYK
HUM Mac-1 (aM)                 CPQQESDIAFLIDGSGSIIPH    DFRRMKEFVSTVMEQL    KKSKTLFSLMQYSEEFR
MOU Mac-1 (aM)                 CPQQESDIVFLIDGSGSINNI    DFQKMKEFVSTVMEQF    KKSKTLFSLMQYSDEFR
HUM p150-95 (ax)               CPRQEQDIVFLIDGSGSISSR    NFATMMNFVRAVISQF    QRPSTQFSLMQYSNKFQ
HUM VLA-1 (a1)                 CST QLDIVIVLDGNSIYP    WDSVTAFLNDLLKRM    DIGPKQTQVGIVQYGENVT
RAT VLA-1 (a1)                 CST QLDIVIVLDGSLSIYP    WESVIAFLNDLLKRM    DIGPKQTQVGIVQYGENVT
CHI VLA-1 (a1)                 CKT QLDIVIVLDGSNSIYP    VESVTAPLNSLLRNM    DIGPQQTQVGIVQYGQTVV
HUM VLA-2 (a2)                 CPS LIDVVVVCDESNSIYP    WDAVKNFLEKFVQGL    DIGPTKTQVGLIQYANNPR
MOU VLA-2 (a2)                 CPS LVDVVVVCDESNSIYP    WEAVKNFLVKFVTGL    DIGPKKTQVALIQYANEPR
POR VLA-2 (a2)                 ..................    WDAVKNFLEKFVQGL    DIGPTKTQVGLIQYANNPR
BOV VLA-2 (a2)                 CPS FIDVVVVCDESNSIYP    WDAVKNFLEKFVQGL    DIGPTKTQMGLIQYANNPR
HUM aE                         EEEAGTEIAIILDGSGSIDP    PDFQRAKDFISNMMRNF    YEKCFECNFALVQYGGVIQ
RAB DHP Ca++ ch.   VDNSRTPNKIDLYDVRRRPWYIQGAASPKDMLILVDVSGSVSG    LTLKLIRTSVSEML    ETLSDDDFVNVASFNSNAQ
RAT DHP Ca++ ch.   VDNSRTPNKIDLYDVRRRPWYIQGAASPKDMLILVDVSGSVSG    LTLKLIRTSVSEML    ETLSDDDFVNVASFNSNAQ
Malarian TRAP          GRDVQNNIVDEIKYSEEVCNDQVDLYLLMDCSGSIRRH    NWVNHAVPLAMKLIQQL    NLNDNAIHLYVNVFSNNAK
Malarian TRAP 2        FLNGQETLDEIKYSEEVCTEQIDIHILMDGSGSIGYS    NWKAHVIPMLNTLVDNL    NISNDEINVSLTLFSTNSR
ETP100 (ex)            ATTSSGQDQVCTSLLDVMLVVDESGSIGTS    NFRKVRQFIEDFVNSM    PISPEDVRVGLITFATRSK
EMP100                 AAASSEADQVCTRLLDVMLVVDESGSIGTS    NYGKVRSFISNFAGTM    PLSPDDVRVGLVTFGTSAV

HUM CMP-1 (ex)             GHLCRTRPTDLVFVVDSSRSVRPV    EFEKVKVFLSQVIESL    DVGPNATRVGMVNYASTVK
CHI CMP-1 (ex)             GTLCRTKPTDLVFIIDSSRSVRPQ    EFEKVKVFLSRVIEGL    DVGPNSTRVGVINYASAVK
HUM CMP-2 (ex)            VCSGGGGSSATDLVFIIDGSKSVRPE    NFELVKKFISQIVDTL    DVSDKLAQVGLVQYSSSVR
CHI CMP-2 (ex)            ACSGGSGS ALDLVFLIDGSKSVRPE    NFELVKKFINQIVESL    EVSEKQAQVGLVQYSSSVR
HUM Co VI a1-N1 (ex)          DCPVDLFFVLDTSESVALRLKPYGALVDKVKSFTKRFIDNLRDRYYRCDRNLVWNAGALHYSDEVE
CHI Co VI a1-N1 (ex)          DCPVDLFVLDTSESVALRVKPFGDLVAQVKDFTNRFIDKLTERYFRCDRFLAWNAGALHYSDSVV
HUM Co VI a2-N1 (ex)          DCPIHVYFVLDTSESVTMQSPTDILLF HMKQFVPQFISQLQNEFYLDQVALSWRYGGLHFSDQVE
CHI Co VI a2-N1 (ex)          DCPISVYFVIDTSESIALQTVPIQSLVDQIKQFIPRFIEKLENEVYQNQVSITWMFGGLHYSDVVE
HUM Co VI a3-N1 (ex)          ACNLDVILGFDGSRDQNV    FVAQKGFESKVDAIL    NRISQMHRVSCSGGRSPTV
MOU Co VI a3-N1 (ex)          ACNLEVILGFDGSRDQNV    FVSQKGLESKVDILL    NRISQIQRISCSGNQLPTV
CHI Co VI a3-N1               DCDLDVILGFDVSDVGAGQN    IFNSQRGLESRVEAVL    NRITQMQKISCTGSRAPSV
HUM Co VI a1-C1    ECEILDIIMKMCSCCECK    CGPIDLLFVLDSSESIGLQ    NFEIAKDFVVKVIDRLSRDELVKFEPGQSYAGVVQYSHSQM
MOU Co VI a1-C1    ECEILDIIMKMCSCCECT    CGPIDLLFVLDSSESIGLQ    NFEIAKDFIIKVIDRLSKDELVKFEPGQSHAGVVQYSHNQM
CHI Co VI a1-C1 (ex) ECEILDIIMKMCSCCECT   CGPVDLLFVLDGSESIGLQ    NFQIAKDFIIKVIDRLSKDERVKFEPGESRVGVVQYSHNNT
HUM Co VI a2-C1 (ex) ECDVMTYVRETCGCCDCEKR CGALDVVFVIDSSESIGYT    NFTLEKNFVINVVNRLGAIAKDPKSETGTRVGVVQYSHEGT
MOU Co VI a2-C1    ....................    ..................AKDPKSETGTRVGVVQYSHEGT
CHI Co VI a2-C1    DCDVMTYVRETCGCCDCEKRCGALDIMFVIDSSESIGYT    NFTLEKNFVVNVVSRLGSIAKDPKSETGARVGVVQYSHEGT
HUM Co VI a3-C1    IDQCALIQSIKDKCPCCYCPLECPVFPTELAFALDTSEGVNQD    TFGRMRDVVLSIVNVL    TIAESNCPTGARVAVVTYNNEVT
MOU Co VI a3-C1    VDQCALIQSIRDKCPCCYGPLECPVLPTELAFALDTSEGVTQD    TFSRMREVLLGIVGDL    TIAESNCPRGARVAVVTYNNEVT
CHI Co VI a3-C1    ISQCALVQNIKDKCPCCYGPKECPVFPTELAFAIDTSSGVGRD    VFNRMKQTVLRVVSNL    TIAESNCPRGARVALVTYNNEVT
HUM Co VI a1-C2    DKKCPDYTCPITFSSPA    DITILLEPPPDVGSH    NFDTTKRFAKRLAERF    LTAGRTDPAHDVRVAVVQYSGTGQ
MOU Co VI a1-C2    DKKCPDYTCPITFSSPA    DITILLDSSASVGSH    NFETTKVFAKRLAERF    LSAGRADPSQDVRVAVVQYSGQGQ
CHI Co VI a1-C2 (ex) EKKCPDYTCPITFANPA   DIMLLVDSSTSVGSK    NFDTTKNFVKRLAERF    LEASKPAEDS VRVSVVQYSGRNQ
HUM Co VI a2-C2 (ex) DPQIVCPDLPCQTELSVAQCTQRPVDIVFLLDGSERLGEQ    NFHKARRFVEQVARRL    TLARRDDDPLNARVALLQFGGPGE
MOU Co VI a2-C2    DPQIVCPELPCQTELYVAQCTQRPVDIVFLLDGSERLGEQ    NFHKVRRFVEDVSRRL    TLARRDDDPLNARMALLQYGSQNQ
CHI Co VI a2-C2 (ex) DPQIVCPELPCQTELAVAQCTQRPVDIVFLLDGSERIGEQ    NFHRAHHFVEQVAQQL    TLARRNDDNMNARIALLQYGSERE
HUM Co VI a3-C2           PSFRDRRAAGSDVDIDMAFILDSAETTLF    QFNEMKKYIAYLVRQLDMSPDPKASQHFARVAVVQHAPSES
MOU Co VI a3-C2           PSFRDRRAAGSDVDIDLAFILDSSEATTLF    QFNEMKKYIGYVIRQL.....................
CHI Co VI a3-C2           PVFRDRRAAPTDVDTDIAFIMDSSASTTPL    QFNEMKKYISHLVSNMEISSEPKISQHHARVAVLQQAPYDH
HUM Co VI a3-N10 (ex)         VKNGAAADIIFLVDSSWTIGEE    HFQLVREFLYDVVKSL    AVGENDFHFALVQFNGNPH
CHI Co VI a3-N10 (ex)         VRNVAVADIIFLVDSSWSIGKE    HFQLVREFLYDVVKAL    DVGGNDFRFALVQFSGNPH
HUM Co VI a3-N9 (ex)          QDSADIIFLIDGSNNTGSV    NFAVILDFLVNLLEKL    PIGTQQIRVGVVQFSDEPR
CHI Co VI a3-N9 (ex)          QESADLIFLIDGSDNIGSV    NFQAIRDFLVNLIESL    RVGAQQIHIGVVQYSDQPR
HUM Co VI a3-N8 (ex)          IEVNKRDIVFLVDGSSALGLA    NFNAIRDFIAKVIQRL    EIGQDLIQVAVAQYADTVR
CHI Co VI a3-N8 (ex)          IEVNKKDIVFLIDGSTALGTG    PFNSIRDFVAKIVQRL    EVGPDLIQVAVAQYADTVR
HUM Co VI a3-N7 (ex)          HSNKRDIIFLLDGSANVGKT    NFPYVRDFVMNLVNSL    DIGNDNIRVGLVQFSDTPV
CHI Co VI a3-N7 (ex)          QVTKRDIIFLLDGSLNVGNA    NFPFVRDFVVTLVNYL    DVGTDKIRVGLVQFSDTPK
HUM Co VI a3-N6 (ex)          ESKRDILFLFDGSANLVGQ    FPVVRDFLYKIIDEL    NVKPEGTRIAVAQYSDDVK
CHI Co VI a3-N6    IVSGGVEEVPLAPTESKKDILFLIDGSANLLGS    FPAVRDFIHKVISDL    NVGPDATRVAVAQFSDNIQ
HUM Co VI a3-N5 (ex)          APVSGEKDVVFLLDGSEGVRSG    FPLLKEFVQRVVESL    DVGQDRVRVAVVQYSDRTR
CHI Co VI a3-N5           QFQPTVVERGEKKDVVFLIDGSDGVRRG    FPLLKTFVERVVESL    DIGRDKVRVAIVQYSNAIQ
HUM Co VI a3-N4 (ex)      PVLQPLPSPGVGGKRDVVFLIDGSQSAGPE    FQYVRTLIRRLVDYL    DVGFDTTRVAVIQFSDDPK
CHI Co VI a3-N4       LAPDLVFTSPSPVGVKRDVVFLVDGSRYAAQE    FYLIRDLIERIVNNL    DVGFDTTRISVVQFSEHPH
HUM Co VI a3-N3 (ex)      ASTRYPPPAVESDAADIVFLIDSSEGVRPD    GFAHIRDFVSRIVRRL    NIGPSKVRVGVVQFSNDVF
CHI Co VI a3-N3       LLGDVTTIPDVSGEEKDVVFLIDSSDSVRSD    GLAHIRDFISRIVQQL    DVGPNKVRIGVVQFSNNVF
HUM Co VI a3-N2 (ex)      GVDTPPPSRPEKKKADIVFLLDGSINFRRD    SFQEVLRFVSEIVDTV    YEDGDSIQVGLVQYNSDPT
MOU Co VI a3-N2           ..................    ................    ...................
CHI Co VI a3-N2    LTVPTTEGPVYPGPEGKKQADIVFLLDGSINLGRD    NFQEVLQFVYSIVDAI    YEDGDSIQVGLAQYNSDVT
HUM Co VII-2 (ex)  EAPRVRAQHRERVTCTRLYAADIVFLLDGSSSIGRS    NFREVRSFLEGLVLPF    SGAASAQGVRFATVQYSDDPR
CHI Co VII-1 (ex)             VCPRGLADVVFLPHATQDNAHR    AEATRRVLERLVLALG    PLGPQAVQVGLLSYSHRPS
CHI Co XII-1       GGPGIPEEKKVEAQIQKCSISAMTDLVFLVDGSWSVGRN    NFRYILDFMVALVSAF    DIGEEKTRVGVVQYSSDTR
CHI Co XII-2       VQVECSRGVDVKADVVFLVDGSYSIGIA    NFVKVRAFLEVIVKSF    EISPRKVQISLVQYSRDPH
CHI Co XII-3       DTTTEPFLSRGLECRTRAEADIVLLVDGSWSIGRP    NFNFISRIVEVFDIGP    DKKTVRVQIGLAQYSGDPR
URO Co XII-3       PSSGLDCTTKAQADIVLLVDGSWSIGRP    NFKIVRNFISRVVEVF    DIGSDRVQIAVSQYSGDPR
CHI Co XII-4       KPTEAPTPPPTPPPPPTIPPARDVCRGAKADIVFLTDASWSIGDD    NFNKVVKFVFNTVGAF    DLINPAGIQVSLVQYSDEAQ
HUM Co XIV-1       ................................    ..............F    DVGSEKTRIGLAQYSGDPR
CHI Co XIV-1           QGNLFTCKTPAIADIVILVDGSWSIGRF    NFRLVRLFLENLVSAF    NVGSEKTRVGLAQYSGDPR
CHI Co XIV-2       LPFPTQPPTSPSTTLPPPTIPPAKEVCKAAKADLVFLVDGSWSIGDD    NFNKIISFLYSTVGAL    DKIGPDGTQVAIIQFSDDPR


SECONDARY STRUCTURE based on Mac-1 I module crystal        ◄──βA──►        ◄───α1───►            ◄─βB─►    ◄βC
SECONDARY STRUCTURE based on Mult.align. prediction        ◄βA►            ◄───α1───►            ◄─βB─►    ◄βC
```

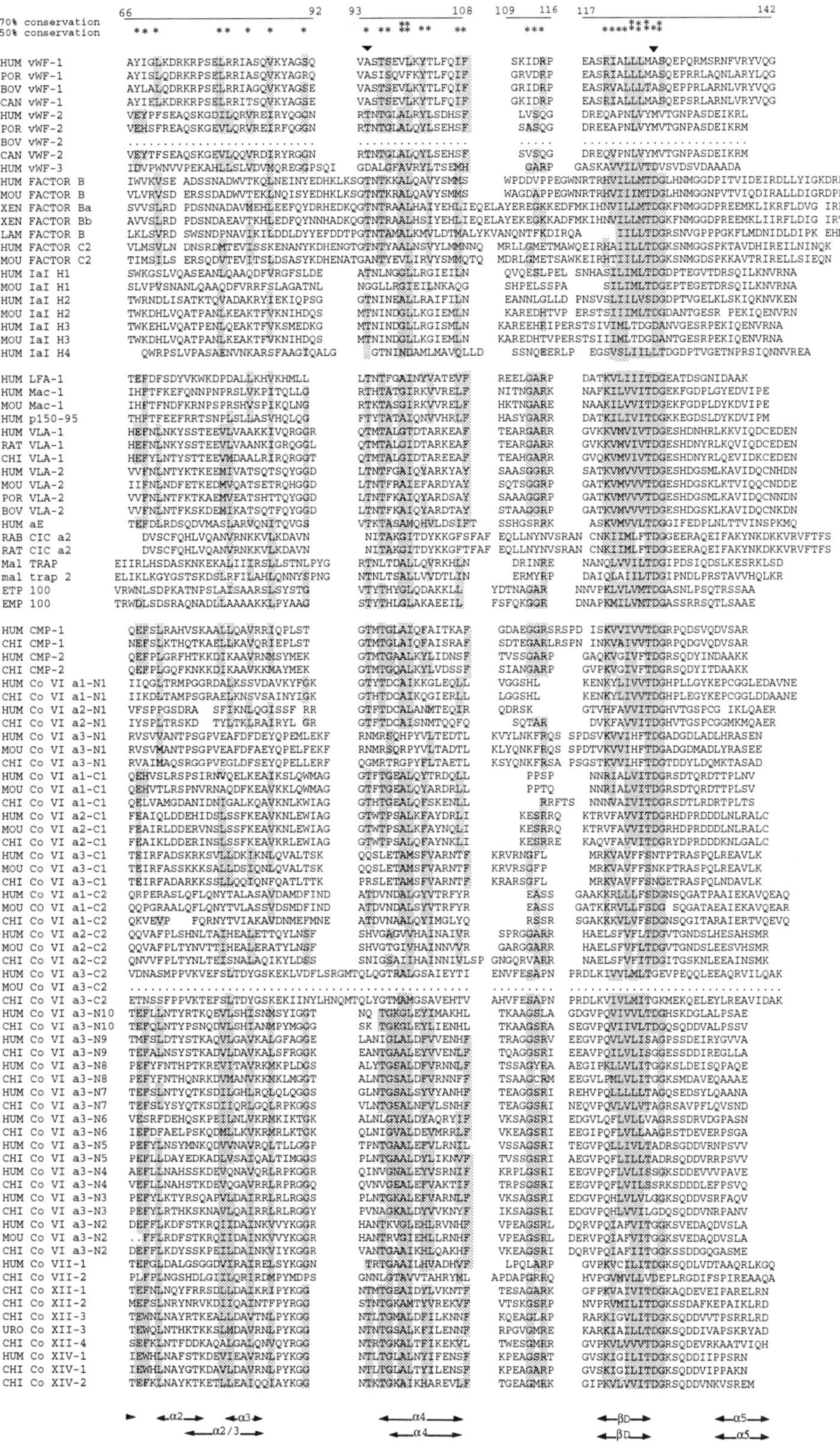

Fig. 1.2 (continued).

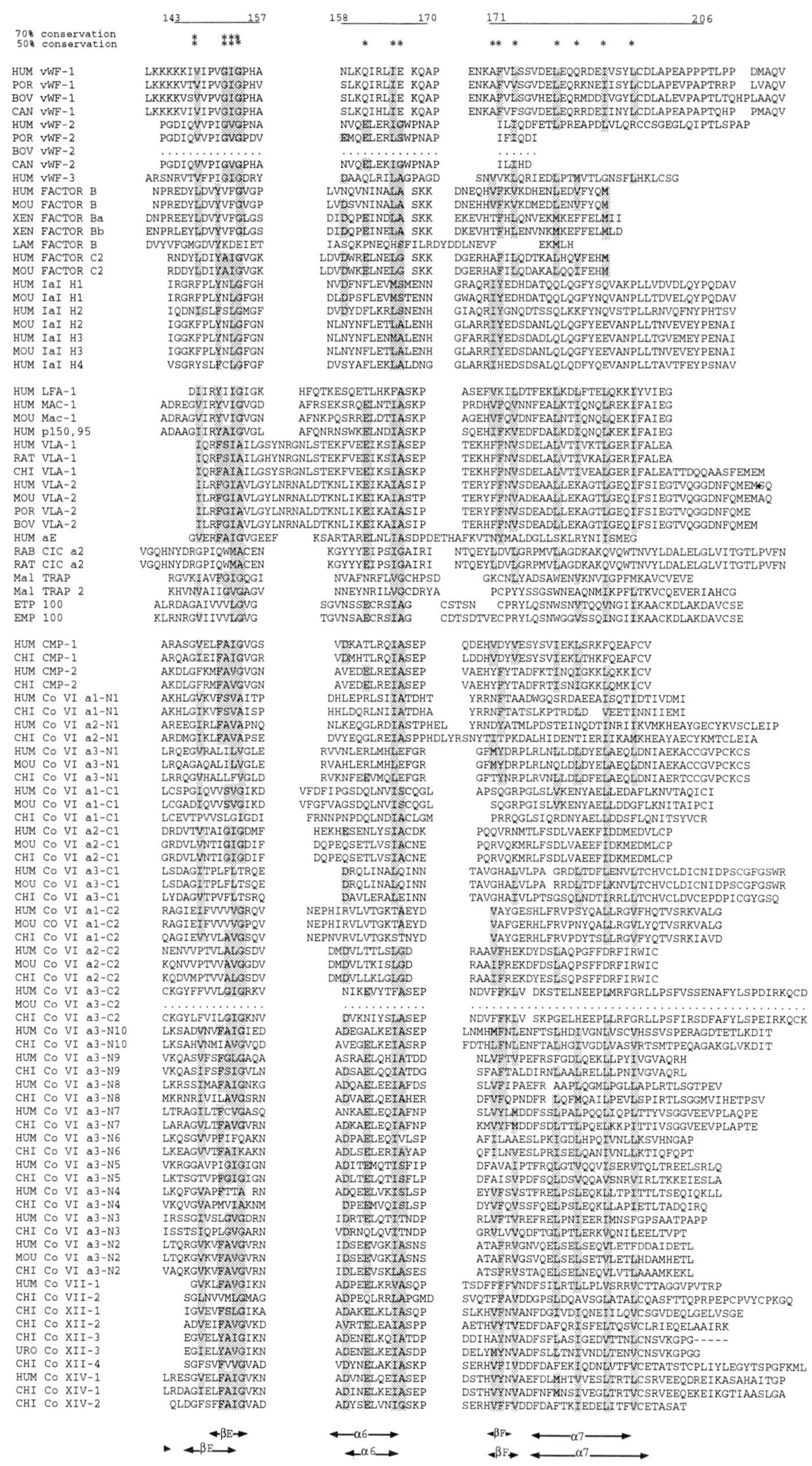

Fig. 1.2 (continued).

cysteines may or may not form disulfide intrachain bonds. For example, the A1 and A3 modules of vWF contain a single intrachain disulfide bond linking C509 and C695 in A1, and C933 and C1109 in A3. In both cases a 185 amino acid residue loop is formed. Other VWFA modules, such as those of the α1β1 and α2β1 integrins, contain two cysteines that are unlikely to form disulfide bridges, as suggested by modeling studies (see below). Conversely it seems likely that only the cysteines located at the extremities, and expecially those closely positioned in space as suggested by the three-dimensional model of Mac-1, might form disulfide bridges. Alignment of the deduced amino acid sequences of all the known VWFA modules shows a framework of short stretches of more conserved subregions separated by sequences of variable length with a very low conservation. The conserved stretches correspond to α helices and β strands at the secondary level. Three of these short sequences, amino acids 15-27, 54-61 and 123-131 (Fig. 1.2.) are remarkably more conserved than the others, showing a similarity above 70%. The length of the sequences with lower homology that separate the three highly conserved stretches is variable ranging from 22 to 36 amino acid residues between the first and the second and from 49 to 66 between the second and the third stretches. The highly conserved sequences can be considered as a mark for the VWFA module, and new candidates of the VWFA family should contain these consensus sequences.

The sequence 15-27 is largely hydrophobic and in absolute is the most conserved. The key role of this short sequence has been highlighted by several mutagenesis studies demonstrating that amino acid substitutions in this region dramatically change the properties of the mutated molecules (see below).[74,91-96]

SECONDARY AND TERTIARY STRUCTURE PREDICTION OF VWFA MODULES

The existence of both α helices and β strands in the secondary structure of VWFA domains was proposed originally by Bonaldo et al,[18] on the basis of a one-sequence Robson prediction. The identification of a large number of VWFA domains together with the improvement of the sequence analysis software, allowed more detailed prediction of the secondary structure of this module. In 1991, Bork put forward a secondary structure model based on multiple alignments of 39 VWFA modules predicting an alternanting pattern of α helices and β strands, in the order BABBABBA.[97] More recently, a very accurate prediction of the secondary and tertiary structure of the VWFA module has been proposed by Edward and Perkins,[16] on the basis of the multiple alignment of 75 amino acid sequences of VWFA modules analysed by the algorithms PHD and SAPIENS (see Fig. 1.2, bottom). Both predictive methods identified a total of 6 α helices and 6 β strands, in the order BABBAABABABA. The first three (BA-BB) and the final six (α4-α7) stuctures show an alternating pattern of α helices and β strands along the VWFA module. These ordered regions, corresponding to well conserved stretches at the primary sequence level, are separated from each other by regions of random coil or turn conformations of variable length (2-13 amino acids). The 8 sequence insertions requested to obtain the best alignment among the VWFA modules are located in these highly variable regions, suggesting that primary structure variations in those connecting segments of the domain do not alter the basic three dimensional structure of the module. Also considering the hydropathic nature for each residue position, the best similarity is found in the 12 predicted α helices and β strands: as calculated by Perkins et al,[16] in 67 positions of the about 200 residues constituting a typical VWFA module the hydropathy is conserved in at least 75% of the aligned sequences, and 53 of these occur in the α helices or β strands. All six predicted β strands are highly hydrophobic, whereas the α helices possess an amphipathic nature. This prediction suggests that the β strands are buried in the domain constituting the hydrophobic core of the VWFA module, whereas the α helices are exposed to water. Almost all potential N-glycosylation sites (a total of 50 located at 27 different positions) in the 75 aligned sequences are inserted in predicted hydrophilic regions, as expected from their presumed exposure to solvent.

Using protein fold recognition procedures, the same authors predicted that the crystal structure of human p21[ras], consisting of a doubly wound open twisted β sheet flanked by α helices, is a good model for representing the three dimensional structure of the VWFA module.[16] This prediction was confirmed by the recently determined crystal structure of a member of this family, the VWFA module from the α subunit of the β2 integrin Mac-1,[17] showing that the two domains differ only in the orientation of two β strands. As the predicted three-dimensional model is built from a consensus secondary structure obtained by comparison of 75 different VWFA modules, we can confidently assume that the main characteristics observed in the crystal of the VWFA module of Mac-1 are likely to be conserved in the vast majority of the VWFA modules.

CRYSTAL STRUCTURE OF THE VWFA/I MODULE OF THE α SUBUNIT OF Mac-1 IN THE PRESENCE OF Mg^{2+}

The crystal structure of the recombinant VWFA module grown in the presence of Mg^{2+} ions was solved at 1,7 A resolution. The model includes the whole module starting from residue D132 and ending at residue K315 (Fig. 1.3).[17] Five parallel and one short antiparallel β strands form an open, twisted β sheet that is surrounded by seven α helices. This arrangement corresponds to a structure called α/β open sheet (also known as "Rossman", "dinucleotide binding" or "doubly wound" fold), representing a common topology that is present in a wide variety of intracellular enzymes. The single cysteine located at the beginning of the module appears disordered in the crystal structure. In the VWFA module of the closely related α1β1 and α2β1 integrins there is a second cysteine buried in the interior unable to form disulfide bridges. In several other VWFA modules, namely those contained in vWF, CMP, type VII, XII and XIV collagens and some of those present in type VI collagen,

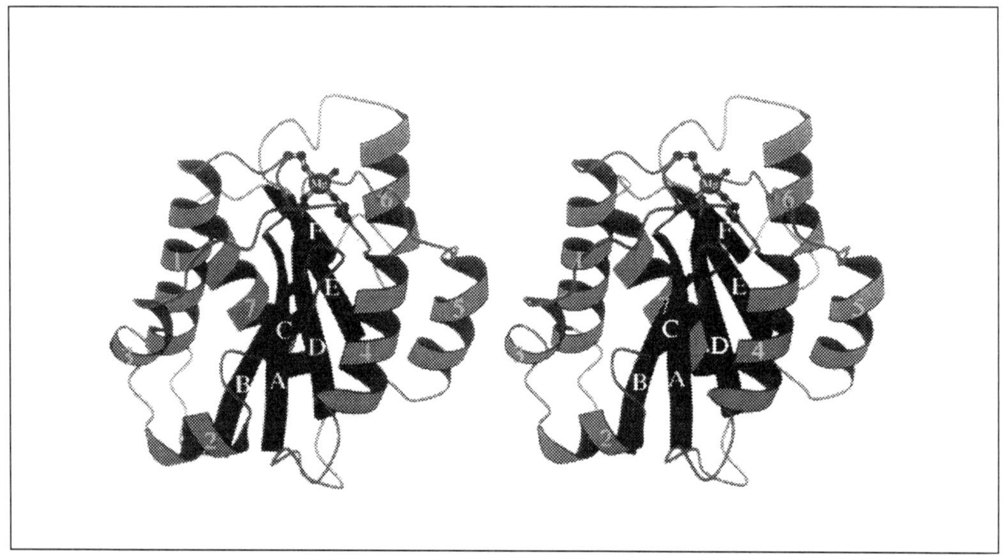

Fig. 1.3. Schematic stereo diagram of the Mac-1 VWFA module. Strand and helix assignments are as in Fig. 1.2. The Mg^{2+} ion is shown as a ball. (With permission from Lee J-O, Rieu P, Arnaout MA, Liddington RC: Crystal structure of the A domain from the a subunit of integrin CR3 (CD11b/CD18). Cell 80:631-638, 1995. Copyright 1995 Cell Press).

all the cysteines are located at the extremities of the domains, where they can be engaged in disulfide bridges as suggested if the coordinates of the crystal structure of the Mac-1 VWFA module are used to build models of the other modules.

Almost all substrate- or cofactor-binding sites in a doubly wound α/β domain are located at a crevice lined by the loops connecting the central β strands with the α helices. A metal ion with a functional or structural role is often present at this site. In the VWFA module of Mac-1, the crevice is located at the top of the β sheet, where the connecting loops from two β strands run in opposite directions, and a Mg^{2+} ion is trapped in this crevice. Usually, stable Mg^{2+} binding by a protein involves six coordination sites, all of them but one or two occupied by functional groups (including at least two negatively charged ligands) from the protein or a cofactor. The free sites are then occupied by water molecules. In this respect, the VWFA module of Mac-1 is highly unusual, as the Mg^{2+} ion coordinates the hydroxyl oxygen atoms of non-charged residues S142, S144 and T209, whereas the remaining positions are occupied by water molecules. D140 and D242 occupy a secondary coordination sphere: each carboxylate group makes hydrogen bonds to water molecule w1 and one hydroxyl side chain (D140 to S142 and D242 to S144). In solution, the sixth Mg^{2+} coordination site is expected to be occupied by a water molecule, but in the crystal structure it is occupied by a carboxylate oxygen atom from residue E314 of a neighboring VWFA molecule. The authors call this Mg^{2+}-binding site with an extra available coordination site "Metal Ion-Dependent Adhesion Site" (MIDAS). The conserved features of this motive are the DxSxS sequence (residues 140-144 in Fig.1.4, x representing any amino acid), a threonine (T209) and an aspartate (D242) from other parts of the chain. The key role of these amino acids in coordinating metal ions and their importance in integrin-ligand interactions has been pointed out by several mutagenesis studies. Recombinant VWFA module of

Mac-1 mutated in D140A and S142A or in D242A, completely loses binding capacity to Mg^{2+} ions and the same mutations in the recombinant entire subunit transfected in COS cells abrogate recognition of the iC3b ligand.[96] These mutations do not affect the integrin heterodimer formation nor cell surface expression. The mutation T195A in Mac-1 blocks binding to iC3b and ICAM-1,[95] and the mutation D242A blocks binding to NIF, iC3b and ICAM-1.[17] Similar mutations in $\alpha2$[93] and αL[92,98] lead to a dramatic reduction of binding of transfected cells to collagen and ICAM-1, respectively. The mutation T253A in integrin $\alpha1$ subunit impairs the ability of the transfected chains to bind to type IV collagen and laminin.[94] Mutations abolishing divalent cation binding also affect the ligand binding capacity suggesting that the divalent-cation may indirectly stabilize a ligand binding conformation, and/or that the cation may directly coordinate with the ligand. The crystal structure and the mutagenesis data indicate that both mechanisms might operate to different extents with the various ligands. Thus, it is possible that the Mg^{2+}-coordination site occupied in the crystal by a carboxylate oxygen atom from residue E314 of neighboring VWFA module is involved in physiological conditions in coordinating an acidic residue of its ligand. In the case of the interaction between Mac-1 and ICAM-1, a good candidate could be E34, which is by far the most important ICAM-1 residue identified so far for binding to the integrin LFA-1.[111] A mutation of this residue greatly reduced the interaction of ICAM-1 with LFA-1. By analogy, alanine mutagenesis of DE752 and E758 in iC3b impair its interaction with Mac-1.[114] Instead, a different binding mechanism should be hypothesized in binding of $\beta1$ integrins to collagens and laminin. In fact, the recombinant VWFA module of the $\alpha2$ chain binds specifically to collagen in a divalent cation-independent manner.[93] Moreover, mutations of D151 and D254 of $\alpha2$ do not significantly alter collagen binding properties, whereas a mutation of T221 results in only a partial inhibition.

Column-group labels: **HIGHLY CONSERVED HYDROPHOBIC STRETCH** (over the ΦΦΦΦΦ and D X S X S columns) and **MIDAS MOTIF** (over the D X S X S Φ and T --33aa-- D columns).

protein	chain	NOTES	D	X	S	X	S	Φ	---50/51aa----	P	14aa	T	--33aa--	D	MUTAGENESIS EFFECTS	REF
Mac-1	α_M	c+m	^{140}A	–	^{142}A	–	–			–		–		^{242}A	abrogate binding to iC3b	96
			–	–	–	–	–			–		–		–	does not reduce binding but shifts the optimal cation concentration required for adhesion of Mac-1 expressing cells to iC3b	95
			–	–	–	–	–			^{195}A		–		–		
		c	–	–	–	–	–			–		^{209}A		–	blocks binding to iC3bi and ICAM-1	
		m	–	–	–	–	–			–		–		^{242}A	abrogates binding to iC3b and NIF and partially abrogates binding to ICAM-1 and fibrinogen	17
LFA-1	α_L	c	^{137}A,K	–	–	–	–			–		–		–	abrogate binding to ICAM-1	92,95
			–	–	–	–	–			–		^{206}A		–		
			–	–	–	–	–			–		–		^{239}A,K		
			–	–	^{139}A	–	–			^{192}A		–		–	inhibition effects linked to an alterate module conformation	
			–	–	–	–	–			–		–		–	no effects	92
VLA-1	α_1	c	–	–	–	–	–			–		^{253}A		–	loss of ligand binding capacity (fragment CB3 of type IV collagen) loss of cell adhesion to type IV collagen and laminin.	94
VLA-2	α_2	c	^{151}A	–	–	–	–					–		^{254}A	abrogates binding to collagen	74,93
			–	–	–	–	–					–		–		
		m	^{151}A	–	–	–	–					–		^{254}A	does not affect (A151), or only partially inhibits (A254) binding to type I collagen	
		m+c	–	–	–	–	–					^{221}A		–	partially abrogates binding to type I collagen	
C2	C2	c	^{240}L	–	–	–	–					–		–	decrease more than 100 fold specific hemolytic activity	91
			–	–	–	–	^{244}A					–		–		

In contrast, a Mac1-VWFA recombinant fragment needs divalent cations to bind to EAiC3b.[99] Thus, even if it is clear that the integrity of the MIDAS motive as well as the divalent cation dependency are critical for the binding activity of VWFA module containing integrins, they seem to use two different molecular mechanisms to bind to their ligands. In $\beta1$ integrins interacting with collagens ($\alpha1\beta1$ and $\alpha2\beta1$), the divalent cation is not directly involved in ligand binding but maintains the three-dimensional structure of the domain in a permissive binding conformation through allosteric effects. A likely explanation for the different cation requirement between the entire molecule and the recombinant fragment might be that the recombinant VWFA module of $\alpha2$, free from the quaternary constraints imposed by the heterodimeric integrin molecule, assumes by default a cation-independent structure able to constitutively bind collagens. On the other hand, the $\beta2$ integrins, which bind to cell-membrane proteins interact with ligands directly via few contact sites as well as via the divalent cation, and this would explain the different cation requirements among recombinant VWFA modules.

It is worth pointing out that the MIDAS motif is not the sole determinant of the integrin-ligand interaction: a recent study based on the species-specific binding between the human LFA-1 and ICAM-1 pair,[98] clearly showed that non-MIDAS residues also are crucial for specific recognition of human ICAM-1. In particular, substitutions of four amino acids of the human VWFA sequence of LFA-1 with the corresponding murine amino acids, impair the binding of this mutated LFA-1 to human ICAM-1. If the coordinates of the Mac-1 α chain VWFA module are used to build a model of the LFA-1 module, these amino acid residues localize at the top of the VWFA module and surround the MIDAS site. Thus it is emerging that in the MIDAS region a ligand-binding interface exists crucial to species-specific ligand recognition. Mapping of integrin-ligand binding sites by means of synthetic peptides spanning the VWFA module indicates a possible role of some other residues surrounding the MIDAS site. Rieu et al,[100] found that two contiguous peptides (A6 and A7) spanning the regions of Mac-1 T213-N232 (TGIRKVVRELFNITNGARKN) and N232-K245 (NALFKILVVITDGEK), respectively, strongly inhibit binding of the neutrophil adhesion inhibitor (NIF) to a recombinant Mac-1 VWFA module. Biotinylated NIF also is able to bind to microplates-immobilized A7 peptide but residue D242 of peptide A7 (one of the MIDAS motif residues), is not involved in peptide inhibition, nor in ligand activity as its mutation does not alter the property of A7. The same peptide and its mutant also are able to inhibit completely and in a cation-independent way the interaction between EAiC3b and the VWFA module of Mac-1.[99] As the mutation does not affect the inhibitory function, and the core of this peptide forms a hydrophobic β structure (βD in the crystal structure of Lee et al)[17] (see Fig. 1.2), the ligand binding activity should reside in the short GEK sequence at the end of peptide. In the crystal structure this short sequence is exposed at the surface and surrounds the Mg^{2+} coordination site. However, several shorter peptides containing the GEK sequence are completely unable to inhibit integrin-ligand interaction and peptide A8 (DATKVLIIITDGEA), containing the corresponding sequence of human LFA-1 in which GEK is substituted by GEA, is not inhibitory. As the A8 sequence is rather different from the sequence of A7, it should be of interest to test the inhibitory effect of peptide A8 on the binding of

LFA-1 to ICAM-1. In fact, the finding of an inhibition could strengthen the idea that these peptides compete in a specific and efficacious manner with the homologous sequences present in the VWFA modules of Mac-1 (A7) and LFA-1 (A8), respectively.

The VWFA module of the complement C2 also harbors a consensus sequence for a MIDAS motife. Dramatic effects have been obtained following mutagenesis of D240A and S242A, leading to a more than 100-fold decrease of specific hemolytic activity of the mutated C2 form compared to the wild form.[91]

CRYSTAL STRUCTURE OF THE VWFA/I MODULE OF THE Mac-1 α SUBUNIT IN THE PRESENCE OF Mn^{2+}

Recently, the recombinant VWFA module of Mac-1 has been crystalized in the presence of Mn^{2+} ions.[101] The resolved structure shows interesting features that could provide some structural explanations of the molecular mechanism involved in regulating integrin activity for their cognate ligands. Crystalization of the module in the presence of Mn^{2+} generates a crystal which is in about two-thirds similar to that produced in the presence of Mg^{2+} (Figs. 1.5 and 1.6).[101] The central β sheet (except for βF) and the α helices (except for $\alpha 1$, $\alpha 5$ and $\alpha 7$), are superimposable, whereas the metal binding site is different in the two structures: in the Mn^{2+} form, the bond to T209 is broken and replaced by a direct bond to D242, with a reduction of the electrophilicity of the metal that does not favor an interaction with an exogenous glutamate. These changes are linked to the structural rearrangements leading to the burial of F302 and F275, which are completely exposed in the Mg^{2+} form. Thus, the crystal structure analyses suggest that the Mg^{2+} form is "liganded" (as there is one highly electrophilic coordination site in Mg^{2+} able to interact with ligands), whereas in the Mn^{2+} form the cation binds directly to D242 lowering the electrophilicity and leading to

an "unliganded" state.

A similar mechanism of changes in metal coordination and correlated protein structure rearrangements occurs, for example, in the human GTPase p21^{ras} that, as mentioned above, has a three-dimensional structure very similar to that of the VWFA module. In the active (GTP-bound) form, the Mg^{2+} ion has an indirect bond with an aspartate that is switched to a direct bond as a consequence of GTP hydrolysis; in this way there is a reduction of the electrophilicity of the metal and changes in the effector region which bury a previously exposed isoleucine and finally lead to an inactive state. This model fails to explain the apparent discrepancy between the crystal inactive form obtained in the presence of Mn^{2+} and the integrin activation promoted by this ion.[102,103] Furthermore, this ion dependent model of double activation state is not extendible to the other VWFA containing integrins, as the crystal of LFA-1 VWFA module grown in the presence of Mg^{2+} or Mn^{2+} adopts the same "unliganded" conformation.[101]

THE MIDAS MOTIF IN THE vWFA SUPERFAMILY

The consensus sequence of the MIDAS motif is constituted by the contiguous sequence DxSxS (residues 140-144 in Mac-1), a threonine (T209) and an aspartate (D242), well separated in the primary sequence, but close to the DxSxS sequence in the three-dimensional structure. Many, VWFA modules exhibit this consensus sequence. The functional relevance of the MIDAS motif has been demonstrated by several site-directed mutagenesis studies, summarized in Fig. 1.4. From most of these studies a consensus has emerged that modifications of the MIDAS residues cause significative alterations of the functional activity of the mutated compared to the non-mutated recombinant fragments. In particular, in all the integrins α chains analyzed there is an almost complete loss of ligand binding capacity irrespective of which of the MIDAS amino acids is mutagenized. This effect has been demon-

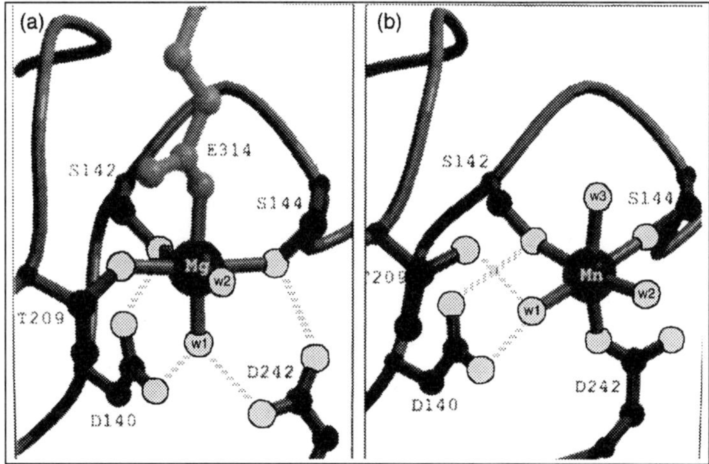

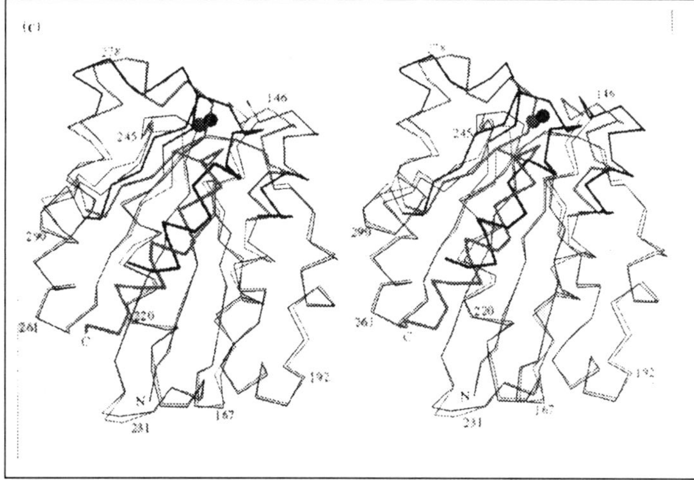

Fig. 1.5. Structural comparison of the VWFA modules of Mac-1 in the presence of Mg^{2+} (a) or Mn^{2+} (b). The color code is grey, protein backbone; outlined in black, coordinating oxygen atom; black, carbon; paler grey, residue from ligand/neighboring molecule. Water molecules are labelled w1-w3 and selected hydrogen bonds are shown as dashed lines. (c) Stereo plot comparing Mg^{2+} (gray) and Mn^{2+} (black) VWFA modules with regions of more relevant changes shown as thicker lines. (d) Stereo close-up view of the plot comparison between the Mg^{2+} (gray) and the Mn^{2+} (black) forms. (With permission from Lee J-O, Banckston LA, Arnaout MA, Liddington RC: Two conformations of the integrin A-domain (I-domain): a pathway for activation? Structure 3: 1333-1340, 1995. Copyright 1995, Current Biol Ltd).

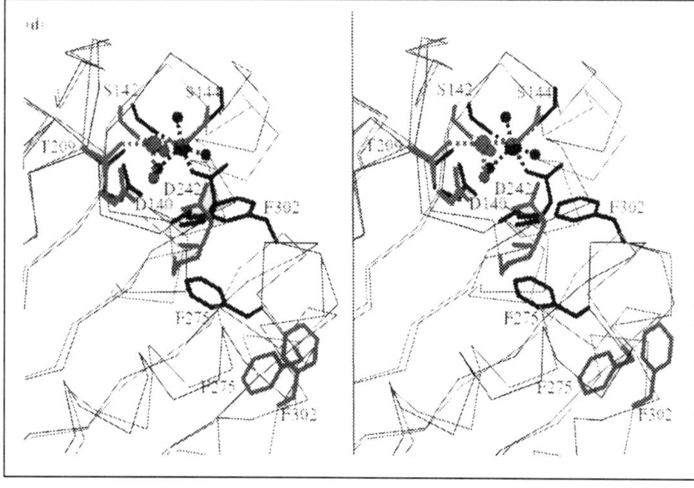

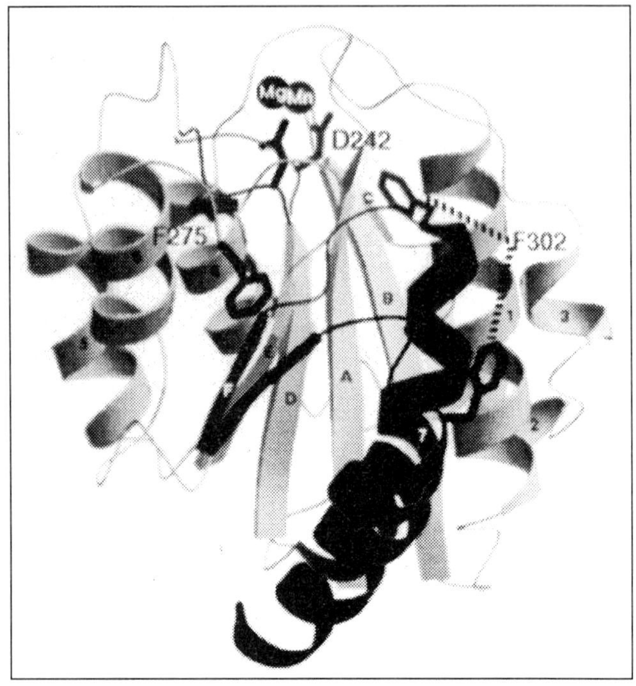

Fig. 1.6 Schematic diagram of the VWFA module of Mac-1 in the presence of Mn²⁺. Major conformational differences are shown in black (Mg²⁺) and dark gray (Mn²⁺) while the backbone is shown in gray. β strands are labelled A-F and α helices 1-7. (With permission from Lee J-O, Banckston LA, Arnaout MA, Liddington RC: Two conformations of the integrin A-domain (I-domain): a pathway for activation? Structure 3: 1333-1340, 1995. Copyright 1995, Current Biol Ltd).

strated in some cases to be related to the loss of the ability to bind divalent cations.

In both the integrin family and the majority of the VWFA superfamily members the MIDAS motif is strictly conserved, though there are some notable exceptions. For instance only 6 out of the 18 VWFA domains of type VI collagen contain a classical MIDAS consensus sequence and none of the three VWFA modules of vWF present the MIDAS sequence. In the VWFA module of type VII collagen only the last Asp is retained. In light of these differences an interesting question arises whether the VWFA modules containing variant MIDAS motifs are indeed able to bind metal ions to the same extent as the VWFA module of Mac-1, and/or whether the corresponding MIDAS motifs still retain a functional role. A partial answer comes from studies on the interaction between the vWF A1 module and its ligand GPIb. Binding of vWF to GPIb in vitro can be induced by the antibiotic ristocetin or by the snake venom protein botrocetin by different mechanisms. An extensive mutagenesis study on the regions involved in vWF-GPIb interaction was reported by

Matsushita and Sadler.[104] Of the 32 mutants raised, two involve amino acids of the variant MIDAS motif, which in the A1 is not perfectly conserved, as the second serine is replaced by an arginine (DxSxR), and the fifth residue is Glu instead of Asp. This variant MIDAS motif seems to maintain an important functional role, as mutations in this area cause dramatic changes in the binding to GPIb as compared to the wild type module. In particular, the double mutant D520A-R524A and the mutant E626A, in which the last Glu of the MIDAS motif is mutated in Ala, exhibit a loss of ristocetin-induced binding to platelets. However, since it is common knowledge that the interaction between vWF and GPIb does not require the presence of metal ions, it is likely that the amino acids of the variant A1 MIDAS motif are not engaged in forming a metal ion binding site, but are nevertheless functionally important. A challenging hypothesis is that two classes of VWFA modules exist: one containing a MIDAS motif constituted by noncontiguous amino acids, which in their three-dimensional architecture coordinate a metal ion able to confer a direct ligand binding activity to the module, and the other in which the corresponding amino acids are part of a metal ion independent functional site.

A MIDAS-LIKE MOTIF IN INTEGRIN β SUBUNITS

Several lines of evidence indicate that both regions within the β and as α subunits of integrins are involved in integrin-ligand interactions.[105] Furthermore, also for integrins lacking a VWFA module in the α chain there is an absolute requirement of divalent cations for ligand binding to occur. In all the integrin β chains there is a conserved sequence of about 250 residues which includes the consensus DxSxS motif, corresponding to that present in many VWFA modules. Moreover, alanine substitution of the D130A in the β1 chain,[106] D134A or S136A in the β2 chain,[107] and D119A, S121A or S123A in the β3 chain,[108-110] all result in defects in ligand binding function. These data strongly suggest that the above amino acids could be part of a divalent cation binding site similar to that present in VWFA modules. Interestingly, sequence alignments of the β chains show that there are absolutely conserved Thr and Asp residues in positions comparable to that found in the MIDAS motifs (for example the T212 and D239 of the β2 subunit). Excluding the region comprising the DxSxS motive, there is no obvious sequence homology between the α subunit VWFA modules and the β subunit conserved sequence using either standard computer algorithms or alignment by eye. If we do not consider the MIDAS-like segment, of the five most conserved amino acids among the VWFA modules, only one appears conserved in integrin β subunits, and of the 78 amino acids conserved in more than 50% VWFA modules only 19 are present in β chains. For comparison, the numbers of amino acids conforming to the VWFA consensus sequence in the individual components of the family vary from 37 in the N1 domain of the α3 chain of type VI collagen, to 70 in the CMP1 domain. In addition, a 20 amino acid long segment has to be inserted in integrin β

chains to maintain the best alignment to VWFA modules. However, although no obvious sequence homology is evident, the hydropathic profiles of integrin α subunit VWFA modules and integrin β subunits conserved sequences aligned from the DxSxS motif are superimposable in the approximately 100 amino acid long sequence comprising the MIDAS motif. It is known that homologies at the three-dimensional structure are very stable regardless of multiple amino acid substitutions. Thus, it is possible that a common evolutionary origin could be detectable only at the three-dimensional level and it would be therefore of great interest to analyze the crystal of this region within the integrin β subunits to confirm whether the cation binding motif possesses a three-dimensional fold similar (common origin or convergence) to that of the VWFA modules.

REFERENCES

1. Bork P, Bairoch A. Extracellular protein modules. Trends Biochem Sci 1995; 3.
2. Doolittle RF. Similar amino acid sequences: Chance or common ancestry? Science 1981; 214:149-159.
3. Verweij CL, Diergaarde PJ, Hart M et al. Full-length von Willebrand factor (vWF) cDNA encodes a highly repetitive protein considerably larger than the mature vWF subunit. EMBO J 1986; 5:1839-1847.
4. Lambowitz AM. Infectious introns. Cell 1989, 56:323-326.
5. Patthy L. Intron-dependent evolution: preferred types of exons and introns. FEBS Lett 1987; 214:1-7.
6. Higgings DG, Labeit S, Gautel M et al. The evolution of titin and related giant muscle proteins. J Mol Evol 1994; 38:395-404.
7. Politou AS, Gautel M, Pfuhl M et al. Immunoglobulin-type domains of titin: same fold, different stability? Biochemistry 1994; 33:4730-4737.
8. Ayme-Southgate A, Vigoreaux J, Benian G et al. *Drosophila* has a twitchin/titin-related gene that appears to encode projectin. Proc Natl Acad Sci USA 1991; 88:7973-7977.
9. Holmgren A, Branden CI. Crystal struc-

ture of chaperone protein PapD reveals an immunoglobulin fold (see comments). Nature 1989; 342:248-251.

10. Bork P. Hundreds of ankyrin-like repeats in functionally diverse proteins: mobile modules that cross phyla horizontally? Proteins 1993; 17:363-374.

11. Bork P, Doolittle RF. Proposed acquisition of an animal protein domain by bacteria. Proc Natl Acad Sci USA 1992; 89:8990-8994.

12. Montelione GT,Wuthrich K, Burgess AW et al. Solution structure of murine epidermal growth fctor determined by NMR spectroscopy and refined by energy minimization with restraints. Biochemistry 1992; 14:236-249.

13. Campbell ID, Baron M, Cooke RM et al. Structure-function relationship in epidermal growth factor (EGF) and transforming growth factor-alpha (TGF-alpha). Biochem Pharmacol 1990; 40:35-40.

14. Davies DR, Wlodawer A. Cytokines and their receptor complexes. 1995, 9:50-56.

15. Handford PA, Baron M, Mayhew M et al. The first EGF-like domain from human factor IX contains a high-affinity calcium binding site. EMBO J 1990; 9:475-480.

16. Edwards YJK, Perkins SJ. The protein fold of the von Willebrand factor type A domain is predicted to be similar to the open twisted b-sheet flanked by α-helices found in human ras-p21. FEBS Letters 1995; 358:283-286.

17. Lee J-O, Rieu P, Arnaout AM et al. Crystal structure of the A domain from the α subunit of integrin CR3 (CD11b/CD18). Cell 1995; 80:631-638.

18. Bonaldo P, Russo V, Bucciotti P et al. α1 chain of chick type VI collagen. cDNA sequence reveals a hybrid molecule made of one short collagen and three von Willebrand factor type A like domains. J Biol Chem 1989; 264:5575-5580.

19. Bonaldo P, Russo V, Bucciotti F et al. Structural and functional features of the α3 chain indicate a bridging role for chicken collagen type VI in connective tissues. Biochemistry 1990; 29:1245-1254.

20. Chu M.-L, Zhang R-Z, Pan T et al. Mosaic structure of globular domains in the human type VI collagen α3 chain: similarity to von Willebrand Factor, fibronectin, actin, salivary proteins and aprotinin type protease inhibitors. EMBO J. 1990; 9:385-393.

21. Doliana R, Bonaldo P, Colombatti A. Multiple forms of chicken α3(VI) collagen chain generated by alternative splicing in type A repeat domains. J Cell Biol 1990; 111:2197-2205.

22. Saitta B, Stokes DG, Vissing H et al. Alternative splicing of the human α2 (VI) collagen gene generates multiple mRNA transcripts which predict three protein variants with distinct carboxyl termini. J Biol Chem 1990; 265:6473-6480.

23. Zanussi S, Doliana R, Segat D et al. The human type VI collagen gene. J Biol Chem 1992; 267:24082-24089.

24. Weil D, Mattei M-G, Passage E et al. Cloning and chromosomal localization of human genes encoding the three chains of type VI collagen. Am J Hum Genet 1988; 42:435-445.

25. Wälchli C, Koller E, Trüeb J. Structural comparison of the chicken genes for α1 (VI) and α2 (VI) collagen. Eur J Biochem 1992; 205:583-589.

26. Trüeb B, Schaeren-Wiemers N, Schreier T et al. Molecular cloning of chicken type VI collagen: primary structure of the subunit α2 (VI)-pepsin. J Biol Chem 1989; 264:136-140.

27. Zhang R-Z, Pan T-C, Timpl R et al. Cloning and sequence analysis of cDNAs encoding the α1, α2, and α3 chains of mouse collagen VI. Biochem J 1993; 291:787-792.

28. Stokes DG, Saitta B, Timpl R. Human α3 (VI) collagen gene. Characterization of exons coding for the amino-terminal globular domain and alternative splicing in normal and tumor cells. J Biol Chem 1991; 266:8626-8633.

29. Saitta B, Timpl R, Chu M-L. Human α2(VI) collagen gene. Heterogeneity at the 5'-untranslated region generated by an alternative exon. J Biol Chem 1992; 267:6188-6196.

30. Hayman AR, Koeppel J, Trüeb B. Complete structure of the chicken α2 (VI) collagen gene. Eur J Biochem 1991; 197:177-184.

31. Bonaldo P, Piccolo S, Marvulli D et al. Murine α1 (VI) collagen chain. Complete

amino acid sequence and identification of the gene promoter region. Matrix 1993; 13:223-233.

32. Christiano AM, Greenspan DS, Lee S et al. Cloning of human type VII collagen. J Biol Chem 1994; 269:20256-20262.

33. Christiano AM, Hoffman GG, Chung-Honet LC et al. Structural organization of the human type VII collagen gene (COL7A1), composed of more exons than any previously characterized gene. Genomics 1994; 21:169-179.

34. Christiano AM, Rosenbaum LM, Chung-Honet LC et al. The large non-collagenous domain (NC-1) of type VII collagen is amino terminal and chimeric. Homology to cartilage matrix protein, the type III domain of fibronectin and the A domain of von Willebrand factor. Hum Mol Genet 1992; 7:475-481.

35. Parente MG, Chung LC, Ryynanen J et al. Human type VII collagen: cDNA cloning and chromosomal mapping of the gene. Proc Natl Acad Sci USA 1991; 88:6931-6935.

36. Gordon MK, Gerecke DR, Dublet B et al. Type XII collagen. A large multidomain molecule with partial homology to type IX collagen. J Biol Chem 1989; 264:19772-19778.

37. Dublet B, van der Rest M. Type XII collagen is expressed in embryonic chick tendons. Isolation of pepsin-derived fragments. J Biol Chem 1987; 262:17724-17727.

38. Yamagata M, Yamada KM, Yamada S et al. The complete primary structure of type XII collagen shows a chimeric molecule with reiterated fibronectin type III motifs, von Willebrand factor A motifs, a domain homologous to a noncollagenous region of type IX collagen, and short collagenous domains with an Arg-Gly-Asp site. J Cell Biol 1991; 115:209-221.

39. Wei Y, Yang EV, Klatt KP et al. Monoclonal antibody MT2 identifies the urodele α1 chain of type XII collagen, a developmentally regulated extracellular matrix protein in regenerating Newt limbs. Developmental Biol 1995; 168:503-513.

40. Just M, Herbst H, Hummel M et al. Undulin is a novel member of the fibronectin-tenascin family of extracellular matrix glycoproteins. J Biol Chem 1991; 266:17326-17332.

41. Gerecke DR, Foley JW, Castagnola P et al. Type XIV collagen is encoded by alternative transcripts with distinct 5' regions and is a multidomain protein with homologies to von Willebrand factor, fibronectin, and other matrix protein. J Biol Chem 1993; 268:12177-12184.

42. Wälchli C, Trüeb J, Kessler B et al. Complete primary structure of chicken collagen XIV. Eur J Biochem 1993; 212:483-490.

43. Agraves WS, Deàk F, Sparks KJ et al. Structural features of cartilage matrix proteins deduced from cDNA. Proc Natl Acad Sci USA 1987; 84:464-468.

44. Kiss I, Deàk F, Holloway RG et al. Structure of the gene for cartilage matrix protein, a modular protein of the extracellular matrix: exon/intron organization, unusual splice sites, and relation to α chains of β2 integrins, von Willebrand factor, complement factors B and C2 and epidermal growth factor. J Biol Chem 1989; 264:8126-8134.

45. Jenkins RN, Osborne-Lawrence SL, Sinclair AK et al. Structure and chromosomal location of the human gene encoding cartilage matrix protein. J Biol Chem 1990; 265:19624-19631.

46. Tondravi MM, Winterbottom N, Haudenschild DR et al. Cartilage matrix protein binds to collagen and plays a role in collagen fibrillogenesis. In: Fallon JF, Goetnick PF, Kelley RO, Stocum DL, eds.Limb Development and Regeneration. New York: Wiley, 515-522.

47. Paulsson M, Heinegard D. Matrix proteins bound to associatively prepared proteoglycans from bovine cartilage. Biochem J 1979; 183:539-545.

48. Winterbottom N, Tondravi MM, Harrington TL et al. Cartilage matrix protein is a component of the collagen fibril of cartilage. Dev Dyn 1992; 193:266-276.

49. Ginsburg D, Handin RI, Bonthron DT et al. Human von Willebrand factor (vWF): isolation of complementary DNA (cDNA) clones and chromosomal localization. Science 1985; 228: 1401-1406.

50. Verweij CL, de Vries CJM, Distel B et al. Construction of cDNA coding for human von Willebrand factor using antibody

probes for colony-screening and mapping of the chromosomal gene. Nucleic Acids Res 1985; 13:4699-4717.

51. Lynch DC, Zimmerman TS, Collins CJ et al. Molecular cloning of cDNA for human von Willebrand factor: authentication by a new method. Cell 1985; 41: 49-56.

52. Bonthron DR, Orr EC, Mitsock LM et al. Nucleotide sequence of pre-pro-von Willebrand factor cDNA. Nucleic Acids Res 1986;14:7125-7127.

53. Shelton-Inloes BB, Titani K, Sadler JE. cDNA sequences for human von Willebrand factor reveal five types of repeated domains and five possible protein sequence polymorphisms. Biochemistry 1986; 25:3164-3171.

54. Mancuso DJ, Tuley EA, Westfield LA et al. Structure of the gene for human von Willebrand factor. J Biol Chem 1989; 264:19519-19527.

55. Koppelman SJ, van Hoeij M, Vink T et al. Requirements of von Willebrand factor to protect factor VIII from inactivation by activated protein C. Blood 1996; 87: 2292-2300.

56. Campbell RD, Porter RR. Molecular cloning and characterization of the gene coding for human complement protein Factor B. Proc Natl Acad Sci USA 1983; 80:4464.

57. Mole JE, Anderson JK, Davison Ea et al. Complete primary structure for the zymogen of human complement factor B. J Biol Chem 1984; 259:3407-3412.

58. Nonaka M, Takahashi M, Sasaki M. Molecular cloning of a lamprey homologue of the mammalian MHC class III gene, complement Factor B. J Immunol 1994; 152:2263-2269.

59. Kato Y, Salter-Cid L, Flajnik MF et al. Isolation of the *Xenopus* complement factor B complementary DNA and linkage of the gene to the frog MHC.

60. Kato Y, Salter-Cid L, Flajnik MF et al. Duplication of the MHC-linked *Xenopus* complement factor B gene. Immunogenetics 1995;42:196-203.

61. Bentley DR. Primary structure of human complement component C2. Homology to two unrelated protein families. Biochem J 1986; 239:339-345.

62. Ishikawa N, Nonaka M, Wetsel RA et al. Murine complement C2 and factor B genomic and cDNA cloning reveals different mechanisms for multiple transcripts of C2 and B. J Biol Chem 1990; 265:19040-19046.

63. Gebhard W, Schreitmller T, Hochstrasser K et al. Complementary DNA and derived amino acid sequence of the precursor of one of the three protein components of the inter-alpha-trypsin inhibitor complex. FEBS Lett 1988; 229:63-67.

64. Gebhard W, Schreitmller T, Hochstrasser K et al. Two out of the three kinds of subunits of inter-alpha-trypsin inhibitor are structurally related. Eur J Biochem 1989; 181:571-576.

65. Bourguignon J, Diarra-Mehrpour M, Thiberville L et al. Human pre-alpha-trypsin inhibitor-precursor heavy chain cDNA and deduced amino-acid sequence. Eur J Biochem 1993; 212:771-776.

66. Saguchi K-I, Tobe T, Hashimoto K et al. Cloning and characterization of cDNA for inter-α-trypsin inhibitor family heavy chain-related protein (IHRP), a novel human plasma glycoprotein. J Biochem (Tokyo) 1995; 117:14-18.

67. Diarra-Mehrpour M, Bourguignon J, Bost F et al. Human inter-alpha-trypsin inhibitor: full-length cDNA sequence of the heavy chain H1. Biochim Biophys Acta; 1992; 1132:114-118.

68. Bost F, Bourguignon J, Martin JP et al. Isolation and characterization of the human inter-alpha-trypsin inhibitor heavy-chain H1 gene. Eur J Biochem 1993; 218:283-291.

69. Ignatius MJ, Large TH, Houde H et al. Molecular cloning of the rat integrin α1-subunit: a receptor for laminin and collagen. J Cell Biol 1990; 111:709-720.

70. Briesewitz R, Epstein MR, Marcantonio EE. Expression of native and truncated forms of the human integrin α1 subunit. J Biol Chem 1993; 268:2989-2996.

71. Kern A, Briesewitz R, Bank I et al. The role of the I domain in ligand binding of the human integrin α1β1. J Biol Chem1994; 269: 22811-22816.

72. Takada Y, Hemler M. The primary structure of the VLA-2/collagen receptor α2 subunit (platelet GPIa): homology to other integrins and the presence of a possible collagen binding domain. J Cell Biol 1989;

109:397-407.

73. Edelman JM, Chan BMC, Uniyal S et al. The mouse VLA-2 homologue supports collagen and laminin adhesion but not virus binding. Cell Adh Comm 1994; 2:131-143.

74. Kamata T, Puzon W, Takada Y. Identification of putative ligand binding sites within I domain of integrin $\alpha 2\beta 1$ (VLA-2, CD49b/CD29). J Biol Chem 1994; 269:9659-9663.

75. Bahou WF, Potter CL, Mirza H. The VLA-2 ($\alpha 2\beta 1$) I domain functions as a ligand-specific recognition sequence for endothelial cell attachment and spreading: molecular and functional characterization. Blood 1994; 11:3734-3741.

76. Larson RS, Corbi AL, Berman L et al. Primary structure of the leukocyte function-associated molecule-1 α subunit: an integrin with an embedded domain defining a protein superfamily. J Cell Biol 1989; 108:703-712.

77. Pytela R. Amino acid sequence of the murine Mac-1 α chain reveals homologuous with the integrin family and an additional domain related to von Willebrand factor. EMBO J 1988; 7: 1371-1378.

78. Corbi AL, Kishimoto TK, Miller LJ et al. The human leukocyte adhesion glycoprotein Mac-1 (complement receptor type 3, CD11b) α subunit. J Biol Chem 1988; 263:12403-12411.

79. Fleming JC, Pahl HL, Gonzales DA et al. Structural analysis of the CD11b gene and phylogenetic analysis of the α-integrin gene family demonstrate remarkable conservation of genomic organization and suggest early diversification during evolution. J Immunol 1993; 150:480-490.

80. Corbi AL, Miller LJ, O'Connor K et al. cDNA cloning and complete primary structure of the α subunit of a leukocyte adhesion glycoprotein, p150,95. EMBO J 1987; 6: 4023-4028.

81. Corbi AL, Garcia-Aguilar J, Springer TA. Genomic structure of an integrin α subunit, the leukocyte p150,95 molecule. J Biol Chem 1990; 265:2782-2788.

82. Danilenko DM, Rossitto PV, Van der Vieren M et al. A novel canine leukointegrin $\alpha_d\beta_2$ is expressed by specific macrophage subpopulations in tissue and a minor CD8$^+$

lymphocyte subpopulation in peripheral blood. J Immunol 1995; 155:35-44.

83. Shaw SK, Cepek KL, Murphy EA et al. Molecular cloning of the human mucosal lymphocyte integrin aE subunit. J Biol Chem 1994; 269:6016-6025.

84. Ellis SB, Williams ME, Ways N et al. Sequence and expression of mRNAs encoding the $\alpha 1$ and $\alpha 2$ subunits of a DHP-sensitive calcium channel. Science 1988; 241:1661-1664.

85. Robson KJH, Hall JRS, Jennings MW et al. A highly conserved amino acid sequence in thrombospondin, properdin and in proteins from sporozoites and blood stage of human malaria parasite. Nature 1988; 335:79-82.

86. Rogers WO, Malik A, Mellouk S et al. Characterization of *Plasmodium falciparum* sporozoite surface protein 2. Proc Natl Acad Sci USA 1992; 89:9176-9180.

87. Tomley FM, Clarke LE, Kawazoe U et al. Sequence of the gene encoding an immunodominant microneme protein of *Eimeria tenella*. Mol Biochem Parasitol 1991; (87)49:277-288.

88. Pasamontes L, Hug D, Humbelin M et al. Sequence of a major *Eimeria maxima* antigen homologous to the *Eimeria tenella* microneme protein Etp 100. Mol Biochem Parasitol 1993; 57:171-174.

89. Craik CS, Sprang S Fletterick R et al. Intron-exon splice junctions map at protein surfaces. Nature 1982; 299:180-182.

90. Perkins SJ, Smith KF, Williams SC et al. The secondary structure of the von Willebrand Factor type A domain in factor B of human complement by fourier transform infrared spectroscopy. J Mol Biol 1994; 238:104-119.

91. Horiuchi T, Macon KJ, Engler JA et al. Site-directed mutagenesis of the region around Cys-241 of complement component C2: evidence for a C4b binding site. J Immunol 1991; 147:584-589.

92. Edwards CP, Champe M, Gonzales T et al. Identification of amino acids in the CD11a I-domain important for binding of the leukocyte function-associated antigen-1 (LFA-1) to intercellular adhesion molecule-1 (ICAM-1). J Biol Chem 1995; 270:12635-12640.

93. Kamata T, Takada Y. Direct binding of

collagen to the I domain of integrin α2β1 (VLA-2, CD49b/CD29) in a divalent cation-independent manner. J Biol Chem 1994; 269:26006-26010.

94. Kern A, Briesewitz R, Bank I et al. The role of the I domain in ligand binding of the human integrin α1β1. J Biol Chem 1994; 269:22811-22816.

95. Kamata T, Wright R, Takada Y. Critical Threonine and aspartic acid residues within the I domains of β2 integrins for interactions with intercellular adhesion molecule 1 (ICAM-1) and C3bi. J Biol Chem 1995; 270:12531-12535.

96. Michishita M, Videm V, Arnaout MA. A novel divalent cation-binding site in the A domain of the β2 integrin CR3 (CD11b/CD18) is essential for ligand binding. Cell 1993; 72:857-867.

97. Bork P, Rohde K. More von Willebrand factor type A domains? Sequence similarities with malaria thrombospondin-related anonymous protein, dihydropyridine-sensitive calcium channel and inter-a-trypsin inhibitor. Biochem J 1991; 279:908-910.

98. Huang C, Springer TA. A binding interface on the I domain of Lymphocyte function-associated antigen-1 (LFA-1) required for specific interaction with intercellular adhesion molecule 1 (ICAM-1). J Biol Chem 1995; 270:19008-19016.

99. Ueda T, Rieu P, Brayer J et al. Identification of the complement iC3b binding site in the β2 integrin CR3 (CD11b/CD18). Proc Natl Acad Sci USA 1994; 91:10680-10684.

100. Rieu P, Ueda T, Haruta I et al. The A-domain of β2 integrin CR3 (CD11b/CD18) is a receptor for the hookworm-derived neutrophil adhesion inhibitor NIF. J Cell Biol 1994; 127:2081-2091.

101. Lee J-O, Bankston LA, Arnaout MA et al. Two conformations of the integrin A-domain (I-domain): a pathway for activation? Structure 1995; 3:1333-1340.

102. Altieri DC. Occupancy of CD11b/CD18 (Mac-1) divalent ion binding site(s) induces leukocyte adhesion. J Immunol 1991; 147:1891-1898.

103. Dransfield I, Cabanas C, Craig A et al. Divalent cation regulation of the function of the leukocyte integrin LFA-1. J Cell Biol 1992; 116:219-226.

104. Matsushita T, Sadler JE. Identification of amino acid residues essential for von Willebrand factor binding to platelet glycoprotein Ib. J Biol Chem 1995; 270:13406-13414.

105. Loftus JC, Smith JW, Ginsberg MH. Integrin-mediated cell adhesion: the extracellular face. J Biol Chem 1994; 269:25235-25238.

106. Takada Y, Ylanne J, Mandelman D et al. A point mutation of integrin β1 subunit blocks binding of α5β1 to fibronectin and invasin but not recruitment to adhesion plaques. J Cell Biol 1992; 119:913-921.

107. Bajt ML, Goodman T, McGuire SL. β2 (CD18) mutations abolish ligand recognition by I domain integrins LFA-1 (aLb2, CD11a/CD18) and MAC-1 (αMβ2, CD11b/CD18). J Biol Chem 1995; 270:94-98.

108. Loftus JC, O'Toole TE, Plow EF et al. A β3 integrin mutations abolishes ligand binding and alters divalent cation-dependent conformation. Science 1990: 249:915-918.

109. Bajt ML, Loftus JC, Gawaz MP et al. Characterization of a gain of function mutation of integrin αIIbβ3 (platelet glycoprotein IIb-IIIa). J Biol Chem 1992; 267:22211-22216.

110. Bajt ML, Loftus JC. Mutation of a ligand binding domain of beta 3 integrin. J Biol Chem 1994; 269:20913-20919.

111. Staunton DE, Dustin ML, Erickson HP et al. The arrangement of the immunoglobulin-like domains of ICAM-1 and the binding sites for LFA-1 and rhinovirus. Cell 1990; 61:243-254.

112. Taniguchi-Sidle A, Isenman DE. Interaction of human complement C3 wiyh factor B and complement receptor type 1 (CR1, CD35) and type 3 (CR3, CD11/CD18) involve an acidic sequence at the N-terminus of C3 a'-chain. J. Immunol 1994; 153:5285-5302.

VON WILLEBRAND FACTOR

In contrast to recirculating leukocytes which migrate through intact endothelium,[1] platelets normally do not interact with endothelial cells. Instead, they interact with damaged blood vessels and attach at sites of injury leading to physiologic hemostasis or at sites of diseased vessels leading to pathologic thrombotic vascular occlusion. The critical event in both conditions is adhesion of platelets to the subendothelium. Platelets therefore have acquired ways to distinguish between a non-thrombogenic endothelium, which is free of platelets, and the exposed subendothelium where platelet deposition is initiated. Rapid formation of the initial platelet layer covering exposed subendothelial surfaces involves bridging between collagens and maybe other components of the subendothelium on one side and platelet membrane receptors and heparin-like glycosaminoglycans on the other side. Hemodynamic forces play a significant role in the process of thrombus formation; as blood moves through a vessel there is a decreasing velocity gradient near the wall that creates a high shear stress opposing platelet adhesion. Platelets, forced toward the vascular lining surface, adhere at sites of vascular damage: this adhesion depends initially on the transient interaction between a receptor on the platelet surface, glycoprotein Ib (GPIb), and von Willebrand factor (vWF) on the vascular surface.

The binding of vWF to GPIb is considered essential for platelet adhesion to damaged vascular wall and for platelet aggregation under high shear stress flow conditions and a deficiency of either one results in abnormal arterial platelet adhesion. This was originally demonstrated by studying platelet adhesion under defined flow conditions from patients with defects in GPIb (Bernard-Soulier syndrome)[2] or von Willebrand Disease (vWD)[3] and in animal models of vWD.[4] At the interface between the blood stream and the vessel wall, shear forces are exerted on both the vascular and platelets' surfaces but vWF-dependent platelet adhesion will not ensue unless sufficient shear rates are present. Therefore, the process of platelet adhesion depends on a mechanical force (shear) affecting specific molecules (GPIb and vWF) and the GPIb-vWF interaction will not occur in the absence of shear or unless either one of the two members is modified. Under static conditions soluble vWF has very low affinity for GPIb unless an appropriate modulator is present, but

The Superfamily with von Willebrand Factor VA Domains, edited by
Alfonso Colombatti and Roberto Doliana. © 1996 R.G. Landes Company.

vWF displays a strong affinity for GPIb either as a surface bound ligand or as a soluble multimeric ligand subjected to rheological conditions producing a high shear stress.[5,6] In particular, binding of vWF to the blood vessel wall exposes "cryptic" binding sites on vWF for GPIb; this event constitutes the initial step in hemostasis but is also instrumental in the pathogenesis of thrombosis. The system is then switched on and platelet adhesion is followed by platelet activation[7] and aggregation.[8] Agonists generated at the site of lesion can act on platelets present in the vicinity and induce an activation state; therefore, adhesive ligands as well as activating soluble molecules contribute to thrombus formation. The process of aggregation, which can be simulated in vitro with the use of an aggregometer, reflects the ability of vWF to support platelet thrombus formation and requires active metabolism. Instead, agglutination, which also can occur with fixed cells, represents an experimental approach to study the vWF-GPIb interaction.

vWF, which plays a key role not only in platelet adhesion and thrombus formation but also in coagulation, is a soluble multimeric protein containing a variable number of subunits.[9] The functions of vWF result from the presence of a series of binding sites for specific ligands and it is not brought about by conformational changes caused by the polymerization into large multimers: the importance of the multimeric nature of vWF for its function is primarily ascribed to its ability to provide a high local density of binding sites by presenting many repeating subunits.

vWD was originally described by Erik von Willebrand in a large family whose members presented with prolonged bleeding times but normal platelet counts and coagulation times.[10] Later on it was recognized that the vWD is an heterogeneous bleeding disorder[11] and the disease, which is the most common congenital bleeding disorder,[12] comprises several distinct clinical subtypes in which the primary abnormality is quantitative (types 1 and 3) or qualitative (type 2) (see below).[13] It is particularly the study of the qualitative vWF defects that has contributed to the understanding of the function of vWF in hemostasis.

MOLECULAR STRUCTURE

vWF has a typical extended multimeric structure[14] with a diameter of 2-3 μm and a variable length which depends on the number of subunits. The repeating unit of vWF, the protomer with a molecular mass of about 500 kD, is composed of two antiparallel subunits linked by disulfide bonds at the C-terminal ends. The globules at the two ends of the protomer interact with other protomers to form the long filamentous structures.[15-17] vWF is stored within platelets and endothelial cell granules. Storage granules contain the largest multimers, while the sizes of the vWF multimers present in the blood are variable.[18]

The human vWF gene, on chromosome 12 (12p12.1-p12.3) has a relatively large size of 180 kb comprising 52 exons.[19] The first exon contains the 5' untranslated sequences, exons 3 through 17 encode the propeptide, and exons 18 to 52 encode the mature protein. Gene duplication and/or exon-shuffling events have generated the structure of vWF gene: this is suggested by the presence of several repetitive modules within the vWF sequence, but the evolutionary history of vWF must have been complex since intron-exon boundaries display limited similarity among homologous modules. In addition, a highly homologous pseudogene corresponding to the central part of the vWF gene (exons 23-34) has been localized to chromosome 22[20] and might be implicated in some vWD type 2A forms by a mechanism of gene conversion.[21,22] The vWF gene demonstrates extensive polymorphism and a large number of single amino acid substitutions have been identified. Many of these substitutions apparently do not impair vWF function and cannot be distinguished from authentic mutations. Amino acids within the mature vWF subunit are numbered 1 to

2,050 with the N-terminal serine set at +1. The mutations are indicated as follows : R611C where R and C represent the wild type and the substitute amino acid residue (in the one letter code), respectively, separated by the amino acid position of the mutation.

Almost the entire coding sequence of vWF is composed of four types of repeating modules designated A (renamed, after Bork and Ames, VWFA or VA in the shortened form)[23] through D (Fig. 2.1).[24-31] In addition, there are few short sequences connecting the different types of modules and other non-repeated sequences in the C-terminal end of the molecule that are required for dimerization.[32] The primary translation product predicted from the cDNA sequence and demonstrated by Northern blotting of endothelial cell mRNA, is about 9 kb in size. It encodes a 2813-residue polypeptide consisting of a signal peptide of 22 residues, a very long propeptide (741 residues) and the mature protein of 2050 residues. vWF has a potential for 22 carbohydrate side chains, 10 of which are O-linked to serine and threonine residues and the content of carbohydrate can be as high as 10% to 19% of the total mass of the mature vWF. The distribution of the carbohydrate side chains along the vWF sequence is not uniform and most of the glycosylated sites are clustered at the N- and C-terminal end regions of the molecule, with a large gap in the central part of the mature vWF where the VWFA modules are located. vWF is characterized by a high content (8.3%) of cysteine residues particularly abundant in the N- and C-terminal regions.[31] The VWFA modules of vWF (defined as A1, A2 and A3) are adjacent and span residues E497-G1111 of the mature vWF subunit. Both A1 and A3 contain an intramolecular disufide bond C509-C695 and C923-C1109, respectively, that generates an identical 187 residue loop.[32-36] The A1 and A3 modules are functionally relevant since they interact with several ligands. The A2

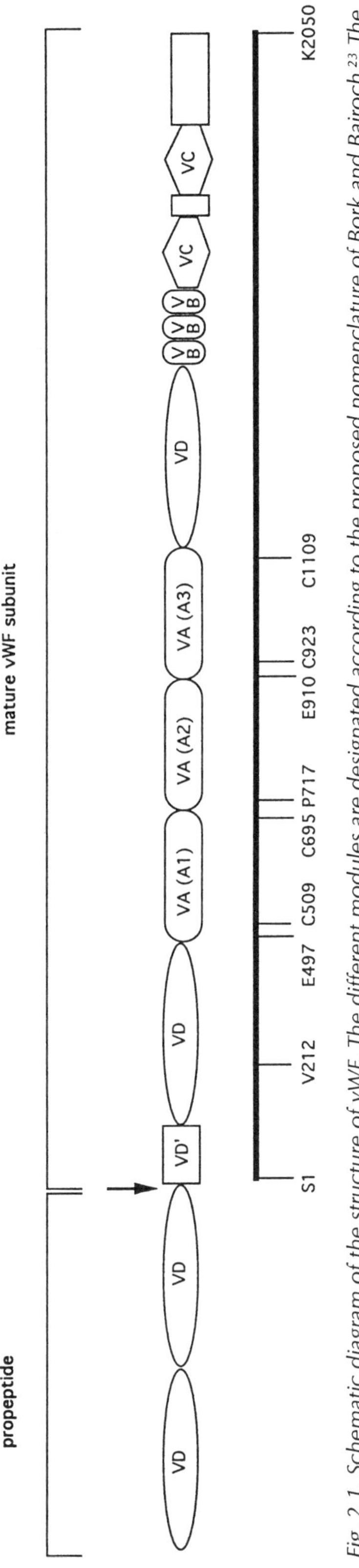

Fig. 2.1. Schematic diagram of the structure of vWF. The different modules are designated according to the proposed nomenclature of Bork and Bairoch.[23] The current designation of the VWFA modules also is included. Numbers refer to the position of relevant residues such as the first residue of each VWFA module (E497, P717 and E910) and the cysteines forming the two loops. The arrow indicates the cleavage site of the furin/PACE serine protease.

module, although similar to A1 and A3 at the primary sequence, apparently is not provided with any binding activity except for the fact that it harbors a proteolytic cleavage site[37] recognized by a specific protease.[38] The three short B modules are adjacent and localize in the C-terminal portion of the mature vWF. Two C modules of about 90 residues each are at the C-terminal end of the polypeptide and share sequence similarity to thrombospondin and type I and III procollagens.[39] The only cell adhesion RGD site present in vWF is located in module C1 and this sequence is recognized by the platelet integrin αIIbβ3.[40,41] The D modules of about 360 residues each, 10% of which are cysteines, constitute the propeptide (D1 and D2) and also are present at the N- (D3 plus a truncated D' domain) and toward the C-terminal end (D4) of the mature vWF. While the position of the cysteine residues are well conserved, only the cysteine residues of module D3 seem to participate in the multimerization process.[42,43]

TISSUE EXPRESSION

vWF is synthesized exclusively in megakaryocytes[44,45] and endothelial cells.[46] Endothelial cells contain membrane-bound elongated granules, called Weibel-Palade bodies.[46] Similar organelles also are present in megakaryocytes and are filled with longitudinally arranged tubular structures of highly organized vWF polymers.[47] Early in vascular development vWF is expressed in a limited subset of endothelial cells,[48] whereas in adults heterogeneous mRNA expression can be found in different vascular beds.[49-52] Consistent with these observations transgenic mice, generated with a chimeric construct including a short segment of the 5' flanking sequence and the first exon fused to *lacZ*, target expression of the reporter gene only to a subpopulation of endothelial cells in the yolk sac and adult brain.[53] Another major site of vWF storage is within the platelet α-granules which are estimated to store up to 20% of the total vWF present in blood.

BIOSYNTHESIS

Depending upon the extent of multimer formation, plasma vWF is composed of a population of molecules that can range up to 50 individual subunits. It is definitively accepted that the extent of vWF multimer formation is directly related to hemostatic efficacy and that the multivalency of the larger multimers confers greater binding affinities[54] and consequently a greater thrombogenic capacity in terms of higher adhesion.[55]

Three cellular model systems have provided most of the current information on the biosynthesis of vWF: megakaryocytes,[44,45,47] endothelial cells[49,50,56] and transfected cells.[32,57-61] These studies have demonstrated that there are two major mechanisms of processing of newly synthesized vWF: a constitutive secretory pathway present in endothelial cells, and a post-translational process leading to storage within Weibel-Palade bodies in endothelial cells and within α-granules in platelets. Similar organelles also are formed in heterologous transfected cells.[60,61] The secretory pathway is the major route in endothelial cells cultured in vitro;[61] in fact, only about 5% of vWF is stored within Weibel-Palade bodies. It is not clear yet whether a constitutive secretion of the same intensity is taking place in vivo or whether the secretion is vectorial toward the lumen or the baso-lateral surface from where vWF is then deposited in the subendothelium.

A schematic representation of the sequence of events during the process of multimeric vWF assembly[62] is the following. In the endoplasmic reticulum and concurrent with the initial glycosylation,[63] pro-vWF monomers dimerize via disulfide bonds and form protomers. The only sequences needed for dimerization are located within the C-terminal 151 amino-acid residues.[32] That the information needed for dimerization is located exclusively in this short segment of the molecule has been convincingly demonstrated using transfected cells: even in the absence of the rest of the molecule the process of dimerization is still takes place.[32] In the Golgi and trans Golgi cisternae, complex N- and O-linked sugars are then added, the sugars are modified by sulfation[63] and the protomers are assembled into large molecular aggregates through the formation of intermolecular bonds among the cysteines in the D3 modules of the mature protein. While several cysteines involved in multimerization have been identified,[42,43] the sequential process of disulfide bond formation has not yet been completely clarified. Furthermore, for the process of multimerization to occur the propeptide must be present; cells transfected with cDNAs of the mature vWF polypeptide do not give rise to multimers[57] unless the cells are cotransfected with the cDNA of the propeptide[58] suggesting that the D1 and D2 modules of the propeptide might promote polymerization via multiple homophilic interactions with other D modules.

Although vWF and its propeptide are present in Weibel-Palade bodies in stoichiometric amounts,[64,65] both the endoproteolytic cleavage and the multimerization process occur early in the trans Golgi apparatus and very likely the propeptide remains noncovalently associated with the mature vWF.[66] The 100 kD propeptide is cleaved by furin/PACE, a calcium-dependent serine protease[38] well before vWF enters the secretory granules but while cleavage is a prerequisite for granule targeting it is not a prerequisite for secretion.[67] Finally, storage is not linked to the formation of multimers, but to the cleavage of the vWF propeptide since a point mutation within the cleavage site of pro-vWF (R763G) leads to complete inhibition of the cleavage of the propeptide without affecting the multimerization process.[68] Once secreted, the propolypeptide might interact with collagen via the collagen binding site in the D2 module[69] and contribute to the wound healing process.

The presence of lateral sugar chains seems very important for protection from proteolysis[70] and for a proper maturation of vWF (both dimerization and multimerization) since treatment with tunic-amycin leads to accumulation of pro-vWF monomers within the endoplasmic reticulum.[71] Furthermore, the carbohydrate side chains can modulate vWF activity: for instance, the removal of terminal sialic acid residues eliminates the need to add ristocetin in order to induce vWF binding to platelets.[70]

After platelets and endothelial cells are activated with agonists such as thrombin, histamine, fibrin and adenosine diphosphate the larger and more thrombogenic multimers generated via the storage pathway and stored in α granules and Weibel-Palade bodies are secreted at sites of injury where hemostasis is needed and vWF is rapidly removed from the circulation. Disappearance of vWF is the consequence of deposition within subendothelial sites where the multimers provide anchorage for platelets, of proteolytic degradation and of controlled proteolysis all of which limit accumulation and reduce the size of vWF multimers in the circulation. This is evidenced by the finding that stored multimers are composed of subunits which are identical in size[72] while circulating vWF is heterogeneous. The controlled proteolysis depends on the presence of one major cleavage site within the A2 module,[37] located between Y842 and M843, that allows the separation of vWF multimers in smaller pieces. This proteolytic process is enhanced by the local rheological conditions.[73]

FUNCTION

The role of vWF in normal hemostasis and blood coagulation is multifaceted: it stabilizes and functions as a carrier of factor VIII[74] and protects factor VIII in the blood from inactivation by protein C;[75] it functions as a cofactor for thrombin-catalyzed cleavage of the factor VIII light chain.[76] vWF interacts with fibrin,[77] predominantly if not exclusively in the venus vascular bed, and participates in the initial formation, propagation and stabilization of thrombi formed by polymerized fibrin and aggregated platelets.[78,79] Since the contribution of vWF to the coagulation process does not seem to involve its VWFA modules it will not be further discussed. Conversely, VWFA modules play a fundamental role in the hemostatic and thrombogenic process under high shear stress conditions by promoting adhesive contacts between platelets and the exposed subendothelial tissue. The events of platelet-vessel wall and platelet-platelet interactions can be summarized in the following temporal sequence: binding of vWF to components of the subendothelium; exposure of vWF "cryptic" sites; binding of vWF to GPIb followed by reversible platelet adhesion; this interaction then generates signal transduction messages that activate αIIbβ3 on platelets; activated αIIbβ3 binds to the vWF RGD recognition sequence and this is followed by irreversible platelet adhesion, spreading and aggregation.

The number of platelets attaching to an injured vessel and the extent of thrombosis are determined by the degree of injury and by the local flow dynamics. In fact, it is the shear rate, which is directly related to the blood flow and inversely to the diameter of the vessel, that modulates platelet-vessel wall interactions. Perfusion experiments have demonstrated that vWF is essential in the process of platelet deposition, in their aggregation, and in thrombus formation, particularly at high shear stress.[80,81] Exposure of de-endothelized vessel wall (a thrombogenic surface) to platelet-rich plasma or blood at high shear stress is sufficient to induce platelet deposition to the vessel wall.[82] However, if fibrillar collagen is present, such as to mimic a more severe damaged vessel wall, significantly more platelets are deposited and fully activated to form a stable thrombus.[83]

To investigate in vitro the role of vWF in contributing to platelet adhesion and aggregation a useful device has been the rotational cone-and-plate viscometer[5,84] equipped with a computerized epifluorescence video microscopy system[85] allowing a direct real-time observation of platelet adhesion and aggregation. With this device, which represents a refinement of the traditional aggregometer, a uniform shear force is applied in the whole chamber and the shear forces generated can be much higher than the forces reached with the aggregometer. Under these conditions stable aggregation can occur in the absence of exogenous agonists provided GPIb is expressed on the platelet surface, soluble multimeric vWF is present in the system and platelet count is between 50,000 and 600,000/ml.[86] It is still not clear how the platelet aggregation phenomenon obtained under high shear forces in the order of 30-100 dynes/cm^2, relates to the *in vivo* conditions where a thrombogenic endothelium interacts with vWF. Nevertheless, there are antibodies against GPIb that block the vWF-GPIb interaction at high shear rate and the resulting platelet aggregation. These same antibodies are not able to inhibit platelet aggregation under low shear rate.[5,87,88] The involvement of vWF in mediating platelet adhesion and thrombus formation is crucial under high shear stress conditions such as those encountered in small vessels and stenosed arteries,[89] because fibrinogen, which is the major ligand for αIIbβ3-mediated platelet irreversible attachment and aggregation, is ineffective under these same conditions.[5,90]

INTERACTION OF vWF WITH THE VESSEL WALL

Platelets and vWF, normally present in the circulation, do not interact since vWF-GPIb binding sites are not functional.[6] For thrombus formation it is necessary that altered endothelial cells or exposed subendothelial tissue come in contact with vWF or that high shear stress forces alter the conformation of vWF or of GPIb leading to their interaction.[5] The participation of vWF in hemostasis is fundamental for thrombus formation under high shear stress conditions such as those present in small arteries or in pathological vessel affections such as stenosed arteries in artheriosclerosis. Once any of the above favoring conditions are present, the initiation of thrombus formation is supported by circulating vWF, which is rapidly absorbed onto the exposed damaged vessel wall, and by insolubilized subendothelial vWF.

Insoluble vWF, by providing adequately exposed GPIb binding sites, supports initial platelet contact.[91,92] However, vWF is not constitutively present in the subendothelium of all vessels; capillaries, for instance, are devoid of subendothelial vWF.[93] In these locations, but this applies also to thrombus formation in small vessels, soluble plasma vWF is necessary in the first steps of the platelet response to the damaged vessel through interactions with constituents of the vessel wall.[6] Newly deposited vWF at any site leads to a rapid increase in the local concentration of insolubilized vWF. Deposited vWF then expresses high affinity binding sites for GPIb and optimal platelet deposition takes place. What are the structures expressed in the subendothelial matrix to which vWF binds? In vitro studies have identified type I collagen, which is present in deeper sites, and type III collagen, which is located immediately underneath the endothelial basement membrane.[94,95] Using complex extracellular matrix (ECM) extracts of vascular tissues and endothelial cells it was concluded that fibrillar collagens are not the only ligands available.[96-98] Furthermore, the relevance of fibrillar collagens was even disputed since collagenase-treated ECM is equally effective in supporting vWF binding.[99] Other constituents of the subendothelium that contribute to vWF initial binding are heparin[100,101] and maybe heparan sulfate proteoglycans.[102] While it is still not conclusively established which ligands are physiologically important for binding of vWF to subendothelial surfaces, type VI collagen is one of the subendothelium components which allow vWF binding[103] after collagenase treatment.[99] Type VI collagen, because of a high content of cysteine residues at the boundaries of the triple helix,[104] is resistant to degradation by collagenases unless this treatment is performed under reducing conditions.[105] This collagen is organized in microfilament structures present also in the subendothelium where it colocalizes with vWF.[106] Recently the role of type VI collagen as a ligand supporting vWF-mediated platelet adhesion has been explored in vitro using both high (40 dynes/cm^2) and low (4 dynes/cm^2) shear stress rates:[107] type VI displays a higher affinity than type I for platelet adhesion at low shear rates in the presence of vWF. Although there might still be functional differences depending upon the species or the tissues from which type VI collagen is obtained (Mazzuccato et al, unpublished results), the present experimental evidence suggests that type VI collagen plays a major role in supporting vWF-mediated initial platelet deposition under shear stress rates that are considerably lower than those required to support type I collagen vWF-mediated platelet adhesion.

INTERACTION OF vWF WITH PLATELETS

Primary hemostasis consists of an interaction between platelets and blood vessels leading to clot formation. Platelets in physiological, but also in pathological, thrombus formation become irreversibly attached at injury sites. Platelets normally circulate in an inactive state, but can be activated by several stimuli. In such cases, the vWF stored in granules is released, raising the local concentration of vWF. This is followed by platelet adhesion, spreading and aggregation. As mentioned above, the role of vWF seems to be most relevant where the shear stress is relatively high, as it is in small arteries.[3] It is likely that vWF takes advantage of its multimeric organization to exert its adhesive function by assuming, under higher shear rates, the extended filament shape observed by transmission electron microscopy following rotary shadowing.[15-17]

vWF interacts with two platelet receptors: GPIb of the GPIb-IX-V complex and the integrin αIIbβ3, the latter being a promiscuous receptor which also recognizes fibrinogen, fibronectin[108] and vitronectin.[109] The binding of vWF to GPIb leads to the initial transient contact of platelets with the subendothelium, i.e. platelet adhesion is initiated. Then, an activation signal is delivered to αIIbβ3 which also binds to vWF via the RGD motif in module C1 and platelet spreading and aggregation takes place.[5,89]

The role of GPIb was first demonstrated by perfusion studies with platelets lacking GPIb.[3] Later GPIb-vWF interactions in platelet aggregation have been studied indirectly with function-blocking antibodies which are able to prevent vWF binding to either GPIb or collagen.[5,87,110] Curiously, some of these antibodies inhibit platelet adhesion only at high shear stress.[5,87,88] In the artificial environment of the modified cone-and-plate viscometer and using shear forces well above those occurring in the circulation (430 dynes/cm^2), GPIb and αIIbβ3 integrin are both involved in the stable and irreversible interaction of platelets with soluble multimeric vWF either in a sequential or concurrent fashion.[86] One conclusion which emerged from those studies is that, in the absence of exogenous modulators, GPIb is not able to support irreversible binding to vWF even if the platelets are exposed to very high shear. The above findings are analogous to those described for adhesion of platelets to insolubilized vWF in a flow chamber,[111] a phenomenon that also relies upon both GPIb and αIIbβ3 to become irreversible.[90] In this case the process of adhesion consists of an initial transient GPIb-mediated attachment until a sufficient platelet activation is reached, followed by αIIbβ3-mediated irreversible arrest. The advantage of the high local density reached when large vWF multimers are deposited is evident: the multivalency of this ligand allows a fast rate of bond formation between GPIb and vWF even if platelets are moving at high speed. For in vitro functional studies and in addition to the cone-and-plate viscometer, the antibiotic ristocetin, which binds to both platelets and vWF, also has been a useful tool for inducing binding of vWF to GPIb and subsequent platelet agglutination.[112,113] Furthermore, botrocetin, a protein isolated from a snake's venom, binds directly to vWF, but not to GPIb, leading to a vWF "conformational" change allowing binding

to GPIb.[114,115] While the precise mechanisms by which these agents promote vWF-GPIb interaction are not entirely known, they have been useful in studying the mechanisms of vWF interactions. However, the conclusions on the mode of action of these modulators should be considered with caution since they do not represent physiological ligands.

STRUCTURE-FUNCTION RELATIONSHIPS

The multifaceted functions of vWF are related to its distinct modular domains which interact with a number of ligands during the process of hemostasis. The extensive functional analysis of the products of limited enzymatic digestion of vWF, the inhibition studies with synthetic peptides and function-blocking antibodies and, more recently, the use of recombinant fragments have allowed the localization of the major functions within the individual domains (Fig. 2.2). With these multiple approaches most of the functions ascribed to vWF have been localized to the A1 and A3 VWFA modules. Some uncertainties remain, but the resolution of the three-dimensional structure of the VWFA modules of Mac-1[116,117] and the ongoing definition of the vWF A1 and A3 modules structure will soon resolve the issues still open. While no specific binding sites for the subendothelium or for platelets have so far been identified within the A2 module, this module plays a relevant role in the regulation of the size and amounts of vWF multimers in circulation through proteolysis at a very specific cleavage site (Y842-M843) approximately in the middle of the A2 module.[37]

INTERACTIONS OF VWF WITH CONSTITUENTS OF THE SUBENDOTHELIUM

FIBRILLAR COLLAGENS

Collagens are the major ligands present in the subendothelium and in vitro direct binding and competition studies with proteolytic fragments of vWF have indicated

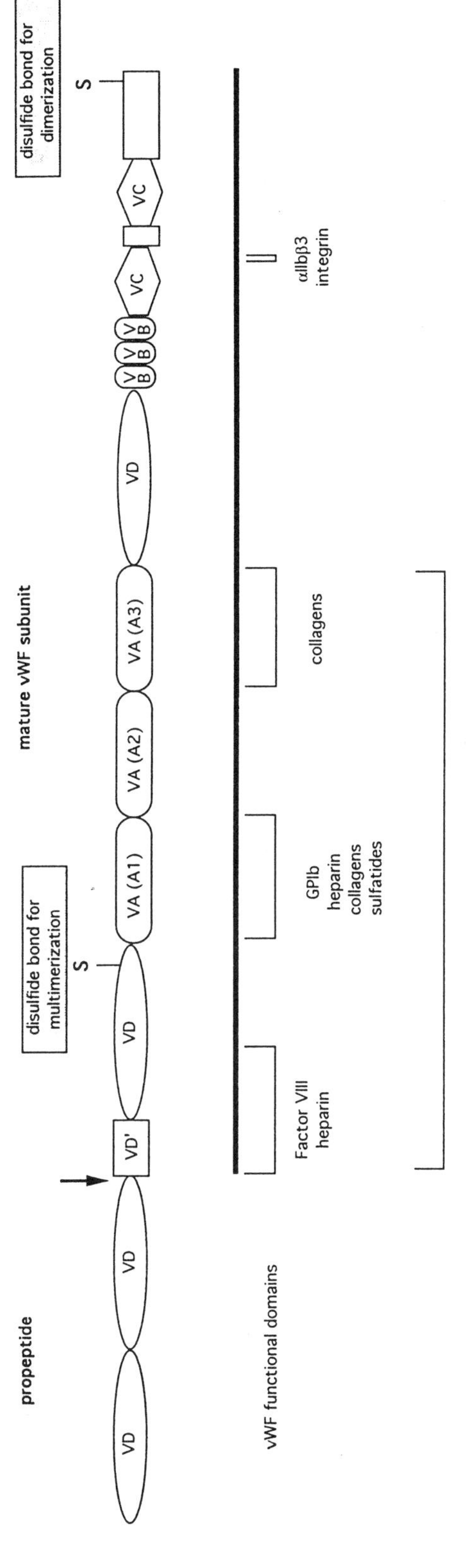

Fig. 2.2. Location of the known functional sites of vWF. The major binding sites for factor VIII, heparin, GPIb, αIIbβ3, collagens, sulfatides, ristocetin and botrocetin are indicated. The arrow indicates the cleavage site of the furin/PACE serine protease.

that there might be at least three potential fibrillar collagen-binding regions. One region is localized in the propeptide[69] and very likely does not play any role in platelet adhesion. Binding studies have localized the major recognition sites for collagen within a tryptic fragment of the vWF subunit spanning the amino acid residues V449-K728.[36,100,110,118] Most of this fragment corresponds to the A1 module (E497-G716). Further, a *Staphylococcus aureus* V8-protease fragment spanning residues G911-E1365 and including the A3 module interacts with type III collagen fibrils.[119] Reduced and alkylated CNBr fragments, localized to sequences E542-L622 in A1 and K948-K988 in A3 modules, respectively, also can compete for vWF binding to collagen.[36,118,119] In addition, several function-blocking antibodies have been described, most of which recognize either the A1 or the A3 modules,[110,120-123] that appear to represent immunodominant portions of the vWF molecule. The high immunogenicity of the VWFA modules of vWF is shared with other modules of vWF superfamily proteins such as Mac-1 and p150,95,[124] LFA-1[125-127] and $\alpha2\beta1$ integrin.[128]

Despite the results obtained with proteolytic fragments,[36,118,129] there is still some uncertainty regarding the existence of a collagen binding site in the A1 module. The relative importance of A1 and A3 recognition sites has not yet been clarified since the different results could depend on the source of vWF, the type of collagen and the binding assay used. In fact, while it was initially found that a recombinant fragment including all the A1 module and few additional flanking sequences bound to collagen,[130] this collagen-binding activity could not be reproduced[131,132] even when a recombinant A1 module was utilized.[133] While galactose moieties in vWF may be critical for the vWF-type I collagen interaction,[134] the inability of the recombinant A1 module to bind collagen seems not to be due to the absence of sugars since a similar glycosylated A1 module secreted by CHO cells still is ineffective.[133]

Recombinant vWF from which the entire A1 module has been deleted still binds to collagen,[135] indicating that the A1 module is not essential for this function and could be replaced by the A3 collagen-binding site. Recent evidence confirms that the A3 module might be more relevant than the A1 for binding to collagen:[136] while a recombinant A3 module binds to immobilized collagen and completely inhibits the binding of multimeric vWF, a recombinant A1 module does not display any competition for vWF binding. There are several possible explanations for the failure of the monomeric recombinant A1 module to compete with intact vWF for binding to type I collagen. First, the A1 module lacks a type I collagen-binding site. Second, the A1 module could still bind to immobilized type I collagen but is sterically or conformationally unable to compete for the binding of vWF. In contrast, both the A3 module and a chimeric A1/A3 molecule (Q475-L598/L1018-R1114) containing the N-terminal half of A1 fused in frame to the C-terminal half of A3, can compete for vWF binding to immobilized type I collagen suggesting that these two recombinant polypeptides assume a proper conformation. The fact that the A1/A3 chimera, but also the A1 module, inhibits ristocetin-induced platelet agglutination in a dose-dependent manner might be direct evidence for the proper folding of both recombinant polypeptides. Third, the affinity of the A1 module binding sites is greatly affected when this domain is isolated from its context. This seems unlikely in light of the results with several function-blocking antibodies raised against the native protein and of the similar results obtained with antibodies against other VWFA-containing proteins such as Mac-1 and p150,95,[124] LFA-1[125-127] and $\alpha2\beta1$.[128] In fact, antibodies raised against the native vWF also recognize the recombinant vWF modules.[122,123] Finally, using the A1/A3 chimera, which lacks part of the reported collagen-binding sequence of the A1 module (E542-L622) and all the collagen-binding sequence of the A3 module

(K948-K988), a significant inhibition of vWF binding to type I collagen can still be obtained. A possible explanation for the lack of function of recombinant A1 might depend on the substrate used in the solid phase assay: acid-soluble monomeric collagen does not represent a proper ligand since either fibers of type I and III collagens or non-fibrillar collagens such as type VI are among the physiological ligands within the subendothelium.[94,95,103,107]

INTERACTION WITH TYPE VI COLLAGEN

Type VI collagen of the vascular subendothelium[106] is a good candidate for vWF binding[103] and, as indicated above, might represent the natural vWF ECM ligand under low shear stress conditions (Fig. 2.3).[107] Proteolytic fragments of vWF, containing either the A1 or the A3 modules, seem to express binding sites for type VI collagen.[129] In view of the significant size of its globular domains, largely constituted by VWFA modules (see chapter 5) and of the supramolecular organization of type VI collagen, it is likely that, in addition to the triple helix, the globular domains play a relevant role in promoting molecular interaction. In fact, the globular domains of type VI collagen have a strong affinity for each other.[137] The VWFA modules of this collagen could interact with the homologous modules of vWF. However, whether the mechanisms leading to vWF recognition of type VI collagen are similar to those at work during the interaction with fibrillar collagens remains to be determined.

INTERACTION WITH OTHER MOLECULES

Two vWF regions have been identified as the ones able to bind heparin: one is at the N-terminus and involves residues S1-V212,[138] and the other, which displays the strongest affinity, is between residues Y565 and A587 in the A1 module.[101,139,140] The A1 binding site is essential for the interaction with heparin as determined by the lack of binding of a recombinant vWF carrying a complete deletion of the A1 module.[135] Sulfated glycolipids, which may be present on the platelet surface and may serve an accessory binding role in vWF-platelet interactions, also bind to positively charged sequences within the A1 module.[141,142] The binding sites for the sulfatides (L512-K673) on A1 module[142] are in part or totally overlapping with those for collagen and heparin, respectively.

INTERACTION OF vWF WITH GPIb

GPIb is a disulfide-bonded heterodimer composed of an α (143 kD) and a β (22 kD) chain noncovalently associated in a tight complex with another glycoprotein (GPIX); this complex is more loosely associated in a hetero-oligomeric complex with GPV.[143] The N-terminal extracytoplasmic domain of GPIbα contains binding sites for vWF[144] and α-thrombin.[145] The binding site for vWF is present on an acidic segment (D251-D287) of the GPIbα chain[144,146,147] with two out of three sulfated Tyr residues (Y276, Y278 and Y279) being necessary for the proper GPIb-vWF interaction.[148] Residues comprised within the sequence 271-284 of GPIbα chain also participate in the binding of α-thrombin.[149]

Soluble plasma vWF has a very low affinity for GPIb,[86] yet as a surface-bound ligand,[6] vWF can bind irreversibly to GPIb. Since GPIb interacts minimally with circulating vWF,[86] the binding might depend upon a specific functional conformation acquired by vWF after its association with components of the subendothelial matrix. In addition, although not yet experimentally proven, the rheological conditions during the thrombogenic process may induce direct and/or indirect conformational changes to GPIb and/or vWF. Exposure of the GPIb-binding site of vWF can be regulated by a series of physiological agonist factors, of which immobilization onto collagen[93,95,103,105] or other subendothelial structures[80] is the most relevant, but the removal of sialic acid from vWF similarly induces its binding to GPIb.[70] On the contrary, antagonists such

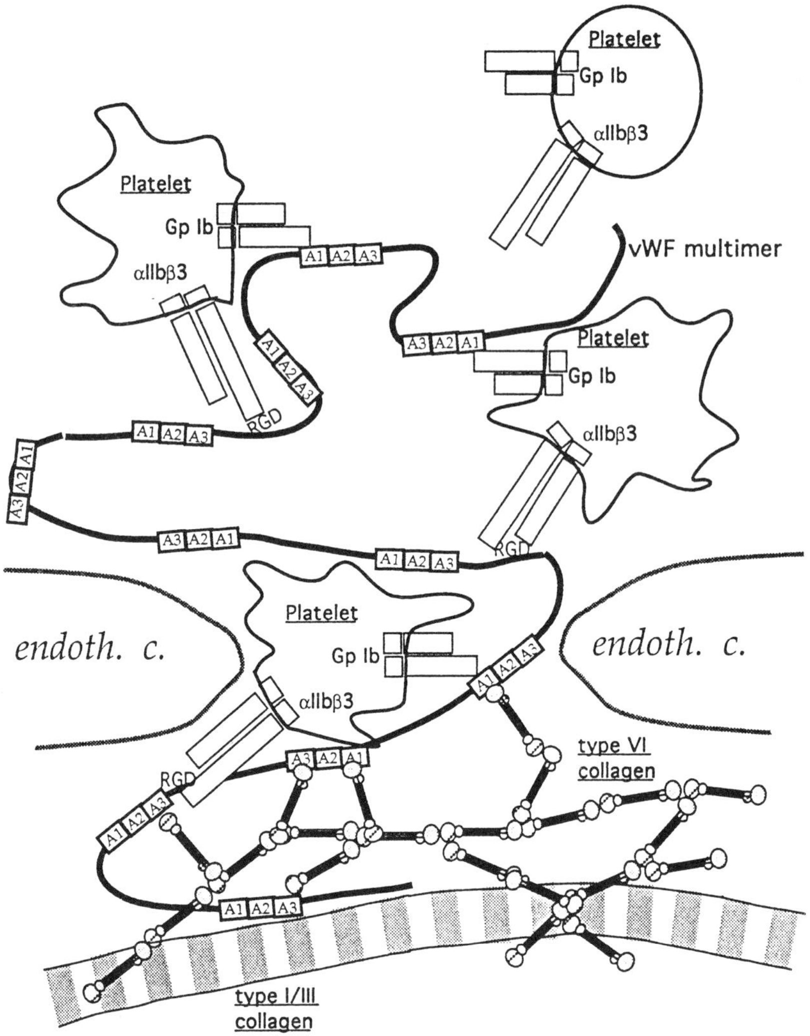

Fig. 2.3. Schematic representation of the proposed role of vWF in hemostasis. A nonactivated platelet expresses both the GPIb and the αIIbβ3 receptors. Under appropriate circumstances of medium to high shear stress and exposure of subendothelial constituents, these platelet receptors interact with vWF multimers. Among the subendothelial constituents a fibril of type I/III collagen and the network of type VI collagen microfilaments are shown. The different components of this scheme are not drawn to scale.

as heparin[150] and polyanionic polyaromatic polymers[151] inhibit vWF interaction with GPIb. The exposure of GPIb-binding sites of vWF also can be enhanced by nonphysiologic modulators: thus, immobilization on solid surfaces,[152] proteolytic degradation,[34,153] or interaction with modulators such as ristocetin[112,113,154] and botrocetin[114,115] are all conditions that promote the binding of GPIb to vWF.

The interaction between the A1 module and GPIb has been demonstrated initially with the use of function-blocking antibodies[35,87,120,122,155] and of proteolytic fragments comprising the A1 module such as the monomeric tryptic- 52/48 kD (V449-K728)[139,153] or dispase-generated 39/34 kD fragments (L480-G718)[34] and the unreduced homodimeric 116 kD fragment (residues V449-K728).[59] While the binding of the unreduced fragments, like that of the native vWF, to GPIb is stimulated by ristocetin or botrocetin, the reduced and alkylated fragments[153,156] bind spontaneously to GPIb. This latter finding suggests that the S-S bond is crucial for the regulation of vWF-GPIb binding and its presence in fragments as well as in native vWF might downregulate the affinity of the interaction. The physiological consequence of the S-S bond between C509 and C695 would thus be to prevent the random binding of native vWF to platelet GPIb in normal circulation. The vWF-GPIb interaction also has been studied by the use of synthetic peptides, and some candidate peptides sequences within this fragment that appear to mediate this interaction have been found.[35,157,158] In addition, by using charged residue to alanine mutagenesis several discontinuous segments of the A1 module were found to mediate interactions with GPIb, ristocetin and botrocetin, but the relative importance of the sequences involved is still controversial.[160] Two peptide sequences, C474-P488 (N-terminal to the A1 module) and L694-P708 (at the C-terminal end of the A1 module) block ristocetin-induced but not botrocetin-induced binding of vWF to platelets.[35,161] These results largely concur with the previous observations of peptide inhibition studies.[35,157,158] The identified sequences do not seem to bind directly to GPIb, instead they interact with ristocetin since recombinant vWF fragments lacking the sequence corresponding to both peptides still bind to GPIb with high affinity.[162] Another peptide, D514-E542,[158] inhibits ristocetin- and botrocetin-induced binding of vWF to GPIb as well as it also inhibits the direct binding of botrocetin to vWF. This peptide corresponds to vWF sequences comprising part of the MIDAS cation binding site.[116] This particular inhibitory peptide might prevent a proper arrangement of the A1 module rather than blocking the binding to GPIb by direct competition. The mechanism by which ristocetin and botrocetin act as modulators of the vWF-GPIb interaction are distinct: ristocetin dimer-

izes in solution and the dimers bridge GPIb with its vWF ligand;[154] botrocetin forms a stoichiometric complex with vWF and this complex then binds to GPIb.[154] This difference has been confirmed by the observation that the lack of O-linked carbohydrate side chains of vWF decreases only ristocetin-dependent binding to GPIb,[156,163] and by the finding that a unique variant of vWF with a G561S point mutation has no ristocetin and normal botrocetin binding.[164] While ristocetin interacts at the level of negatively charged proline-rich peptide sequences,[158,165] botrocetin binds to peptide sequences having net positive charges.[157,158] The positive charges are important in regulating the proper exposure of the GPIb-binding sites of vWF since their interaction is inhibited by polyanionic and polyaromatic polymers.[166]

Functional studies with soluble recombinant fragments corresponding to the A1 module have confirmed that this module contains recognition sites for GPIb.[59,130-132] A bacterial recombinant fragment comprising the whole A1 module and few additional N- and C-terminal sequences (S445-V733) in which the cysteine residues (C509 and C695) were reduced and alkylated binds to GPIb within the same sites involved in binding of the native vWF molecule.[131] Very likely because of the lack of the disulfide bond and/or of the carbohydrate side chains, the binding of this recombinant vWF molecule can occur even in the absence of ristocetin, suggesting that the proper sites might have been exposed already following the reduction and alkylation procedures. However, even though this recombinant fragment has an inherent ability to interact with GPIb, botrocetin can still increase the activity of this interaction by 10-fold.[131] The conformation of the C509-C695 loop may be important to juxtapose the non-contiguous sequences involved in the interaction with GPIb.[133] The fact that recombinant fragments containing the C509-C695 loop bind more tightly after reduction and alkylation[162] suggests that the disulfide bond per se is not within the GPIb binding site, but it might be required for the normal regulation of vWF-GPIb binding, as are three successive proline residues at positions 702-704.[165] However, contrasting evidence as obtained by other authors using a similar approach with a recombinant A1 module, i.e., after reduction of the C509-C695 disulfide bond no binding to platelets could be measured.[133] The relevance of the A1 module is further underscored by the functional abnormalities found in type 2B vWD in which an increased reactivity of vWF with GPIb is detected.[167,168] Most of the point mutations so far identified are located within residues M540 and R578 in one of the regions implicated in inhibition of vWF function.[160] Curiously, the sequences of porcine[169] and bovine[170] vWF diverge from the human sequence at a few of the positions associated with type 2B vWD and vWF from both of these species binds spontaneously to GPIb. These findings suggest that segments comprising the residues affected by vWD type 2B mutations may normally prevent the binding of soluble vWF to GPIb. The type 2B mutations would alter the local structure and relieve this inhibition leading to spontaneous binding of soluble vWF to GPIb.

DISEASE ASSOCIATION

vWD is defined in major categories in terms of quantitative or qualitative defects.[13] Quantitative defects comprise partial deficiencies (vWD type 1) and severe deficiencies (vWD type 3). Among the qualitative defects (vWD type 2) two are more common: type 2A includes variants with decreased platelet function associated with the loss of large multimers and type 2B includes variants with increased affinity for platelet GPIb.

The type 1 variant is the most common form, but little is known of the molecular defects. It should be mentioned that murine vWD is caused by a defect in a gene distinct from the murine vWF gene[171] Nevertheless, it seems that at least a subset of type 1 variant is associated with the vWF gene by linkage analysis.[172] Type 3 variant, which presents the most severe quantitative deficiency of vWF, is very rare and in a number of families it is associated with large deletions in the vWF gene.[173]

Type 2A is an heterogeneous frequent qualitative variant accounting for about 10% of vWD patients.[173-180] The characteristics of this variant is the decrease of the high molecular weight multimers that are replaced very frequently by a 176 kD fragment associated with a reduced platelet function. Virtually all type 2A mutations cluster within the A2 module, between G742 and P875 although a distinct C509R mutation preventing the formation of the C509-C695 disulfide loop[181] and other mutations in the A1 module (R611C/H) that resemble type 2A vWD have been reported.[182] Expression of vWF mutants with type 2A molecular defects in mammalian cells have identified two groups of mutations. Group 1 results in defective intracellular transport[183] leading to intracellular retention without storage. Since larger multimers have a greater chance of containing mutant monomers, they are preferentially retained. In group 2 the whole spectrum of multimers is present in the protected environment of storage granules, but not in plasma. It seems that these mutated forms are grossly normal as long as they are stored in granules, but once secreted, the mutant monomers embodied in large multimers are cleaved by as yet unidentified proteases and hence large multimers are not detected in blood.[37,184] While increased sensitivity to proteolysis has not yet been directly demonstrated in vitro, normal appearing vWF can be obtained from type 2A patients if several protease inhibitors are added to blood samples during the purification steps.[175,185,186] These variants are associated with a lack of large multimers and a decreased reactivity with GPIb. Functional studies with mutated recombinant vWF have shown that the decreased reactivity of type 2A vWF for GPIb is not directly related to the mutations per se, but to the lack of multimer formation.[183,187,188]

The relatively rare type 2B variant is characterized by an increased affinity of the mutant vWF for GPIb[189-193] leading to a loss of the largest vWF multimers, clearance of vWF-platelet complexes and thrombocytopenia.[194] When patients with 2B vWD have vascular lesions they bleed since the GPIb receptor is blocked by soluble vWF and can no longer support platelet adhesion on insolubilized vWF in the vessel wall. The type 2B phenotype is easily identified by the increased platelet agglutination induced by low concentrations of ristocetin. In addition, platelet aggregation induced by low shear stress is enhanced in type 2B patients compared to controls.[195] Most mutations which cause type 2B vWD are included in a short sequence (M540-R578) within the disulfide loop comprised by C509 and C695, although more recent mutations have been detected in short segments flanking both sides of the loop (Fig. 2.4).[196-198] The 2B variants provide unique natural examples of mutations which relieve the inhibition of soluble vWF function, analogous to those induced experimentally by point mutations.[160,199]

Finally, a case of acutely acquired vWD has been described recently caused by an autoantibody that inhibits the interaction of vWF with collagen by binding apparently to both A1 and A3 modules.[200]

CONCLUSIONS

While the precise localization of collagen binding sites within the VWFA A1 and A3 modules remains undetermined, there are residues (E596 and K599 in A1 module) which appear to be important in the direct interaction of vWF with platelet GPIb.[160] There are then some negatively and positively charged segments which function as activators and contain ristocetin and botrocetin binding sites. Finally there are segments, comprised within the A1 module, that prevent the binding of soluble vWF to GPIb; one of these segments corresponds to the locations of several vWF 2B mutations.[160] Therefore, a model can be proposed in which the binding to vWF of certain modulators, the interaction of vWF with components of the subendothelium and artificial[160,199] or natural[13] modulators might relieve the binding inhibition. vWF in the circulation, which is unable to bind to GPIb unless very high shear forces are exerted, adopts primarily an "off" conformation and switches to the "on" conformation if the appropriate stimuli are present that modulate the A1 module conformation. Structural evidences for two conformations of Mac-1 VWFA module likely representing the active and the inactive states of this integrin have been reported[117] and are in agreement with the suggestion on the different conformations of the A1 module in vWF. GPIb binding sites might be located in the $\alpha 4$ helix and in the loop connecting the βD sheet and $\alpha 5$ helix if the coordinates of the Mac-1 α chain VWFA module (see Fig. 1.3, chapter 1)[116] are used to build a model of the A1 module. Using the same approach, the inhibitory (residues corresponding to several 2B vWD) and activatory (binding sites for ristocetin and botrocetin, reduction of the S-S bond between C509 and C695) sequences are distantly positioned from the proposed location of the GPIb binding sites. An effect of even more distantly located sequences has been suggested by the recent finding of an antibody mapping in the N-terminal region of mature vWF that increases ristocetin induced platelet aggregation.[201] Therefore, although residues within the VWFA modules contribute to the direct interaction with their ligands, it appears also that sequences outside and distantly located can affect the actual functional role of VWFA modules.[201-204] Finally, it is worth mentioning that all the in vitro interactions with collagens, heparin, sulfatides and GPIb mediated by the VWFA modules of vWF and irrespectively of whether intact vWF, proteolytic or recombinant fragments are used, do not require further addition of divalent cations nor are they inhibited by EDTA. This is in agreement with findings showing that Echovirus 1 binds to the $\alpha 2 \beta 1$ integrin in

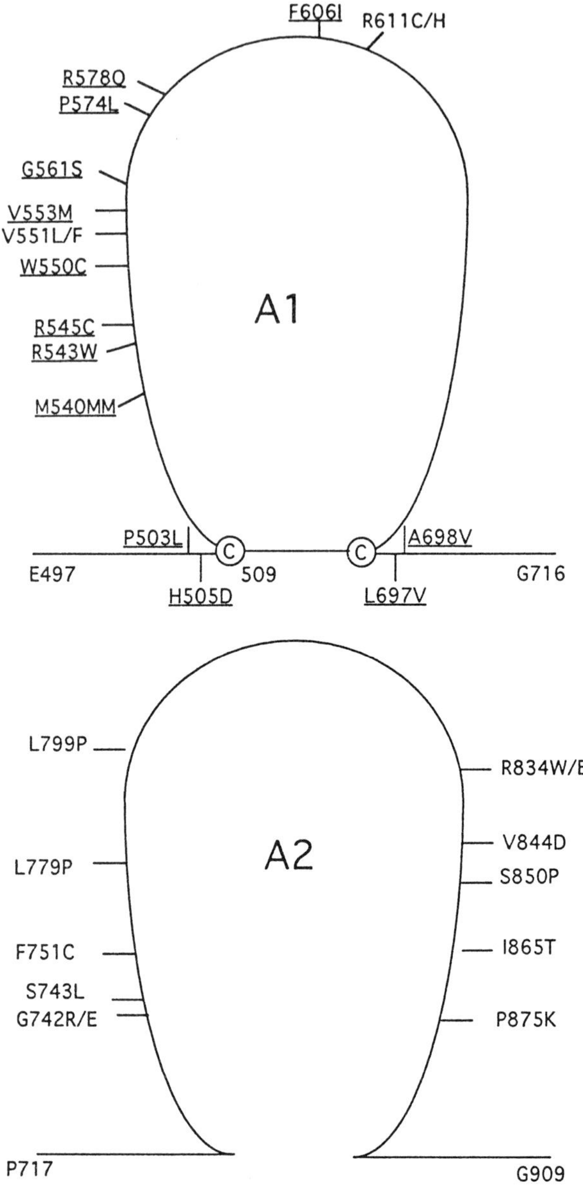

Fig. 2.4. Schematic representation of vWF A1 and A2 VWFA modules with the location of the type 2A and type 2B mutations. Mutations resulting in type 2B vWD are underlined.

the absence of cations,[205] but it is at variance with the findings of several other proteins of the VWFA superfamily[203,206-210] whose function strictly depends on the presence of cations. This apparent cation-independent binding might depend upon the fact that the A1 module has a variant MIDAS motif in which a conserved Ser is substituted by an Arg and the last Asp by an Ala.

REFERENCES

1. Carlos TM, Harlan JM. Leukocytes-endothelial adhesion molecules. Blood 1994; 84:2068-2101.

2. Weiss HJ, Turitto VT, Baumgartner HR. Platelet adhesion and thrombus formation on subendothelium in platelets deficient in glycoproteins IIb-IIIa, Ib and storage granules. Blood. 1986; 67:322-330.

3. Weiss HJ, Turitto VT, Baumgartner HR. Effect of shear rate on platelet interaction with subendothelium in citrate and native

blood. I. Shear rate-dependent decrease of adhesion in von Willebrand's disease and the Bernard-Soulier syndrome. J Lab Clin Med 1978; 92:750-764.

4. Nichols TC, Bellinger DA, Reddick RL et al. Role of von Willebrandfactor in arterial thrombosis. Studies in normal and von Willebrand disease pigs. Circulation 1991; 83:56-64.

5. Ikeda Y, Handa M, Kawano K et al. The role of von Willebrand factor and fibrinogen in platelet aggregation under varying shear stress. J Clin Invest 1991; 87:1234-1240.

6. Sakariassen KS, Bolhouis PA, Sixma JJ. Human blood platelet adhesion to artery subendothelium is mediated by factor VIII/ von Willebrand factor bound to the subendothelium. Nature 1979; 279:636-638.

7. Chow TW, Hellums JD, Moake JL et al. Shear stress-induced von Willebrand factor binding to platelet glycoprotein Ib initiates calcium influx associated with aggregation. Blood 1992; 80:113-120.

8. Ikeda Y, Handa M, Kamata T et al. Transmembrane calcium influx associated with von Willebrand factor binding to GP Ib in the initiation of shear-induced platelet aggregation. Thromb Haemostasis 1993; 69: 496-502.

9. Chopek MW, Girma JP, Fujikawa K et al. Human von Willebrand factor: a multivalent protein composed of identical subunits. Biochemistry 1986; 25:3146-3155.

10. von Willebrand EA. Hereditaer Pseudohemofili. Finska Laekarsaeallskapetes 1926; 67:7-112.

11. Weiss HJ, Pietu G, Rabinowitz R et al. Heterogeneous abnormalities in the multimeric structure, antigenic properties, and plasma-platelet content of factor VIII/ von Willebrand factor in subtypes of classic (type I) and variant (type IIa) von Willebrand's disease. J Lab Clin Med 1983; 101:411-425.

12. Rodeghiero F, Castaman G, Dini E. Epidemiological investigation of the prevalence of von Willebrand's disease. Blood 1987; 69:454-459.

13. Sadler JE. A revised classification of von Willebrand disease. Thromb Haemost 1994; 71:520-525.

14. Hoyer LW, Shainoff JR. Factor VIII-related protein circulates in normal human plasma as high molecular weight multimers. Blood 1980; 55:1056-1059.

15. Slayter H, Loscalzo J, Bockenstedt P et al. The native conformation of human von Willebrand protein-analysis by electron microscopy and quasielastic light scattering. J Biol Chem 1985; 260:8559-8563.

16. Fowler WE, Fretto LJ. Electron microscopy of von Willebrand factor. In: Zimmerman TS, Ruggeri ZM, eds. Coagulation and Bleeding Disorders. The Role of Factor VIII and von Willebrand Factor. New York: Marcel Dekker, 1989: 181-193.

17. Fowler WE, Fretto LJ, Hamilton KK et al. Substructure of human von Willebrand factor. J Clin Invest 1985; 76:1491-1500.

18. Sporn LA, Marder VJ, Wagner DD. Inducible secretion of large biologically potent von Willebrand factor multimers. Cell 1986; 46:185-190.

19. Mancuso DJ, Tuley EA, Westfield LA et al. Structure of the gene for human von Willebrand factor. J Biol Chem 1989; 264:19519-19527.

20. Mancuso DJ, Tuley EA, Westfield MA et al. Human von Willebrand factor gene and pseudogene: structural analysis and differentiation by polymerase chain reaction. Biochemistry 1991; 30:253-269.

21. Eikenboom JCJ, Vink T, Brieet E et al. Multiple substitutions in the von Willebrand factor gene that mimic the pseudogene sequence. Proc Natl Acad Sci USA 1994; 91:2221-2224.

22. Perez-Casal M, Daly M, Peake J. A de novo mutation in exon 28 of the von Willebrand factor gene in a patient with type IIA von Willebrand's disease coincides with an MboI polymorphism in the von Willebrand pseudogene. Hum Mol Genet 1993; 2:2159-2161.

23. Bork P, Bairoch A. Extracellular protein modules. Trends Biochem Sci 1995; 3.

24. Ginsburg D, Handin RI, Bonthron DT et al. Human von Willebrand factor (vWF): isolation of complementary DNA (cDNA) clones and chromosomal localization. Science 1985; 228:1401-1406.

25. Verweij CL, de Vries CJM, Distel B et al. Construction of cDNA coding for human von Willebrand factor using antibody probes for colony-screening and mapping of the chromosomal gene. Nucleic Acids Res 1985; 13:4699-4717.

26. Lynch DC, Zimmerman TS, Collins CJ et al. Molecular cloning of cDNA for human von Willebrand factor: authentication by a new method. Cell 1985; 41:49-56.

27. Sadler JE, Shelton-Inloes BB, Sorace JM et al. Cloning and characterization of two cDNAs coding for human von Willebrand factor. Proc Natl Acad Sci USA 1985; 82:6394-6398.

28. Verweij CL, Diergaarde PJ, Hart M et al. Full-length von Willebrand factor (vWF) cDNA encodes a highly repetitive protein considerably larger than the mature vWF subunit. EMBO J 1986; 5:1839-1847.

29. Bonthron DR, Orr EC, Mitsock LM et al. Nucleotide sequence of pre-pro-von Willebrand factor cDNA. Nucleic Acids Res 1986; 14:7125-7127.

30. Shelton-Inloes BB, Titani K, Sadler JE. cDNA sequences for human von Willebrand factor reveal five types of repeated domains and five possible protein sequence polymorphisms. Biochemistry 1986; 25:3164-3171.

31. Titani K, Kumar S, Takio K et al. Amino acid sequence of human von Willebrand factor. Biochemistry 1986; 25:3171-3184.

32. Voorberg J, Fontijn R, Calafat J et al. Assembly and routing of von Willebrand factor variants: the requirements for disulfide-linked dimerization reside within the carboxy-terminal 151 amino-acids. J Cell Biol 1991; 113:195-205.

33. Marti T, Roesselet S, Titani K et al. Identification of disulfide-bridge substructure within human von Willebrand factor. Biochemistry 1987; 26:8099-8109.

34. Andrews RK, Gorman JJ, Booth WJ et al. Cross-linking of a monomeric 39/34-kDa dispase fragment of von Willebrand factor (Leu-480/Val-481-Gly-718) to the N-terminal region of the α-chain of membrane glycoprotein Ib on intact platelets with bis (sulfosuccinimidyl) suberate. Biochemistry 1989; 28:8326-8336.

35. Mohri H, Fujimura Y, Shima M et al. Structure of the von Willebrand factor domain interacting with glycoprotein Ib. J Biol Chem 1988; 263:17901-17904.

36. Roth GL, Titani K, Hoyer LW et al. Localization of binding sites within human von Willebrand factor for monomeric type III collagen. Biochemistry 1986; 25:8357-8361.

37. Dent JA, Berkowitz SD, Ware J et al. Identification of a cleavage site directing the immunochemical detection of molecular abnormalities in type IIA von Willebrand factor. Proc Natl Acad Sci USA 1990; 87:6306-6310.

38. Wise RJ, Barr PJ, Wong PA et al. Expression of a human proprotein processing enzyme: correct cleavage of the von Willebrand factor precursor at a paired basic amino acid site. Proc Natl Acad Sci USA 1990; 87: 9378-9382.

39. Hunt Lois T, Barker WC. von Willebrand factor shares a distinctive cystein-rich domain with thrombospondin and procollagen. Biochem Biophys Res Commun 1987; 144:876-882.

40. Ruggeri ZM, Bader R, De Marco L. Glanzmann thrombasthenia: deficient binding of von Willebrand factor to thrombin-stimulated platelets. Proc Natl Acad Sci USA 1982; 79:6038-6041.

41. Ruggeri ZM, De Marco L, Gatti L et al. Platelets have more than one binding site for von Willebrand factor. J Clin Invest 1983; 72:1-12.

42. Azuma H, Hayashi T, Dent JA et al. Disulfide bond requirements for assembly of the platelet glycoprotein Ib-binding of von Willebrand factor. J Biol Chem 1993; 268:2821-2827.

43. Dong Z, Thoma RS, Crimmins DL et al. Disulfide bonds required to assemble functional von Willebrand factor multimers. J Biol Chem 1994; 268:6753-6758.

44. Nachman RL, Levine R, Jaffe EA. Synthesis of factor VIII antigen by cultured guinea pig megakaryocytes. J Clin Invest 1977; 60:914-921.

45. Sporn LA, Chavin SI, Marder VJ et al. Biosynthesis of von Willebrand protein by human megakaryocytes. J Clin Invest 1985; 76: 1102-1106.

46. Wagner DD, Olmsted JB, Marder VJ. Immunolocalization of von Willebrand protein in Weibel-Palade bodies of human endothelial cells. J Cell Biol 1964; 23: 101-112.

47. Cramer EM; Breton-Gorius J, Beesley JE et al. Ultrastructural demonstration of tubular inclusions coinciding with von Willebrand factor in pig megakaryocytes. Blood 1988; 71: 1533-1538.

48. Coffin JD, Harrison J, Schwartz S et al. Angioblast differentiation and morphogenesis of the vascular endothelium in the mouse embryo. Dev Biol 1991; 148:51-62.

49. Wu QY, Drout L, Carrier JL et al. Differential distribution of von Willebrand factor in endothelial cells. Comparison between normal pigs and pigs with von Willebrand disease. Arteriosclerosis 1987; 7:47-54.

50. Bahnak BR, Wu Q-Y, Coulombel L et al. Expression of von Willebrand factor in porcine vessels: heterogeneity at the level of von Willebrand factor mRNA. J Cell Physiol 1989; 138:305-310.

51. Rand J, Badimon L, Gordon RE et al. Distribution of von Willebrand factor in porcine intima varies with blood type and location. Arteriosclerosis 1987; 7:287-292.

52. Page C, Rose M, Yacoub M et al. Antigenic heterogeneity of vascular endothelium. Am J Pathol 1992;141:673-683.

53. Aird WC, Jahroudi N, Weiler-Guettler H et al. Human von Willebrand factor gene sequences target expression to a subpopulation of endothelial cells in transgenic mice. Proc Natl Acad Sci USA 1995; 92:4567-4571.

54. Federici AB, Bader R, Pagani S et al. Binding of von Willebrand factor (vWF) to glycoproteins (GP) Ib and IIb-IIIa complex: affinity is related to multimeric size. Br J Haematol 1989; 73:93-99.

55. Sixma JJ, Sakariassen KS, Beeser-Visser NH et al. Adhesion of platelets to human artery subendothelium: effect of factor VIII-von Willebrand factor of various multimeric composition. Blood 1984; 63:128-139.

56. Wagner DD, Lawrence SO, Ohlsson-Wilhelm BM et al. Topology and order of formation of interchain disulfide bonds in von Willebrand factor. Blood 1987; 69:27-32.

57. Verweij CL, Hart M, Pannekoek H. Expression of von Willebrand factor (vWF) cDNA in heterologous cells: requirement of the pro-polypeptide in vWF multimer formation. EMBO J 1987; 6:2885-2890.

58. Wise RJ, Pitmann DD, Handin RI et al. The propeptide of von Willebrand factor independently mediates the assembly of von Willebrand multimers. Cell 1988; 52:229-236.

59. Azuma H, Dent JA, Sugimoto M et al. Independent assembly and secretion of a dimeric adhesive domain of von Willebrand factor containing the glycoprotein Ib-binding site. J Biol Chem 1991; 266: 12342-12347.

60. Wagner DD, Saffaripour S, Bonfanti R et al. Induction of specific storage organelles by von Willebrand factor propolypeptide. Cell 1991; 64:403-413.

61. Voorberg J, Fontijn R, Calafat J et al. Biogenesis of von Willebrand factor-containing organelles in heterologous transfected CV-1 cells. EMBO J 1993; 12:749-758.

62. Mayadas TN, Wagner DD. von Willebrand factor biosynthesis and processing. Ann NY Acad Sci 1991; 614:153-166.

63. Carew JA, Browning PJ, Lynch DC. Sulfation of von Willebrand factor. Blood 1990; 76:2530-2539.

64. Wagner DD, Fay PJ, Sporn LA et al. Divergent fates of von Willebrand factor and its propolypeptide (von Willebrand antigen II) after secretion from endothelial cells. Proc Natl Acad Sci USA 1987; 84:1955-1959.

65. Ewenstein BM, Warhol MJ, Handin RI et al. Composition of the von Willebrand factor storage organelle (Weibel-Palade body) isolated from cultured human umbilical vein endothelial cells. J Cell Biol 1987; 104: 1423-1433.

66. Vischer UM, Wagner DD. von Willebrand factor proteolytic processing and multimerization precede the formation of Weibel Palade Bodies. Blood 1994; 83:3536-3544.

67. Bonthron DT, Handin RI, Kaufman RJ et al. Structure of pre-pro von Willebrand factor and its expression in heterologous cells. Nature 1986; 324:270-273.

68. Journet AM, Saffaripour S, Cramer EM et al. von Willebrand factor storage requires intact prosequence cleavage site. Eur J Cell Biol 1993; 60:31-41.

69. Takagi J, Sekiya F, Kasahara K. et al. Collagen-binding domain within bovine propolypeptide of von Willebrand factor. J Biol Chem 1989; 264:6017-6020.

70. Federici AB, De Romeuf C, De Groot PG et al. Adhesive properties of the carbohydrate-modified von Willebrand Factor (CHO-vWF). Blood 1988; 71:947-952.

71. Wagner DD, Mayadas T, Marder VJ. Initial glycosylation and acid pH in the Golgi apparatus are required for multimerization of von Willebrand factor. J Cell Biol 1986; 102:1320-1324.

72. Dent JA, Galbusera M, Ruggeri ZM et al. Heterogeneity of plasma von Willebrand factor multimers resulting from proteolysis of the constituent subunit. J Clin Invest 1991; 88:774-782.

73. Tsai H-M, Sussman II, Nagel RL. Shear stress enhances the proteolysis of von Willebrand factor in normal plasma. Blood 1994; 83:2171-2179.

74. Foster PA, Fulcher CA, Marti T et al. A major factor VIII binding domain resides within the aminoterminal 272 amino acid residues of von Willebrand factor. J Biol Chem 1987; 262:8443-8446.

75. Koppelman SJ, van Hoeij M, Vink T et al. Requirements of von Willebrand factor to protect factor VIII from inactivation by activated protein C. Blood 1996; 87: 2292-2300.

76. Hill-Eubanks DC, Lollars P. von Willebrand factor is a cofactor for thrombin-catalyzed cleavage of the factor VIII light chain. J Biol Chem 1990; 265:17854-17858.

77. Parker RI, Gralnick HR. Fibrin monomer induces binding of endogenous vWF to the glycocalycin portion of platelet glycoprotein Ib. Blood 1987; 70:1589-1594.

78. Loscalzo J, Inbal A, Handin RI et al. von Willebrand protein facilitates platelet incorporation into polymerizing fibrin. J Clin Invest 1981; 68:321-328.

79. Hantgan RR, Hindriks G, Taylor RG et al. Glycoprotein Ib, von Willebrand factor, and glycoprotein IIb/IIIa are all involved in platelet adhesion to fibrin in flowing whole blood. Blood 1990; 76:345-353.

80. Baruch D, Denis C, Marteaux C et al. Role of von Willebrand factor associated to extracellular matrices in platelet adhesion. Blood 1991; 77:519-527.

81. Weiss HJ. von Willebrand factor and platelet function. Ann NY Acad Sci 1991; 614:125-137.

82. Badimon L, Badimon JJ, Galvez A et al. Influence of arterial damage and wall shear rate on platelet deposition. Ex vivo study in a swine model. Arteriosclerosis 1986; 6:312-320.

83. Badimon L, Badimon JJ, Turitto VT et al. Platelet thrombus formation on collagen type I. A model of deep vessel injury-influence of blood rheology, von Willebrand factor and blood coagulation. Circulation 1988; 78:1431-1442.

84. Fukuyama M, Sakai K, Itagaki I et al. Continuous measurement of shear-induced platelet aggregation. Thromb Res 1989; 54:253-260.

85. Alevriadou BR, Moake JL, Turner NA et al. Real-time analysis of shear-dependent thrombus formation and its blockade by inhibitors of von Willebrand factor binding to platelets. Blood 1993; 81:1263-1276.

86. Goto S, Salomon DR, Ikeda Y et al. Characterization of the unique mechanism mediating the shear-dependent binding of soluble von Willebrand factor to platelets. J Biol Chem 1995; 270:23352-23361.

87. Fressinaud E, Baruch D, Girma JP et al. von Willebrand factor mediated platelet adhesion to collagen involves platelet membrane glycoprotein IIb/IIIa as well as glycoprotein Ib. J Lab Clin Med 1988; 112:58-67.

88. Peterson DM, Stathopoulos NA, Giorgio TD et al. Shear-platelet aggregation requires von Willebrand factor and platelet membrane glycoproteins Ib and IIb-IIIa. Blood 1987; 69:625-628.

89. Weiss HJ, Hawiger J, Ruggeri ZM et al. Fibrinogen-independent platelet adhesion and thrombus formation on subendothelium mediated by glycoprotein IIb-IIIa complex at high shear rate. J Clin Invest 1989; 83:288-297.

90. Savage B, Saldivar E, Ruggeri ZM. Initiation of platelet adhesion by arrest onto fibrinogen or translocation on von Willebrand factor. Cell 1996; 84: 289-297.

91. Stel HV, Sakariassen KS, de Groot PG et al. von Willebrand Factor in the vessel wall mediates platelet adherence. Blood 1985; 65:85-90.

92. Turitto VT, Weiss HJ, Zimmermann TS et al. Factor VIII/von Willebrand factor in subendothelium mediates platelet adhesion. Blood 1985; 65:823-831.

93. van der Kwast TH, Stel HV, Cristen E et al. Localization of factor VIII-procoagulant antigen: an immunohistological survey of the human body using monoclonal antibodies. Blood 1986; 67:222-227.

94. Nyman D. Interaction of collagen with the factor VIII antigen activity-von Willebrand factor complex. Thromb Res 1977; 12:433-438.

95. Scott DM, Griffin B, Pepper DS et al. The binding of purified factor VIII/von Willebrand factor to collagens of different type and form. Thromb Res 1981; 24:467-472.

96. Legrand YL, Fauvel F, Gutman N et al. Microfibrils (MF) platelet interaction: requirement of von Willebrand Factor. Thromb Res 1980; 19:737-739.

97. Fauvel F, Grant ME, Legrand YJ et al. Interaction of blood platelets with a microfibrillar extract from adult bovine aorta: requirement for von Willebrand factor. Proc Natl Acad Sci USA 1983; 80:551-554.

98. De Groot PG, Ottenhof-Rovers M, van Mourik JA et al. Evidence that the primary binding site of von Willebrand factor that mediates platelet adhesion on subendothelium is not collagen. J Clin Invest 1988; 82:65-73.

99. Wagner DD, Urban-Pickering M, Marder VJ. von Willebrand protein binds to extracellular matrices independently of collagen. Proc Natl Acad Sci USA 1984; 81:471-475.

100. Mohri H, Yoshioka A, Zimmerman TS et al. Isolation of the von Willebrand factor domain interacting with platelet glycoprotein Ib, heparin, and collagen, and characterization of its three distinct functional sites. J Biol Chem 1989; 264:17361-17367.

101. Sobel M, Soler DF, Kermode JC et al. Localization and characterization of a heparin binding domain peptide of human von Willebrand factor. J Biol Chem 1992; 267:8857-8862.

102. Iozzo RV, Cohen IR, Grassel S et al. The biology of perlecan: the multifaceted heparan sulphate proteoglycan of basement membranes and pericellular matrices. Biochem J 1994; 302:625-639.

103. Rand JH, Patel ND, Schwartz E et al. 150-kD von Willebrand factor binding protein extracted from human vascular subendothelium is type VI collagen. J Clin Invest 1991; 88:253-259.

104. Chu M-L, Conway D, Pan T-C et al. Amino acid sequence of the triple-helical domain of human collagen type VI. J Biol Chem 1988; 263: 18601-18606.

105. Kuo H-J, Keene DR, Glanville RW. Orientation of type VI collagen monomers in molecular aggregates. Biochemistry; 1989; 28:3757-3762.

106. Rand JH, Wu X-X, Potter BJ et al. Co-localization of von Willebrand factor and type VI collagen in human vascular subendothelium. Am J Pathol 1993; 142:843-850.

107. Ross JM, McIntire LV, Moake JL et al. Platelet adhesion and aggregation on human type VI collagen surfaces under physiological flow conditions. Blood 1995; 85: 1826-1835.

108. Plow EF, Srouji AH, Meyer D et al. Evidence that three adhesive proteins interact with a common recognition site on activated platelets. J Biol Chem 1984; 259: 5388-5391.

109. Thiagarajan P, Kelly KL. Exposure of binding sites for vitronectin on platelets following stimulation. J Biol Chem 1988; 263: 3035-3038.

110. Girma JP, Kalafatis M, Pietu G et al. Mapping of distinct von Willebrand Factor domains interacting with platelet GPIb and GPIIb/IIIa and with collagen using monoclonal antibodies. Blood 1986; 67:1356-1366.

111. Usami S, Chen HH, Zhao Y et al. Design and construction of a linear shear stress flow chamber. Ann Biomed Eng 1993; 21: 77-83.

112. Howard MA, Firkin BG. Ristocetin-a new tool in the investigation of platelet aggregation. Thromb Diath Haemorrh 1971; 76:362-369.

113. Weiss HJ, Rogers J, Brand H. Defective ristocetin-induced platelet aggregation in von Willebrand's disease and its correction by factor VIII. J Clin Invest 1973; 52:2697-2707.

114. Read MS, Smith SV, Lamb MA et al. Role of botrocetin in platelet agglutination: formation of an activated complex of botrocetin and von Willebrand factor. Blood 1989; 74: 1031-1035.

115. Andrews RK, Booth WJ, Gorman JJ et al. Purification of botrocetin from Bothrops Jararaca venom. Analysis of the botrocetin-mediated interaction between von Willebrand factor and the human platelet membrane glycoprotein Ib-IX complex. Biochemistry 1989; 28:8317-8326.

116. Lee J-O, Rieu P, Arnaout AM et al. Crystal structure of the A domain from the a subunit of integrin CR3 (CDllb/CD18). Cell 1995; 80:631-638.

117. Lee J-O, Bankston LA, Arnaout MA et al. Two conformations of the integrin A-domain (I-domain): a pathway for activation? Structure 1995; 3:1333-1340.

118. Pareti FI, Niiya K, McPherson JM et al. Isolation and characterization of two domains of human von Willebrand factor that interact with fibrillar collagen types I and III. J Biol Chem 1987; 262:13835-13841.

119. Kalafatis M, Takahashi Y, Girma JP et al. Localization of a collagen-interactive domain of human von Willebrand factor between amino acid residues Gly^{911} and Glu^{1365}. Blood 1987; 70:1577-1583.

120. Meyer D, Zimmermann TS, Obert B et al. Hybridoma antibodies to human von Willebrand factor. I. Characterization of seven clones function. Br J Haematol 1984; 57:597-608.

121. Stel HV, Sakariassen KS, Scholte BJ et al. Characterization of 25 monoclonal antibodies to factor VIII-von Willebrand factor: relationship between ristocetin-induced platelet aggregation and platelet adherence to subendothelium. Blood 1984; 63:1408-1415.

122. Pietu G, Ribba A-S, Cherel G et al. Epitope mapping of inhibitory monoclonal antibodies to human von Willebrand factor by using recombinant cDNA libraries. Thromb Haemost 1994; 71:788-792.

123. Christophe O, Rouault C, Obert B et al. A monoclonal antibody (B724) to von Willebrand factor recognizing an epitope within the A1 disulphide loop (Cys509-Cys695) discriminates between type 2A and type 2B von Willebrand disease. Br J Haematol 1995; 90:195-203.

124. Diamond MS, Garcia-Aguilar J, Bickford JK et al. The I domain is a major recognition site on the leukocyte integrin Mac-1 (CD1 lb/CD18) for four distinct adhesion ligands. J Cell Biol 1993; 120: 1031-1043.

125. Landis RC, Bennett RI, Hogg N. A novel LFA-1 activation epitope maps to the I domain. J Cell Biol 1993; 120: 1519-1527.

126. Randi AM, Hogg N. I domain of β2 integrin lymphocyte function associated antigen-1 contains a binding site for ligand intercellular adhesion molecule-1. J Biol Chem 1994; 269:12395-12398.

127. Huang C, Springer TA. A binding interface on the I domain of Lymphocyte function-associated antigen-1 (LFA-1) required for specific interaction with intercellular adhesion molecule 1 (ICAM-1). J Biol Chem 1995; 270:19008-19016.

128. Kamata T, Puzon W, Takada Y. Identification of putative ligand binding sites within I domain of integrin α2β1 (VLA-2, CD49b/CD29). J Biol Chem 1994; 269:9659-9663.

129. Denis C, Baruch D, Kielty CM et al. Localization of von Willebrand factor binding domains to endothelial extracellular matrix and to type VI collagen. Arterioscler Thromb 1993; 13:396-406.

130. Pietu G, Meulien P, Cherel G et al. Production in *Escherichiae coli* of a biologically active subfragment of von Willebrand factor corresponding to the platelet glycoprotein Ib, collagen and heparin binding domains. Biochem Biophys Res Commun 1989; 164:1339-1347.

131. Sugimoto M, Ricca G, Hrinda ME et al. Functional modulation of the isolated glycoprotein Ib-binding domain of von

Willebrand factor expressed in *Escherichia coli*. Biochemistry 1991; 30:5202-5209.

132. Gralnick HR, Williams S, McKeown L et al. A monomeric von Willebrand factor fragment, Leu-504-Ser-728, inhibits von Willebrand factor interaction with glycoprotein Ib-IX. Proc Natl Acad Sci USA 1992; 89: 7880-7884.

133. Cruz Ma, Handin RI, Wise RJ. The interaction of von Willebrand factor-A1 domain with platelet glycoprotein Ib-IX. J Biol Chem 1993; 268:21238-21245.

134. Kessler CM, Floyd CM, Frantz SC et al. Critical role of the carbohydrate moiety in human von Willebrand factor protein for interactions with type I collagen. Thromb Res 1990; 57:59-76.

135. Sixma JJ, Shiphorst ME, Verweij CL et al. Effect of deletion of the A1-domain of von Willebrand factor on its binding to heparin, collagen and platelets in the presence of ristocetin. Eur J Biochem 1991; 196:369-375.

136. Cruz MA, Yuan H, Lee JR et al. Interaction of the von Willebrand Factor (vWF) with collagen. J Biol Chem 1995; 270:10822-10827.

137. Kuo H-J, Keene D, Glanville RW. The macromolecular structure of type-VI collagen. Formation and stability of filaments. Eur J Biochem 1995; 232:364-372.

138. Fretto LJ, Fowler WE, McCaslin DR et al. Substructure of human von Willebrand factor. Proteolysis by V8 and characterization of two functional domains. J Biol Chem 1986; 261:15679-15689.

139. Fujimura Y, Titani K, Holland LZ et al. A heparin-binding domain of human von Willebrand factor. Characterization and localization to a tryptic fragment extending from amino acid residue Val-449 to Lys-728. J Biol Chem 1987; 262:1734-1739.

140. Sobel M, Soler DF, Kermode JC et al. Localization and characterization of a heparin binding domain peptide of human von Willebrand Factor. J Biol Chem 1992; 267:8857-8862.

141. Roberts DD, Williams SB, Gralnick HR et al. von Willebrand factor binds specifically to sulfated glycolipids. J Biol Chem 1986; 261:3306-3309.

142. Christophe O, Obert B, Meyer D et al. The binding domain of von Willebrand factor to sulfatides is distinct from those interacting with glycoprotein Ib, heparin and collagen and resides between amino acid residues Leu512 and Lys673. Blood 1991; 78:2310-2317.

143. Modderman PW, Admiraal LG, Sonnenberg A et al. Glycoproteins V and Ib-IX form a noncovalent complex in the platelet membrane. J Biol Chem 1992; 264:364-369.

144. Vicente V, Houghten RA, Ruggeri ZM. Identification of a site in the a chain of platelet glycoprotein Ib that participates in von Willebrand Factor binding. J Biol Chem 1990; 265:274-280.

145. De Marco L, Mazzuccato M, Masotti A et al. Function of glycoprotein Iba in platelet activation induced by α-thrombin. J Biol Chem 1991; 266:23776-23783.

146. Murata M, Ware J, Ruggeri ZM. Site-directed mutagenesis of a soluble recombinant fragment of platelet glycoprotein Ibα demonstrating negatively charged residues involved in von Willebrand factor binding. J Biol Chem. 1991; 266:15474-15480.

147. Vicente V, Kostel PJ, Ruggeri ZM. Isolation and functional characterization of the von Willebrand factor-binding domain located between residues His-Arg293 of the alpha-chain of glycoprotein Ib. J Biol Chem 1988; 263:18473-18479.

148. Marchese P, Murata M, Mazzuccato M et al. Identification of three tyrosine residues of glycoprotein Iba with distinct roles in von Willebrand factor and α-thrombin binding. J Biol Chem 1995; 270:9571-9578.

149. De Marco L, Mazzuccato M, Masotti A et al. Localization and characterization of an α-thrombin-binding site on platelet glycoprotein Iba. J Biol Chem 1994; 269: 6474-6484.

150. Sobel M, Mcneill PM, Carlson PL et al. Heparin inhibition of von Willebrand factor-dependent platelet function in vitro and in vivo. J Clin Invest 1991; 87:1787-1793.

151. Weinstein M, Vosburgh E, Phillips M et al. Isolation from commercial aurin tricarboxylic acid of the most effective polymeric inhibitors of von Willebrand factor. Interaction with platelet glycoprotein Ib. Com-

parison with other polyanionic and polyaromatic polymers. Blood 1991; 78:2291-2298.

152. Savage B, Shattil SJ, Ruggeri ZM. Modulation of platelet function through adhesion receptors - A dual role for glycoprotein IIb-IIIa (integrin-alpha(IIb)beta(3) mediated by fibrinogen and glycoprotein von Willebrand factor. J Biol Chem 1992; 267:11300-11306.

153. Fujimura Y, Titani K, Holland LZ et al. von Willebrand factor. A reduced and alkylated 52/48 kDa fragment beginning at amino acid residue 449 contains the domain interacting with platelet glycoprotein Ib. J Biol Chem 1986; 261:381-385.

154. Scott JP, Montgomery RR, Retzinger GS. Dimeric ristocetin flocculates proteins, binds to platelets, and mediates von Willebrand factor-dependent agglutination of platelets. J Biol Chem 1991; 266:8149-8155.

155. Miura S, Fujimura Y, Sugimoto M et al. Structural elements influencing von Willebrand factor (vWF) binding affinity for platelet glycoprotein Ib within a dispase-digested vWF fragment. Blood 1994; 84:1553-1558.

156. Sugimoto M, Mohri H, McClintock RA et al. Identification of discontinous von Willebrand factor sequences involved in complex formation with botrocetin: a model for the regulation of von Willebrand factor binding to platelet glycoprotein Ib. J Biol Chem 1991; 266:18172-18178.

157. Fujimura Y, Usami Y, Titani K et al. Studies on anti-von Willebrand factor (vWF) monoclonal antibody NMC-4, which inhibits both ristocetin- and botrocetin-induced vWF binding to platelet glycoprotein Ib. Blood 1991; 77:113-120.

158. Berndt MC, Ward CM, Booth WJ et al. Identification of aspartic acid 514 through glutamic acid 542 as a glycoprotein Ib-IX complex receptor recognition sequence in von Willebrand factor-Mechanism of modulation of von Willebrand factor by ristocetin and botrocetin. Biochemistry 1992; 31:11144-11151.

159. Knott HM, Berndt MC, Kralicek AV et al. Determination of the solution structure of a platelet-adhesion peptide of von Willebrand factor. Biochemistry 1992; 31:11152-11158.

160. Matsushita T, Sadler JE. Identification of amino acid residues essential for von Willebrand factor binding to platelet glycoprotein Ib. J Biol Chem 1995; 270:13406-13414.

161. Girma JP, Takahashi Y, Yoshioka A et al. Ristocetin and botrocetin involve two distinct domains of von Willebrand factor for binding to platelet membrane glycoprotein Ib. Thromb Haemostas 1990; 64:326-332.

162. Sugimoto M, Dent J, McClintock R et al. Analysis of structure function relationships in the platelet membrane glycoprotein Ib binding domain of von Willebrand's factor by expression of deletion mutants. J Biol Chem 1993; 268:12185-12192.

163. Carew JA, Quinn SM, Stoddart JH et al. O-linked carbohydrate of recombinant von Willebrand factor influences ristocetin-induced binding to platelet glycoprotein Ib. J Clin Invest 1992; 90:2258-2267.

164. Rabinowitz I, Tuley EA, Mancuso DJ et al. von Willebrand disease type B-A missense mutation selectively abolishes ristocetin-induced von Willebrand factor binding to platelet glycoprotein Ib. Proc Natl Acad Sci USA 1992; 89:9846-9849.

165. Azuma H, Sugimoto M, Ruggeri ZM et al. A role of von Willebrand factor proline residues 702-704 in ristocetin-mediated binding to platelet glycoprotein Ib. Thromb Haemostas 1993; 69:192-196.

166. Girma JP, Fressinaud E, Christophe O et al. Aurin tricarboxylic acid inhibits platelet adhesion to collagen by binding to the 509-695 disulfide loop of von Willebrand factor competing with glycoprotein Ib. Thromb Haemostas 1992; 68:703-713.

167. Kroner PA, Klussendorf ML, Scott JP et al. Expressed full-length von Willebrand factor containing missense mutation linked to type IIB von Willebrand disease shows enhanced binding to platelets. Blood 1992; 79:2048-2055.

168. Randi AM, Jorieux S, Tuley EA et al. Recombinant von Willebrand factor Arg(578) - Gln: A type IIB von Willebrand disease mutation effects binding to glycoprotein Ib but not to collagen or heparin. J Biol Chem

1992; 267:21187-21192.

169. Bahnak BR, Lavergne JM, Ferreira V et al. Comparison of the primary structure of the functional domains of human and porcine von Willebrand factor that mediate platelet adhesion. Biochem Biophys Res Commun 1992; 182:561-568.

170. Bakhshi MR, Myers JC, Howard PS et al. Sequencing of the primary adhesion domain of bovine von Willebrand factor. Biochem Biophys Acta 1992; 1132:325-328.

171. Nichols WC, Cooney KA, Mohlke KL et al. von Willebrand disease in the RIIIS/J mouse is caused by a defect outside of the von Willebrand factor gene. Blood 1994; 83:3225-3231.

172. Standen GR, Bignell P, Bowen DJ et al. Family studies in von Willebrand diseases by analysis of restriction fragment length polymorphisms and an intragenic variable number tandem repeat (VNTR) sequence. Br J Haematol 1990; 76:242-249.

173. Ginsburg D, Sadler JE. von Willebrand disease: a database of point mutations, insertions, and deletions. Thromb Haemost 1993; 69: 177-184.

174. Berkowitz SD, Dent J, Roberts J et al. Epitope mapping of the von Willebrand factor subunit distinguishes fragments present in normal and type IIA von Willebrand disease from those generated by plasmin. J Clin Invest 1987; 79:524-531.

175. Battle J, Lopez Fernandez MF, Campos M et al. The heterogeneity of type IIA von Willebrand's disease: studies with protease inhibitors. Blood 1986; 68: 1207-1212.

176. Verweij CL, Quadt R, Briet E et al. Genetic linkage of two intragenic restriction fragment length polymorphisms with von Willebrand's disease type IIA. J Clin Invest 1988; 81: 1116-1121.

177. Iannuzzi MC, Hikada N, Boehnke ML et al. Analysis of the relationship of von Willebrand disease (vWD) and hereditary hemorrhagic telangiectasia and identification of potential type IIA vWD mutation (Ile865 to Thr). Am J Hum Genet 1991; 48:757-763.

178. Ginsburg D, Konkle BA, Gill JC et al. Molecular basis of human von Willebrand disease: analysis of platelet von Willebrand factor mRNA. Proc Natl Acad Sci USA 1989; 86:3723-3727.

179. Gaucher C, Hanss M, Dechavanne M et al. Substitution of cysteine for phenylalanine 751 in mature von Willebrand factor is a novel candidate mutation in a family with type IIA von Willebrand disease. Thromb Haemost 1992; 67:612-617.

180. Inbal A, Eglender T, Kornbrot N et al. Identification of three candidate mutations causing type IIa von Willebrand disease using a rapid, nonradioactive, allele-specific hybridization method. Blood 1993; 82:830-836.

181. Lavergne JM, de Paillette L, Bahnak BR et al. Defects in type IIA von Willebrand disease-A cysteine 509 to arginine substitution in the mature von Willebrand factor disrupts a disulfide loop involved in the interaction with platelet glycoprotein Ib-IX. Br J Haematol 1992; 82:66-72.

182. Hilbert L, Gaucher C, Mazurier C. Identification of two mutations (Arg611Cys and Arg611His) in the A1 loop of von Willebrand factor (vWF) responsible for type 2 von Willebrand disease with decreased platelet-dependent function of vWF. Blood 1995; 86:1010-1018.

183. Lyons SE, Bruck ME, Bowie EJW et al. Impaired intracellular transport produced by a subset of type IIA von Willebrand disease mutation. J Biol Chem 1992; 267: 4424-4430.

184. Dent JA, Galbusera M, Ruggeri ZM. Heterogeneity of plasma von Willebrand factor multimers resulting from proteolysis of the constituent subunit. J Clin Invest 1991; 88:774-782.

185. Gralnick HR, Williams SB, McKeown LP et al. In vitro correction of the abnormal multimeric structure of von Willebrand factor in type IIa von Willebrand's disease. Proc Natl Acad Sci USA 1985; 82:5968-5972.

186. Zimmermann TS, Dent JA, Ruggeri ZM et al. Subunit composition of plasma von Willebrand factor. J Clin Invest 1986; 77:947-951.

187. Ribba AS, Voorberg J, Meyer D et al. Characterization of recombinant von Willebrand factor corresponding to mutations in type

IIA and type IIB von Willebrand disease. J Biol Chem 1992; 267:23209-23215.

188. Christophe O, Ribba AS, Baruch D et al. Influence of mutations and size of multimers in type II von Willebrand disease upon the function of von Willebrand factor. Blood 1994; 83:3553-3561.

189. De Marco L, Girolami A, Zimmerman TS et al. Interaction of purified type IIb von Willebrand factor with the platelet membrane glycoprotein Ib induces fibrinogen binding to the glycoprotein IIb/IIIa complex and initiates aggregation. Proc Natl Acad Sci USA 1985; 82:7424-7428.

190. Ware J, Dent JA, Azuma H et al. Identification of a point mutation in type IIB von Willebrand disease illustrating the regulation of von Willebrand factor affinity for the platelet membrane glycoprotein Ib-IX receptor. Proc Natl Acad Sci USA 1991; 88:2946-2950.

191. Randi AM, Rabinowitz I, Mancuso DJ et al. Molecular basis of von Willebrand disease type IIb. Candidate mutations cluster in one disulfide loop between proposed platelet glycoproteins Ib binding sequences. J Clin Invest 1991; 87:1220-1226.

192. Cooney KA, Nichols WC, Bruck ME et al. The molecular defect in type IIb von Willebrand disease. Identification of four potential missense mutations within the putative GPIb binding domain. J Clin Invest 1991; 87:1227-1233.

193. Cooney KA, Lyons SE, Ginsburg D. Functional analysis of a type IIB von Willebrand disease missense mutation: increased binding of large von Willebrand factor multimers to platelets. Proc Natl Acad Sci USA 1992; 89:2869-2872.

194. Ruggeri ZM, Pareti FI, Mannucci PM et al. Heightened interaction between platelets and factor VIII/von Willebrand factor in a new subtype of von Willebrand's disease. N Engl J Med 1980; 302:1047-1051.

195. Murata M, Fukuyama M, Satoh K et al. Low shear stress can initiate von Willebrand factor-dependent platelet aggregation in patients witn type IIB and platelet-type von Willebrand disease. J Clin Invest 1993; 92: 1555-1558.

196. Holmberg L, Dent JA, Schneppenheim R et al. von Willebrand factor mutation enhancing interactions with platelets in patients with normal multimeric structure. J Clin Invest 1993; 91:2169-2177.

197. Rabinowitz I, Randi AM, Shindler KS et al. Type IIB mutation His 505——>Asp implicates a new segment in the control of von Willebrand factor binding to platelet glycoprotein Ib. J Biol Chem 1993; 268:20497-20501.

198. Hilbert L, Gaucher C, de Romeuf C et al. Leu697—>Val mutation in mature von Willebrand factor is responsible for type IIB von Willebrand disease. Blood 1994; 83:1542-1550.

199. Cooney KA, Ginsburg D. Comparative analysis of type 2b von Willebrand disease mutations: implications for the mechanism of von Willebrand factor binding to platelets. Blood 1996; 87: 2322-2328.

200. van Genderen PJJ, Vink T, Michiels JJ et al. Acquired von Willebrand disease caused by an autoantibody selectively inhibiting the binding of von Willebrand factor to collagen. Blood 1994; 84:3378-3384.

201. Tornai I, Arnout J, Deckmyn H et al. A monoclonal antibody recognizes a von Willebrand factor domain within the amino-terminal portion of the subunit that modulates the function of the glycoprotein IB- and IIB/IIIA-binding domain. J Clin Invest 1993; 91:273-279.

202. Champe M, McIntyre W, Berman PW. Monoclonal antibodies that block the activity of leukocyte function-associated antigen 1 recognize three discrete epitopes in the inserted domain of CD11a. J Biol Chem 1995; 270:1388-1394.

203. Huang C, Springer TA. A binding interface on the I domain of Lymphocyte function-associated antigen-1 (LFA-1) required for specific interaction with intercellular adhesion molecule 1 (ICAM-1). J Biol Chem 1995; 270:19008-19016.

204. Zhou L, Lee DHS, Plescia J et al. Differential ligand binding specificities of recombinant CD11b/CD18 integrin I-domain. J Biol Chem 1994; 269:17075-17079.

205. Bergelson JM, Chan BMC, Finberg RW et al. The integrin VLA-2 binds Echovirus 1 and extracellular matrix ligands by differ-

ent mechanisms. J Clin Invest 1993; 92:232-239.

206. Horiuchi T, Macon KJ, Engler JA et al. Site-directed mutagenesis of the region around Cys-241 of complement component C2: evidence for a C4b binding site. J Immunol 1991; 147:584-589.

207. Kamata T, Takada Y. Direct binding of collagen to the I domain of integrin α2β1 (VLA-2, CD49b/CD29). J Biol Chem 1994; 269:26006-26010.

208. Kern A, Briesewitz R, Bank I et al. The role of the I domain in ligand binding of the human integrin α1β1. J Biol Chem1994; 269:22811-22816.

209. Ueda T, Rieu P, Brayer J et al. Identification of the complement iC3b binding site in the β2 integrin CR3 (CD11b/CD18). Proc Natl Acad Sci USA 1994; 91:10680-10684.

210. Moyle M, Foster DL, McGrath DE et al. A hookworm glycoprotein that inhibits neutrophil functions is a ligand of the integrin CD11b/CD18. J Biol Chem 1994; 269:10008-10015.

β1 Integrins

INTRODUCTION ON INTEGRINS

Several cellular processes such as proliferation, migration, hemostasis and tissue morphogenesis depend upon communication between cells and the extracellular matrix (ECM). Integrins, heterodimeric receptors composed of noncovalently associated α and β subunits, form a major group of adhesion molecules mediating cell-ECM interactions.[1-4] To date, 16 α subunits (Mr 130 to 210 kD) and 9 β subunits (Mr 90 to 110Kd) have been identified and sequenced (Fig. 3.1). Individual subunits do not associate freely and the diversity and the repertoire generated is limited since α and β subunits are found to associate only with the complementary subunit. However, some of the subunits are polygamous and pair with more than one subunit and this results in an integrin family consisting of 22 αβ heterodimers. The α and β chain association can be facilitated by chaperones in the endoplasmic reticulum. Calnexin, a membrane-bound chaperone facilitating the assembly of several membrane protein complexes such as MHC class I, the T cell receptor complex and the membrane bound Ig complex, plays a dual role in integrin processing and assembly.[5] It retains a large pool of β1 subunits in the endoplasmic reticulum ready for assembly with any nascent α subunit and it keeps the β1 and α chains in an assembly competent conformation thereby facilitating their assembly process. The specificity of receptor-ligand interaction is provided by both the α and β subunits, as shown by the αv-containing integrins which recognize different ligands depending upon the β subunit (β1 or β3) present,[6-8] and by the α4β1 and α5β1[9,10] integrins which recognize different sites on fibronectin (FN).

Electron microscopic (EM) and/or immuno EM images of integrins indicate that the two subunits protrude out of the cell membrane with two stalks of about 18 nm in length and form a globular head of about 8 x 12 nm. This head is thought to contain the seven homologous repeats of the α subunit and the conserved N-terminal region of the β subunit. The two stalks are formed by the cysteine rich repeats of the β subunit and the pleated sheet portion of the α subunit.[11-14] Largely based on biochemical and biophysical data, including the distance constraints imposed by the disulfide bonding patterns, cross-linking and controlled

The Superfamily with von Willebrand Factor VA Domains, edited by Alfonso Colombatti and Roberto Doliana. © 1996 R.G. Landes Company.

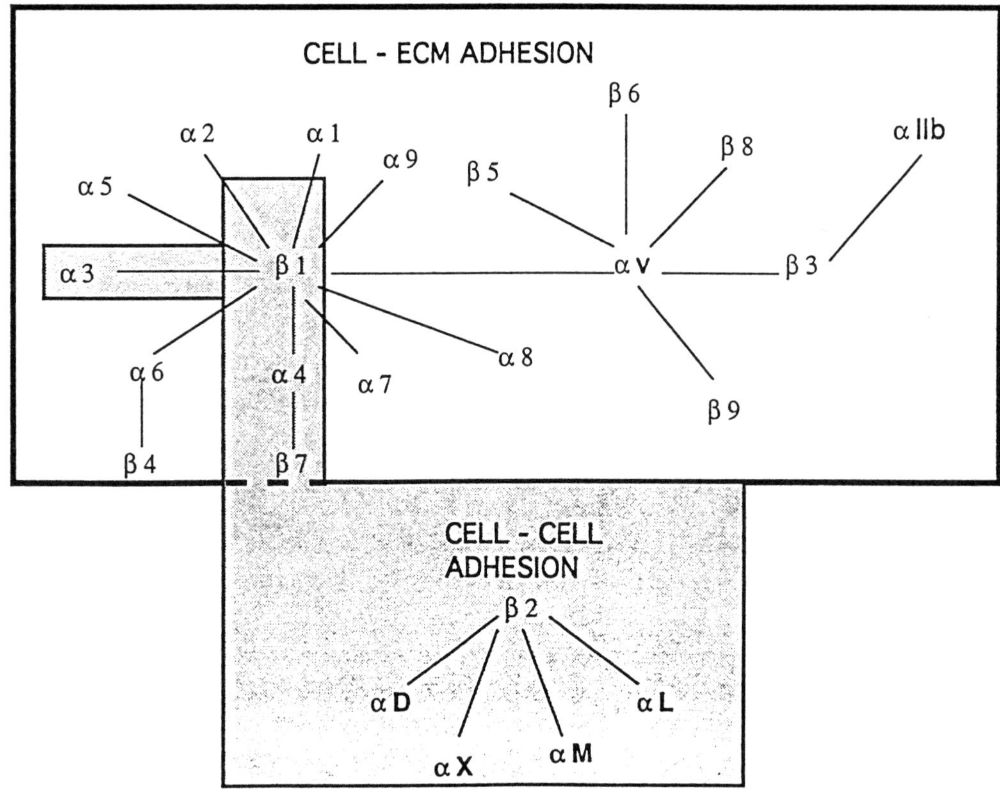

Fig. 3.1. Overview of the currently known integrins involved in cell-cell and cell-ECM interactions.

proteolysis studies, as well as antibody epitope mapping, an alternative model, in which the αIIbβ3 integrin exhibits a very compact structure, also has been suggested.[15-17] By applying a low resolution modeling procedure in which the two integrin subunits are represented as an array of nonoverlapping and interconnected beads of defined sizes, a third model has been proposed that attempts to reconcile the model derived from the analysis of the EM images, the biochemical data and the behavior of the integrin complex in detergent solution.[18] Based on this model, the αIIbβ3 integrin assumes a conformation that is more compact than that suggested by EM and both its putative binding sites are located on the same solvent exposed face in a close spatial relationship to allow simultaneous interaction of the ligand(s) with two integrin recognition sites.

Most of the subunits have been cloned and their sequences determined. The predicted amino acid sequences of the integrin α and β subunits indicate that both subunits possess a large extracellular domain, a single transmembrane region, and a short cytoplasmic tail at the C-terminus; the integrin β4 subunit is the only exception as its cytoplasmic domain is much larger.[19,20]

Integrin α subunits have about 900-1000 amino acid long extracellular domains and fall into four categories on the basis of their structural motifs (Fig. 3.2). Some members (αIIb, α3, α5, α6, α7, α8, α9, αv) consist of seven repeats of about 50-60 amino acid residues. Repeats IV-VII contain motifs similar to the divalent cation binding EF hand-like present in other proteins such as calmodulin.[21] It is believed that the cations bound to these motifs serve

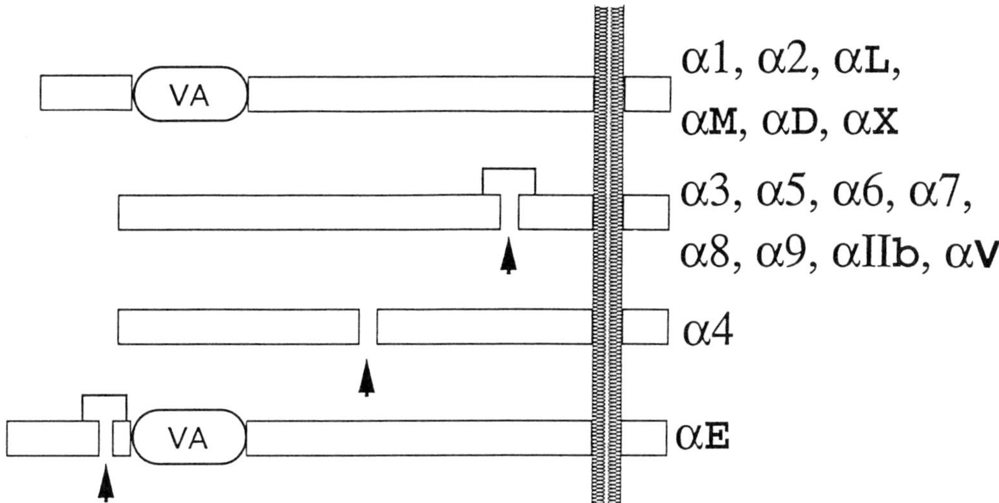

Fig. 3.2. Schematic diagram of the structural features of integrin α chains. The α chains that associate with the β1 subunit, integrins α1β1, α2β1 and those associated with the β2 integrins LFA-1, Mac-1, p150,95 and αDβ2 integrins, contain an inserted VWFA/I module designated VA, according to the proposed nomenclature of Bork and Bairoch,[247] but lack a disulfide linked cleavage site. Most α chains, including α3, α5, α6, α7, α8, α9, αv and αIIb have a disulfide linked (shown as square braket) cleavage site (indicated by an arrow) near the C-terminus of the extracellular domain. The αE has an unusual disulfide linked cleavage site, which occurs in the acidic sequence upstream of the VWFA module. Finally, the α4 subunit has a non-disulfide linked cleavage site, which occurs in the middle of the extracellular portion.

to stabilize the tertiary structure of the individual subunits. In addition, they are necessary for the interaction of the heterodimeric receptors with their respective ligands.[22] These integrin chains have a protease cleavage site near the cell membrane. Other members (αM, αL, αX, αD, α1, α2) (see chapter 4) also have three putative divalent-cation binding sites, lack a protease cleavage site and include one VWFA module. The α4 subunit has three putative divalent cation binding sites and a distinct protease cleavage site.[23] Finally, the αE subunit (see chapter 7) has three putative divalent cation binding sites and a cleavage site distinct from that of all other integrins.[24] It contains one VWFA module and an additional sequence of 55 amino acid residues that includes the cleavage site located just N-terminally to the VWFA module. The cytoplasmic domains of α subunits are short (ranging from 15 to 77 amino acids) and not closely related to one another except for the GFFKR sequence motif,[25] conserved among all α subunits and thought to participate in signal

transduction and to play a critical role in regulating inside-out signal transduction[26,27] and post-ligand binding outside-in signaling.[28,29]

One or more integrins are expressed at any given time on the surface of every cell type except for mature erythrocytes which are devoid of integrins. All integrins require divalent cations for binding to their ligands, consistent with the presence of multiple cation-binding sites (EF hand-like motifs)[21] and metal ion dependent adhesion sites (MIDAS)[30] motifs for the VWFA module containing integrins, in the extracellular portion of their α subunits. The α subunits EF hand-like motifs differ from the classic EF hand in that they lack the glutamic acid at position 12, which functions as a sixth obligatory metal-coordinating residue. This has led to the speculation that either these cation binding sites are functional as such, or that the missing residue must be contributed by the ligand or alternatively by a noncontiguous segment of the α subunit, or by the associated β chain. Some general rules for the sensitivity of integrins to divalent cations and the relationships between ligand and cation binding have been proposed,[31] but the individual requirements differ among different integrins and appear to depend upon specific integrin ligand interactions. Furthermore, integrin sites involved in ligand recognition have been found in both α and β subunits.[32-35] A region highly conserved in all β subunits,[36] which is likely to contain a MIDAS motif[30] contributes to the structure of ligand and cation binding sites.[37]

The existence of alternatively spliced forms of integrin subunits adds to the complexity of this family of receptors and provides the potential for the generation of wider ligand specificities and of distinct functional activities and for changes of the strength and quality of signaling. In fact, splice variants of the cytoplasmic tail[38-46] and extracellular portion[42,47,48] have been described for both subunits.

Integrin β subunits have a 675-700 amino acid long extracellular domain with a four-fold repeat of a cysteine rich region with internal disulfide bonds and a cytoplasmic tail of varying length (ranging from 40-60 amino acids to more than 1000 in the case of β4). The extracellular domain contains a region of about 200 residues that is highly conserved among all β subunits and might include a variant MIDAS like motif. Naturally occurring[37] and experimentally induced[36,49-51] point mutations in this area, and in particular in the MIDAS aspartic and serine residues, reveal that this region is important for α/β association and ligand recognition.

A wide variety of proteins serve as ligands for integrin receptors. These include ECM proteins such as collagen, FN, laminin and others that function as ligands for several integrins including all the β1 subunit containing integrins; plasma proteins such as fibrinogen, von Willebrand factor, factor X, and vitronectin; cell bound complement iC3b and adhesion molecules on cell surfaces such as ICAM-1,-2,-3, VCAM-1, MAdCAM-1, and fertilin; proteins of pathogenic microorganisms, such

as invasin; and surface proteins of viruses.[4,52-59] Many integrins bind to more than one of the above ligands, and some ligands bind to more than one integrin,[4] the result being that cell adhesion can be strengthened by these overlapping ligand/integrin recognition mechanisms.

In the case of cell adhesion to ECM, the availability of multiple integrins with the selective ability to recognize defined regions of ECM components suggests that the effects of a given ECM molecule may be mediated by distinct ligand-receptor pairs acting via multiple and distinct intracellular signaling pathways.[60] This is particularly relevant taking into account the fact that ECM constituents can vary in structure, as a consequence of alternative splicing and association with other ECM constituents.[61-64] In addition, mechanical forces generated via integrin-ECM interactions result in activation of at least five different classes of chemical signaling pathways that share common downstream targets with the growth factor signaling mechanisms.[65] These include tyrosine kinases, serine/threonine kinases, inositol lipid turnover, G proteins, ion transporters (Ca2+ channels and the Na+/H+ antiporter)[60] and cytoskeletal rearrangements leading to changes in the nuclear matrix.[66] These signaling pathways are thought to ultimately affect gene expression.[64,67-69]

Studies on cell binding to FN, the prototype ECM adhesive molecule, led to the first molecular identification of a specific linear peptide site for an integrin. The linear sequence Arg-Gly-Asp (RGD), in the tenth type III module, is an essential motif for cell adhesion to FN,[10] and ligand binding can be inhibited if molar concentrations of RGD-containing peptides (i.e., several orders of magnitude higher than that of the ligand) are added. The RGD sequence is a putative recognition site in many different adhesive proteins. However, while the integrin α5β1 interacts in a rather specific way only with FN, the other RGD-specific integrins have a much broader ligand specificity.[2] These observations and the finding that several proteins contain RGD sequences led to the proposal that integrins recognized their ligands mostly via a linear RGD motif.[2] Later on it was found that other integrins do not bind, at least primarily, to the linear RGD sequence but instead they bind to other residues. The α4β1 integrin, which mediates attachment to VCAM-1 expressed on activated endothelium and to FN, binds to the LDV sequence on FN[72] as well as to the RGD-containing region[73] and to the QIDSPL sequence on VCAM-1.[74] One of these sequences, QAGDV on the γ chain of fibrinogen, is recognized by αIIbβ3,[70] and appears anyhow to mimic the RGD site since its binding to the αIIbβ3 integrin is inhibited by RGD peptides.[71] Finally, other integrins such as the α6β1, α7β1, α1β1 and α2β1[75,76] bind to their respective ligands, collagens and laminins, in a conformation-dependent manner. However, most integrin-binding sequence motifs share an aspartic acid,[77] and this oxygenated residue may be important because of its potential contribution to divalent cation binding. One hypothesis regarding the recognition of ligands by integrins postulates that the glutamic acid at position 12 of the classic EF hand is missing on the EF hand-like cation binding motifs of integrins and that the missing coordination site is provided by the ligand. The aspartic acid of the RGD motif and of the other adhesion motifs containing an aspartic acid residue might substitute for the missing coordination site when an integrin binds to its ligand.[78]

Members of the integrin family have the ability to dynamically regulate their ligand affinity and to modulate their binding efficiency even in the absence of any quantitative change in their cell surface expression. Following ligand binding, "outside-in" signals are triggered inside the cell[60] and in a process called "activation" or "inside-out" signaling, integrins increase their affinity for the ligand and strengthen cellular adhesion. The β subunit cytoplasmic sequences are particularly involved in this bi-directional signaling, although the α subunit cytoplasmic tails may also play a role in cellular regulatory events.[26-29] Recently Yamada and coworkers were able to demonstrate synergistic roles for integrin clustering and receptor occupancy in integrin transmembrane function[79] and suggested that only the combination of both clustering and ligand occupancy delivers a complete downstream signal.

MOLECULAR STRUCTURE OF THE THIRD α1 AND α2 SUBUNITS

Since the α1 and α2 subunits are the only α subunits of the β1 integrin family that include a VWFA module, the remainder of this chapter will be focused on the functional role of the α1β1 and α2β1 integrins (Fig. 3.3).

Neither the genomic organization nor the promoter elements regulating the transcriptional activation of the α1 and α2 subunit genes are known. The only information available concerns the regulation of megakaryocytic differentiation of K562 cells by phorbol esters. In this system the expression of the α2β1 integrin is greatly enhanced as a consequence of the increased steady state levels of mRNA due to a 20-fold increase in transcription rate.[80]

The cDNA cloning of the α1 subunit was initially accomplished in the rat[81] and later in human.[82] The full length cDNA encodes a mature polypeptide consisting of a total of 1152 amino acid residues with three potential divalent cation binding motifs. Comparison between the two sequences shows that there is nearly complete identity in the transmembrane and cytoplasmic domains, while numerous substitutions are detected in the extracellular domain. The α1 sequence diverges in the extracellular portion from other integrin α subunits since it presents, in both rat and human, the VWFA module and a stretch of 38 residues, inserted between two EF hand-like cation binding motifs, that contains four cysteines. There is also a unique cluster of charged residues right after the conserved GFFKR cytoplasmic sequence. A partial sequence

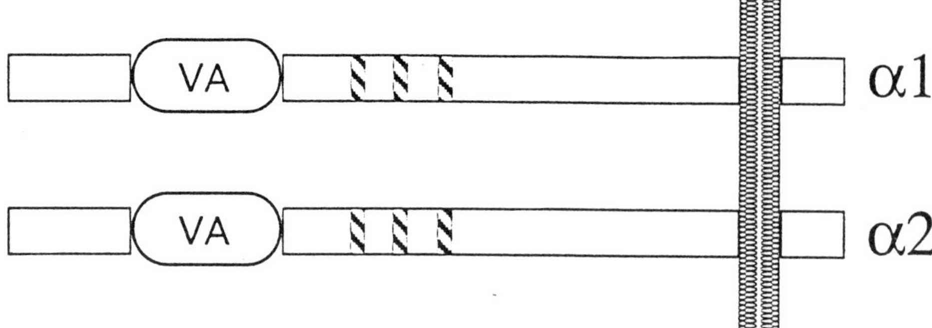

Fig. 3.3. Schematic diagram of the α1 and α2 integrin subunit structure. The striped boxes represent the EF hand-like cation binding sites.

of the chicken[83] α1 subunit, including the VWFA module, indicates that in this portion of the molecule there is amino acid identity with the human cDNA of 84-88% depending upon whether conservative substitutions are considered.

The full length cDNA of the human α2 encodes a mature protein of 1152 amino acid residues[84] with three potential divalent cation binding motifs and a VWFA module of 191 amino acid residues. The murine sequence[85] has an overall 84% amino acid residue identity, but in two functionally important regions, the cytoplasmic tail and the VWFA module, it exhibits significant sequence divergence from the human molecule. The cytoplasmic tail is only 70% identical in the sequences following the conserved GFFKR motif. The VWFA module of mouse,[85] and also of pig,[86] is nearly identical in its C-terminal one-third. The N-terminal two-thirds of the α2 subunit show only 64% sequence identity in the segment that is flanked by a short highly conserved stretch of residues. The bovine α2 subunit sequence has an overall 86% identity at the amino acid residue level that rises to 92% in the VWFA module.[87]

The α1 subunit immunoprecipitated from T lymphocytes,[88] neural cells[89-91] and fibroblasts[92] migrates in SDS-PAGE under nonreducing conditions with an apparent molecular mass between 200 and 210 kD. After reduction the subunit migrates faster at about 170 kD. Correspondingly, the α2 subunit from T lymphocytes,[93,94] platelets,[95] endothelial cells[96-98] and fibroblasts[92] migrates under nonreducing conditions with an apparent molecular mass of about 150-160 kD, which is decreased about 10 kD after reduction.

TISSUE EXPRESSION

EXPRESSION ON LYMPHOCYTES

Normal resting peripheral blood T cells express relatively high levels of α4β1, α5β1 and α6β1 integrins while these cells are negative for the α1β1 and α2β1 integrins. After about four weeks of in vitro cell activation with mitogens or alloantigens the levels of these latter integrins increase dramatically.[88,93,94,99] However, following T cell activation, integrin upregulation can be very specific for certain subpopulations. Maintaining T cell lines for long term in vitro cultures in the presence of a feeder cell layer and IL-2 results in significantly higher levels of α1β1 in CD8+ TCR αβ and CD4−CD8− TCR γδ lymphocytes compared to CD4+ TCR αβ cells. α1β1 might be envisioned to provide a major contribution also during lymphocyte extravasation or for homing in epithelia.[100] In agreement with this hypothesis are the data indicating that α1β1 is highly expressed on intra-epithelial T lymphocytes of the gut[101] and lung.[102]

Circulating lymphocytes continuously migrate through the microenvironment of peripheral lymphoid tissues where, upon encountering exogenous antigens,[103,104] are activated, proliferate, undergo differentiation and acquire α1β1 and α2β1 integrins. T lymphocytes of patients with systemic lupus erythematosus express high levels of α1β1.[105] Similarly, high levels of α1β1 are found on all T cells isolated from synovial tissues and synovial fluid of patients with rheumatoid arthritis.[106] In these patients α1β1 is not found on peripheral blood T cells and it is likely that expression of α1β1 is important for the migration to and the compartmentalization of T cells in the inflamed synovium. T cell expression of α1β1 in vivo (including the expression in intraepithelial lymphocytes) is related to chronic antigenic stimulation and the role of this integrin might be to allow activated post-mitotic T lymphocytes to attach to type IV collagen and to migrate through basement membranes within inflammatory sites.

Both α1β1 and α2β1 function in vitro as costimulatory molecules in the activation of T lymphocytes in the presence of submitogenic amounts of anti-CD3 antibodies and promote attachment of activated T lymphocytes to type IV collagen and to laminin.[107] Furthermore, the increased secretion of the inflammatory mediator TNF-α following α1β1- or α2β1-mediated cell adhesion to type IV collagen is not observed unless submitogenic amounts of anti- CD3 antibody are present. This suggests that these integrins contribute to leukocyte emigration into inflammatory sites and are involved in maintaining the inflammatory responses.[104-106,108] At variance with the finding of polyclonal T cell cultures,[106] activation of CD4⁻CD8⁻ TCR γδ cells can be induced by cross-linking of α1β1 even in the absence of a submitogenic costimulation with anti-CD3 antibodies, suggesting that, at least in some subsets of T lymphocytes, activation signals can be induced solely through the engagement of the α1β1 integrin.[100]

Cell adherence to ECM constituents can result in the production and release of cytokines and therefore, modulation of integrin function represents a mechanism whereby the inflammatory response induced by ECM recognition can be regulated.[109] In addition, secretion of IL-1 induced by α2β1-mediated attachment to type I collagen is potentiated when monocytes adhere to the 120 kD cell binding fragment of FN via the α5β1 integrin.[110,111] Ligand binding to α5β1 generates a PKC-dependent "inside-out" signal that modulates the functional status of α2β1 leading to an increased binding activity of α2β1 without upregulated expression.[111]

EXPRESSION ON NONHEMATOPOIETIC CELLS

Apart from lymphocytes, α1β1 and α2β1 also are present on several other cell types. Among the cells constituting the lymphoid microenvironment, fibroblastic reticular stromal cells, follicular dendritic cells, endothelial cells, macrophages and interdigitating dendritic cells, only reticular and endothelial cells express α1β1 and α2β1.[112,113] These cells are associated with reticular fibers composed of type I and III collagens surrounded by a basement membrane-like layer of laminin and type IV collagen with which they can selectively interact.

While α1β1 and α2β1 integrins are expressed on smooth muscle cells of several organs,[114,115] within the gut the expression of α1β1 is restricted to muscularis propria, muscularis mucosae and to the smooth muscle cells of villi, with α2β1 being expressed exclusively in this last site.[101] α1β1 is present at very high levels on smooth muscle cells but its expression changes dramatically during development and during the transition from a synthetic (low expression) to a contractile state (high expression).[116] This suggests that the α1β1 integrin, by interacting with specific ligands expressed in a developmental manner (laminins?), might play an important regulatory role in the control of smooth muscle development.[116]

α1β1 also is present in some specialized sites such as neural crest cells,[117] astroglia,[118] mesangial cells[119-121] and human articular chondrocytes.[122,123] Neural crest cells attach to laminin by at least two integrin-mediated mechanisms one of which is mediated by α1β1. This integrin recognizes a conformation that laminin assumes when coated in the presence of Ca^{2+} cations and this cell attachment functions in the absence of added soluble divalent cations.[117] Some caution is necessary in interpreting these data since the MIDAS cation binding motif has a ten-fold higher affinity for cations compared to the EF hand-like motifs present in other integrins[124] and it might be that even minute amounts of cations present in the system are sufficient for an adequate cell attachment in the presence of an optimal ligand. This may explain why cation independent neural crest cell binding to laminin occurs only when this molecule is coated onto plastic in the presence of Ca^{2+}.[117,125] This cation-independent attachment is displayed by α1β1 as a function of development and is lost at a time when the neural crest cells have ceased their migration.

α2β1 is expressed on platelets,[126,127] where it also is known as the platelet complex Ia/IIa,[127-129] on megakaryocytes[130] and on primary keratinocytes.[131] In fibroblasts, α2β1 is expressed at high levels and α1β1 is present in very low amounts.[126-128,132,133] Both α1β1 and α2β1 are present on epithelial cells including hepatocytes,[134,135] but α2β1 is present primarily at cell contacts with the basement membrane and its expression is more elevated at sites of proliferating epithelium, such as the basal layer in fetal skin,[131] the nonkeratinizing epithelium of the tonsil,[101,134] and at the base of the crypts of Lieberkuhn of the colon mucosa.[101] α1β1 is expressed on most crypt epithelial cells with a different intensity: cells in the central part of the crypts are stained more intensely than the nonmigratory Paneth cells at the base of the crypts.[101]

Most endothelial cells including human umbilical vein endothelial cells (HUVECs) express α2β1.[97,98,113,136] In HUVECs α2β1 is present at sites of intercellular contacts and contributes to the regulation of the integrity and the permeability of the cell monolayer.[137] Disruption of the tight adhesion of HUVECs to a collagen matrix by an antibody against α2β1 converts the cells from a proliferative to a differentiated phenotype and promotes Ca^{2+} independent migration[138] and angiogenesis manifested by the formation of capillary-like structures.[139,140] α1β1 is selectively expressed by endothelial cells of the microvasculature of several organs including skeletal muscle, foreskin, dermis, brain, and kidney both in situ and in cultured cells.[141,142] However, the lack of α1β1 is not constitutive as its expression can be induced in endothelial cells from large vessels (aorta, femoral vein, umbilical arteries and veins) by inflammatory cytokines such as TNF-α and by PMA or retinoic acid.

It should be mentioned that among the integrin α subunits immunoprecipitated from *C. elegans* by an anti-β1-like antibody at least one, based on mobility under reduced and nonreduced gel conditions, might well correspond to an α subunit containing a VWFA module.[143]

Retinoids[144] but also several cytokines and growth factors such as IL-1β, TGF-β, TNF-α, or NGF can rapidly upregulate the expression of α1β1 in fibroblasts, endothelial and smooth muscle cells.[142,145-149] TNF-α is even more effective in increasing the expression of α2β1 in dermal fibroblasts,[150] while the ability of TGF-β1 to upregulate the expression of α1β1 is seen only in cells already expressing a certain amount of this integrin such as fibroblasts[151] and tumor cell lines.[152] On the other hand, a combined treatment with IL-1β and TNF-α induces the de novo expression of α1β1 in MG63 osteosarcoma cells that are negative for this integrin.[146] In this case the increased expression of α1β1 is correlated with a selective increased ability of MG63 cells to attach to laminin, while there is no increased attachment to type I collagen.[146]

NGF upregulates protein synthesis and expression of α1β1 in PC12 pheochromocytoma cells,[149] and this increased expression correlates with an increased adhesion and neurite formation on type I collagen[149] and laminin.[153] NGF is known to induce common immediate early genes (i.e., transcription factors) and late genes which are specifically induced in PC12 cells by a long term treatment with NGF. EGF, which induces in PC12 cells most of the same immediate early genes as NGF, does not induce α1β1 expression which appears to play an essential and rate-limiting role in NGF induced neurite outgrowth on type I collagen substrata.[149]

FUNCTION

When plated on type IV collagen in the presence of Mg^{2+}, CD8[+] TCR αβ and CD4[-]CD8[-] TCR γδ cells spread and form dendritic extensions and this morphological change from spherical to elongated shape is prevented by antibodies against α1β1 integrin.[100] In contrast, although the α2β1 integrin can mediate attachment of several leukocytes to type IV collagen,[154] antibodies to α2β1 only have a marginal effect on the attachment of CD8[+] TCR αβ or CD4[-]CD8[-] TCR γδ cells to type IV collagen.[100] This suggests that α1β1 and α2β1 might play quite distinct roles in the interaction of specific T cell subpopulations with collagen substrata.

In addition, the ligand specificity of integrins may be altered by as yet undefined cell type specific modulators. One of the most striking examples involves the α2β1 integrin, which is a collagen receptor on platelets, fibroblasts and melanoma cells[127,128,155-158] and a collagen and laminin receptor on endothelial cells but also on many other cell types.[159-163] Although α2β1 integrin isolated from platelets and endothelial cells are indistinguishable by immunological and biochemical means, the distinct ligand specificity is retained in the detergent solubilized receptor[159] which maintains the same Mg^{2+} dependence[127] for its ligand binding, as in the case of intact platelets, after incorporation into liposomes. Subtle structural modifications or a strong association with cell-type specific lipids/proteins has been hypothesized as an explanation for this dual binding activity. This means that different cell types may

receive and/or convey different intracellular signals through ligation to the same receptor of different ECM substrates and further suggests that the binding specificity of an integrin is not defined solely by the association of one particular α to a defined β subunit, but also by the cellular environment in which the heterodimer is expressed. Divalent cations also are considered fundamental for integrin function: for instance α2β1-mediated changes in cation ratios can affect migration of fibroblasts[164] or keratinocytes[165] on type I collagen, with Mg^{2+} exerting a supportive and Ca^{2+} an inhibitory effect.

Collagen is considered an important constituent for the support of cell/platelet adhesion and thrombus formation following vascular injury (see chapter 2). The α2β1 integrin is a minor component in platelets[126-129,155,166] but its importance in hemostasis is stressed by the observation that human platelets, which fail to express the α2 subunit[167,168] or have α2 autoantibodies bound to the cell surface,[169] fail to bind collagen and display hemostatic defects. Moreover, function-blocking antibodies against α2β1 not only inhibit adhesion of unactivated platelets to type I and type III collagens[128] under static conditions, but do so also under more physiological conditions of continuous flow. In this case, α2β1 integrin behaves as a major receptor for various native triple helical collagens.[170-172] Under flow conditions the process of α2β1-mediated platelet adhesion to collagens is extremely fast (with exponential halftimes as short as 0.2 seconds) and is nearly complete within 1 second.[170] This adhesion, which causes a rapid tyrosine phosphorylation of several proteins including pp125[FAK173] is dependent upon the shear rate and the type of collagen substrates: adhesion to types I, II, III and IV collagens is independent of shear rates above 75 dynes/cm²; adhesion to type VI collagen is shear-rate dependent and optimal at about 75 dynes/cm², whereas type V, VII and VIII collagens are largely ineffective in supporting platelet adhesion.[172]

The number of α2β1 molecules expressed by human platelets as estimated by different antibodies against the α2 subunit varies in different individuals between 800 and 1800.[126,166] Nevertheless, these minor quantitative variations are reflected in up to a 20-fold difference in functional activity when adhesion assays are performed with type I collagen substrata and in a 5-fold difference if the substratum is type III collagen.[166] The wide range of functional activity displayed by α2β1 is not justified by the minor quantitative differences in expression levels nor by the clinically relevant polymorphism as defined by the Br alloantigen system.[174-176] Furthermore, it is unlikely that differences in carbohydrate composition account for this functional heterogeneity since the two-dimensional isoelectric focusing properties of the α2 subunits isolated from platelets which display different functional activities seem identical. Whether the 20-fold difference in α2β1 function underscores a natural clinical condition characterized by a higher α2β1-dependent thrombotic risk remains to be determined.

Expression of a single α2 cDNA construct in two different cell lines can yield an α2β1 integrin with three stable but distinct patterns of binding specificities, which are independent of stimulation by PMA and type of cation available.[177] Only the addition of a stimulatory anti-β1 subunit antibody can convert a nonfunctional, or a collagen-specific α2β1, to an integrin capable to attach to both collagen and laminin substrata. Thus, by inducing a conformational change of the integrin through the β1 subunit, the spectrum of ligand specificities can be varied. Therefore, the ligand specificity of α2β1 is controlled by the cellular environment and by the conformational changes imposed on the integrin. The interconvertible α2β1 forms detected in transfected cell lines[177] might then represent an in vitro experimental correlate of the wide range of α2β1 integrin functional activities in platelets as detected in clinical samples.[166]

Integrins are transducers of information from the extracellular environment to the cell:[60] cells receive and transmit "outside

in" and "inside out" signals via integrins that can ultimately affect the microenvironment in its three-dimensional structure. Contracting three-dimensional hydrated collagen lattices mimic soft-tissue matrices during remodeling: when fibroblasts are embedded in this lattice they change morphology and can exert forces sufficient to contract these hydrated gels and form a densely organized, tissue-like structure resembling dermis or scars and granulation tissue.[178] After transfection with an α2 subunit both dermal fibroblasts and rhabdomyosarcoma cells acquire the ability to reorganize the collagen matrix in an Mg^{2+} dependent manner.[179,180] Vascular smooth muscle,[181] fibroblasts,[182] and other cells[183] use α2β1 rather than α1β1 to reorganize a collagen gel.[179] Increasing the expression of the α2β1 integrin by treatment with TGF-β[153] leads to increased gel contraction,[183] suggesting that there is a direct correlation between the levels of α2β1 expressed at the cell surface and the collagen gel contraction activity.[184] Instead, in the same collagen gel retraction model α1β1 expression seems to be correlated with down regulation of collagen production.[184] Furthermore, the ability to contract a collagen gel (a function related with α2β1 expression levels) distinguishes highly invasive from less invasive melanoma cell clones.[184] α2β1 is the major candidate in another function coupled with a putative invasion mechanism: it mediates cellular responses to extracellular collagens by increasing collagenase (MMP-1) production[184,185] and thereby promoting degradation of ECM.

Finally, the integrin α2β1 functions as a specific receptor for Echovirus 1.[59] Echoviruses are human picornaviruses responsible for an illness characterized by fever and sometimes meningitis.

STRUCTURE-FUNCTION RELATIONSHIPS

Before considering in more detail the role of the α1 and α2 subunit extracellular portions and of their VWFA modules in particular, a brief comment on the critical function of the cytoplasmic tail of the α1 and α2 in determining cell adhesion will be given. Studies with chimeric integrin subunits were performed to investigate whether the cytoplasmic domain of the α1 subunit exerts a negative effect in the recruitment of the α1β1 integrin to focal contact sites. While in cells transfected with wild type α1 and plated onto FN only α5 localizes to focal contacts, in cells transfected with an α1 subunit deleted in its cytoplasmic domain and plated onto FN both α5 and α1 localize to focal contacts. The same results are obtained if the cells are plated on vitronectin.[186] In contrast with the results on FN and vitronectin, a deletion of the cytoplasmic domain of the α1 subunit allows cell adhesion and focal contact formation on type IV collagen. This strongly suggests that deleting the cytoplasmic tail of α1 might remove inhibitory sequence signals allowing the localization of a ligand-free α1β1 integrin (i.e., cells plated onto FN or vitronetin) to focal contacts.

Similar chimeras have shown that there are important differences in adhesion strengthening between integrin cytoplasmic domains: α2β1 supports integrin-mediated collagen gel contraction but is less able than α4β1 to support random cell migration.[187] In addition, under conditions of linear flow shear, chimeras with an α2β1 cytoplasmic tail support initial tethering to ICAM or to the 38 kD chymotryptic fragment of FN to the same extent as α4β1 and α5β1.[188] However, the strength of attachment to VCAM-1 is regulated by the α2 cytoplasmic tail to a much greater extent than by the α4 cytoplasmic tail.[188] In addition, the α2 tail in an α4β1 chimera markedly increases the localization of the chimeric receptor into focal adhesion-like complexes.[189] The increased ability of α2β1 to localize into focal adhesion-like complexes indicates a higher propensity of this integrin to interact with cytoskeletal components such as α-actinin, vinculin and talin, all known to localize at focal adhesion sites and to mediate association of integrin with the cytoskeleton. Therefore,

the augmented strengthening of adhesion and the cytoskeletal interactions mediated by the α2 cytoplasmic tail makes the α2β1 integrin well suited for strong and firm adhesion. This is in agreement with the known strong attachment mediated by α2β1 on collagen and laminin[190] on both of which it promotes growth rather than locomotion and differentiation of endothelial cells.[139]

The known ECM ligands for α1β1 and α2β1 are collagen and laminin: these molecules have their three constituent polypeptides (denominated α chains in collagens and α, β and γ chains in laminin) arranged in globular as well as in domains with triple helical and coiled-coil structures, respectively. In triple helices of collagens the three-dimensional structure is characterized by a continuous repeating tripeptide unit, Gly-Xaa-Yaa, where glycine residues are in the center of the helix and the side chains of Xaa and Yaa residues (very often proline and hydroxyproline) project outward of the helix.[191] A more detailed description of collagens is provided in chapter 6. The term laminin, which is considered one of the major constituents of basement membranes,[192] defines and includes at present several molecules (eleven have been described until now)[193,194] that consist of a combination of distinct isoforms of the three subunits (α, β, and γ) (Table 3.1) arranged to form an asymmetric cross- or Y-shaped molecule with three or two short arms, respectively, in which globular domains are separated by EGF-like motifs and one long arm of heptad repeats arranged in a coiled-coil domain of all three chains interwined[195,196] (Fig. 3.4). As will be more evident from the following examples, it appears that the interaction of α1β1 and α2β1 integrins with collagens and laminins is largely conformation-dependent.

INTERACTION OF α1β1 AND α2β1 INTEGRINS WITH LAMININS

An important approach to identify the multiple integrin recognition sites on laminins has been the use of fragments generated by limited proteolytic digestion

Table 3.1. Laminin isoforms

Name	Subunit composition	Previous name
Laminin-1	α1β1γ1	EHS/standard
Laminin-2	α2β1γ1	Merosin
Laminin-3 [a]	α1β2γ1	S-laminin
Laminin-4	α2β2γ1	S-merosin
Laminin-5 [b]	α3β3γ2	Kalinin/nicein/epiligrin
Laminin-6 [c]	α3β1γ1	K-laminin
Laminin-7	α3β3γ1	KS-laminin
Laminin-8	α4β1γ1	
Laminin-9	α4β2γ1	
Laminin-10	α5β1γ1	Dros. like
Laminin-11 [a]	α5β2γ1	Dros. like

a Laminin 3 and 11 have not yet formally been isolated
b Does not bind nidogen/entactin
c Covalent association

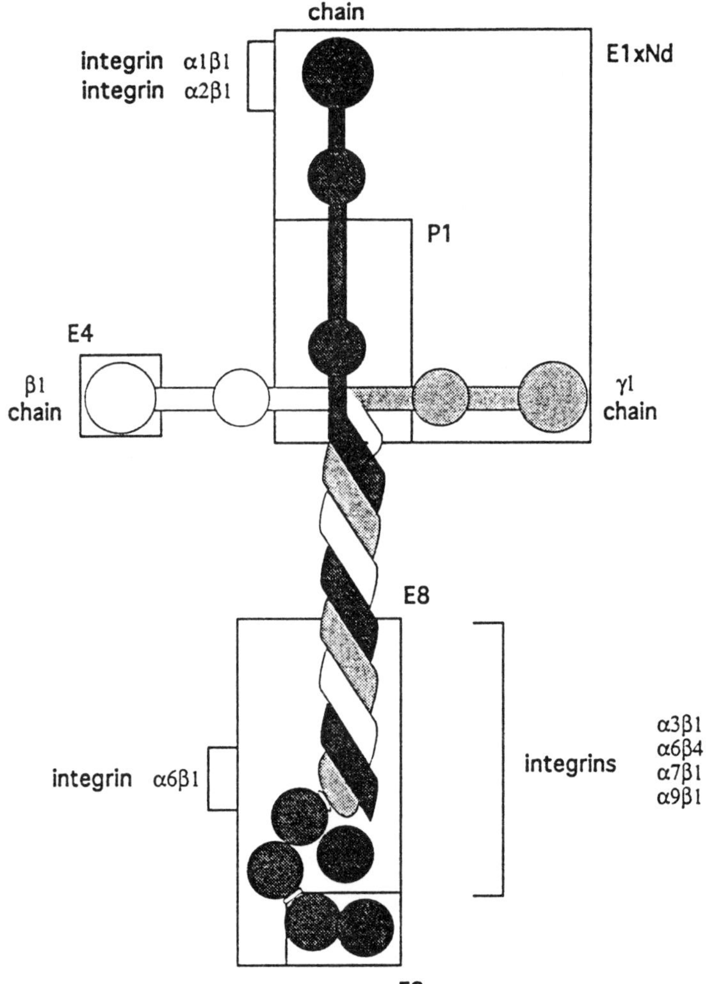

Fig. 3.4. Schematic diagram of the Laminin-1 structure. The major elastase (E) and pepsin (P) proteolytic fragments are boxed. The short arm of the α1 chain contains the recognition site for the α1β1 and α2β1 integrins. The recognition site for the α6β1 is at the end of the coiled-coil structure of the E8 fragment, whereas the α3β1, α7β1, α9β1 and α6β4 recognition sites have not been more precisely mapped within the E8 fragment.

and of cell lines expressing different integrins. These fragments have been tested as ligands in cell adhesion, as inhibitors of cell attachment to the intact laminin molecule and to specifically elute the ligand or the receptor from affinity chromatography columns. The most investigated laminin isoform, isolated from the EHS murine tumor[192] and now defined as Lam 1, consists of the α1, β1 and γ1 subunits. In the Lam 1 molecule, the β and γ chains are connected by a disulfide bridge near to their C-termini at the end of the coiled-coil domain and all three chains are disulfide-linked at the N-terminus of the coiled-coil domain. These cysteine bonds stabilize the coiled-coil region which is maintained in a flexible conformation[197] by weak non-covalent interactions.[196] Using Lam 1 and the proteolysis approach, several fragments (E8, E1XNd, P1, E3) have been generated. The E8 fragment, comprising about one-third of the coiled-coil domain and the globular domain at the C-terminus of the Lam 1 α1 chain, is the major region promoting cell adhesion and migration.[198,199] This fragment functions by virtue of the native quaternary structure maintained by the proper interaction of all three subunit chains.[200,201] Several integrins bind to the E8 fragment including α3β1,[202] α6β1,[89,203,204] α7β1[205] and α6β4.[206] In addition, one cryptic RGD site becomes exposed after pepsin digestion and is recognized by αvβ3.[207-209] The major binding site for the α1β1 integrin is present in the cross structure of laminin formed by the short arms with a fundamental contribution of the N-terminus (domain VI) of the α1 chain (fragment E1XNd).[89,202,210-212] The binding site of α2β1 also has been determined and found to correspond to that of the α1β1.[209] Notable is the negligible binding by both α1β1 and α2β1 integrins to Lam 2 (subunit composition α2β1γ1) and Lam 4 (subunit composition α2β2γ1). Since these latter laminins are recognized by α6β1 and more weakly by α3β1,[213,214] these results demonstrate that distinct integrins can bind specifically to different laminin isoforms and this may be important for selective integrin- and substrate-dependent

signals. Others have identified a peptide sequence within the β1 chain of Lam 1 that inhibits α2β1 integrin-mediated HUVEC endothelial cell attachment to both Lam 1 and type IV collagen[215] while the same peptide is only weakly effective in inhibiting attachment to type I collagen. This peptide, whose sequence is similar to the FYFDLR peptide sequence in CB3(IV) endowed with α1β1- and α2β1-dependent cell attachment activity,[216] is not able to promote cell attachment even after conjugation to BSA. However, the work of Timpl and collaborators with native Lam 1 fragments[209] is not consistent with the supposed function of the laminin β1 chain peptide since only Lam 1 but not Lam 2, both of which contain the β1 laminin chain, supports an α2β1-mediated cell attachment. Using correctly folded recombinant fragments of Lam 1, others have reached the conclusion that the major α1β1 integrin binding site is located in domain VI of the α1 chain of laminin.[210] There is no evidence at the moment to suggest that α1β1 and α2β1 bind to the other laminins identified except in the avian system where α1β1 recognizes Lam 1, 2, 4 and a still uncharacterized new laminin.[211]

INTERACTION OF α1β1 AND α2β1 INTEGRINS WITH COLLAGENS

α1β1 and α2β1 have been shown to interact not only with laminin but also with collagens[216-219] in a conformation-dependent manner. The apparently contrasting observation that platelet α2β1 binds to both native and denatured fibrillar collagen,[220] may be explained by the tendency of triple-helical structures to refold after denaturation.[218,221,222] While a number of studies have employed CNBr fragments of collagens to identify cell binding sites, the use of these fragments might lend itself to potential artifacts since the melting point of these shorter triple helices is reduced compared to that of the whole collagen molecule and under several experimental conditions could lead to denaturation of the fragment. In addition, the ultimate structure of the CNBr fragments in the cell adhesion assays performed has not been always determined. An antibody against the α1β1 integrin completely inhibits HeLA cell adhesion to types I, IV and V collagens[223] and a similar antibody inhibits hepatocyte attachment to α1(I)CB3 and α1(I)CB8,[217] which are two of the fragments generated by CNBr treatment of acid-soluble type I collagen. α2β1-mediated platelet adhesion to type I collagen is inhibited by the CNBr peptide α1(I)CB3, in which the sequence DGEA has been recognized as an essential peptide motif for collagen binding.[224] However, cell adhesion is observed not only to the α1(I)CB3 but also to other CNBr peptides such as α1(I)CB7, CB8, α2(I)CB4, CB3.5 but not to the synthetic DGEA peptide.[222] To complicate this matter even further, it has been shown that at least in the case of the attachment of chondrosarcoma cells to both denatured fibrillar collagen and to its CNBr fragments, binding is mediated by an α5β1-FN bridge and is therefore quite distinct from the α2β1-mediated binding to native fibrillar collagens. [225]

At variance with the inconclusive results obtained with fibrillar collagens the recognition site(s) on native type IV collagen were successfully investigated[75] also because this study was facilitated by the presence of interchain disulfide bonds in the triple helical CB3(IV) CNBr peptide which contains the α1β1 and the α2β1 recognition sites:[218] binding of both α1β1 and α2β1 to type IV collagen is completely inhibited only by CB3(IV). Further proteolysis of CB3(IV) allowed the fine localization of the α1β1 and α2β1 binding sites to two distinct but closely spaced areas. In addition, a C-terminal portion of this peptide is needed to allow a good α2β1-dependent adhesion. This latter sequence, FYFDLR, is located in the more exposed and less protected area of the triple helix in a part of the molecule readily accessible to cells.[226] The essential residues of the recognition site of α1β1 are spatially distributed on different collagen polypeptide chains and occur only once in the entire type IV collagen molecule (Fig. 3.5). Rather interestingly, the two essential residues for α1β1 and α2β1 collagen recognition are R and D, which are two of the three residues representing the major linear RGD motif of the recognition site of several integrins including α5β1, αvβ1, αvβ3, αvβ5, αIIbβ3, αvβ6 and αvβ8. In the case of type IV collagen, the location of these two residues onto different collagen chains results in a spatially different arrangement compared to the arrangement of the linear RGD peptide. Native collagens, despite the frequent presence of linear RGD motifs in their constituent chains, are not recognized by the RGD-dependent integrins because linear RGD motifs are buried within the triple helical arrangement of the polypeptide chains. For instance, type VI collagen, which contains 13 linear RGD motifs buried into the triple helix, is recognized with a high affinity by αvβ3 and αIIbβ3 only after denaturation and unfolding, while in its native conformation it is recognized in an RGD-independent manner by both α1β1 and α2β1 integrins.[227] While a common feature of most integrin ligand active sites is a critical aspartate residue within a short linear peptide, i.e., RGD,[10] LDV,[72] QAGDV,[70] the triple helical structures constrain the conformation of any binding site and it is quite evident that the rigid conformation-dependent recognition site on type IV collagen is structurally different from the flexible RGD recognition site of fibronectin.[228]

Given the above evidence how can we explain that α1β1 and α2β1 also recognize types I, II, III and VI collagens, although they might not necessarily contain the spatial R and D arrangement found in type IV collagen, and that both α1β1 and α2β1 interact with laminin, although the native structure of the collagen triple-helix and of the short arm of the α1 chain of laminin are rather different? One possibility is that these two integrins have a weaker reactivity for conformation-dependent triple helical and non-triple helical native recognition sites compared to the classical integrins recognizing linear peptide sequences. It is obvious that the conformation-dependent nature of the α1β1 and

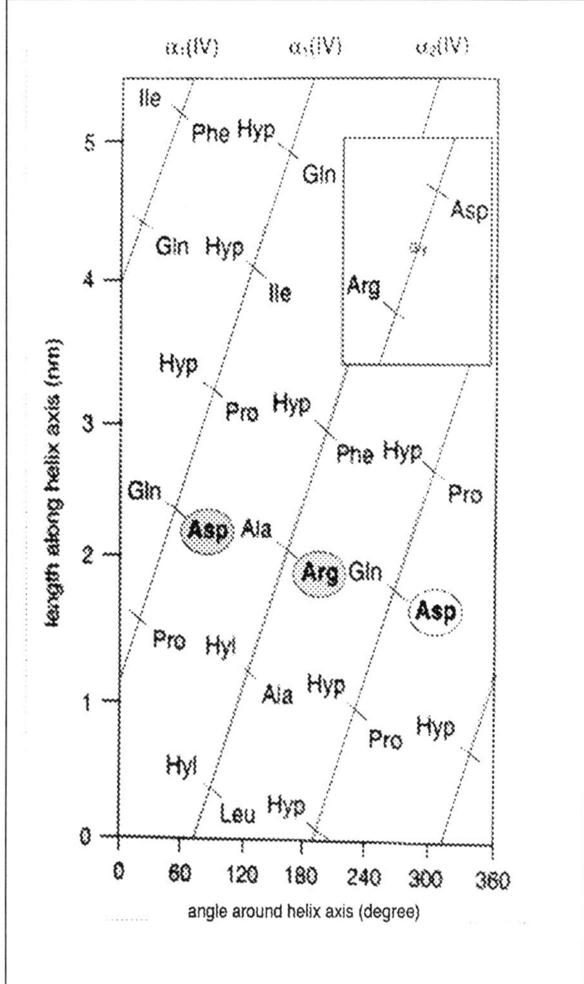

Fig. 3.5. Schematic diagram of the recognition site of α1β1 integrin on the triple helix of type IV collagen. The three α chains are shown in the order α1 (IV), α2 (IV) and α1 (IV) although the actual alignment order in the triple helix is not known. The residues Arg and Asp, fundamental for the recognition of type IV collagen by the α1β1, are arranged along the flat left-handed screw formed by the ridge of the side of Xaa and Yaa residues of the tripeptides Gly-Xaa-Yaa. Arg and Asp of the linear sequence Arg-Gly-Asp would be arranged differently along the steep screw (see inset). (With permission from Kuhn K, Eble J: The structural bases of integrin-ligand interactions. Trends Cell Biol 4: 256-261, 1994. Copyright 1994 Elsevier Science Ltd).

α2β1 interaction makes it difficult to identify the ligand binding sites using, for instance, linear peptides as competitors since they do not provide appropriate native structures. Nevertheless, it was reported that cyclic peptides can be designed that apparently possess the proper "native" conformation: inhibition of cell adhesion to type I collagen and specific elution of α2β1 from a collagen Sepharose affinity matrix was achieved with a cyclic RGD peptide.[229]

The VWFA Modules of β1 Integrin α Subunits Mediate Their Functions

Known collagen-binding proteins such as cartilage matrix protein[230,231] and vWF[232,233] possess VWFA modules that mediate collagen binding. Also the VWFA modules of α1β1 and α2β1 integrins have been hypothesized to be putative collagen-binding domains (Fig. 3.6).[83,84] Notably, all the known α2β1 function-blocking antibodies recognize a small region (residues L173-D259) within the recombinant VWFA module, whereas nonfunctional antibodies bind to other sites.[234] This suggests that the recombinant module is properly folded and maintains an overall native conformation similar to that found in the a subunit of the heterodimeric α2β1 integrin present at the cell membrane. Since function-blocking antibodies map to residues L173-D259, the sequence might represent the putative ligand binding site of α2. This α2 sequence corresponds to the sequence of the peptide fragments of vWF, included in the A1 (E542-L622) and A3 (K948-E988) modules and generated by CNBr treatment, that inhibit vWF binding to fibrillar collagens[232,233] (see chapter 2). In agreement with the above hypothesis the module has been shown to function as the major ligand-recognition sequence of the α2β1 integrin: endothelial cell adhesion and spreading onto collagen and gelatin, but not onto other known endothelial cell ligands such as FN and fibrinogen, is prevented by preincubating the cells with a polyclonal antiserum raised against a GST-fusion protein of the human α2 VWFA module.[235] Intriguingly, attachment to laminin also is prevented suggesting that the same domain of the α2 subunit can confer ligand-binding specificity for distinct ECM ligands of the endothelial α2β1 integrin. One cautionary note in interpreting these latter data relates to the fact that endothelial cells were allowed to adhere to coated microplates for 16 hrs. With this long incubation time cells can and in fact do produce a large amount of their own ECM and this might affect the interpretation of the data on inhibition of cell adhesion.

Further, mutations D151A and D254A, while not affecting the reactivity of func-

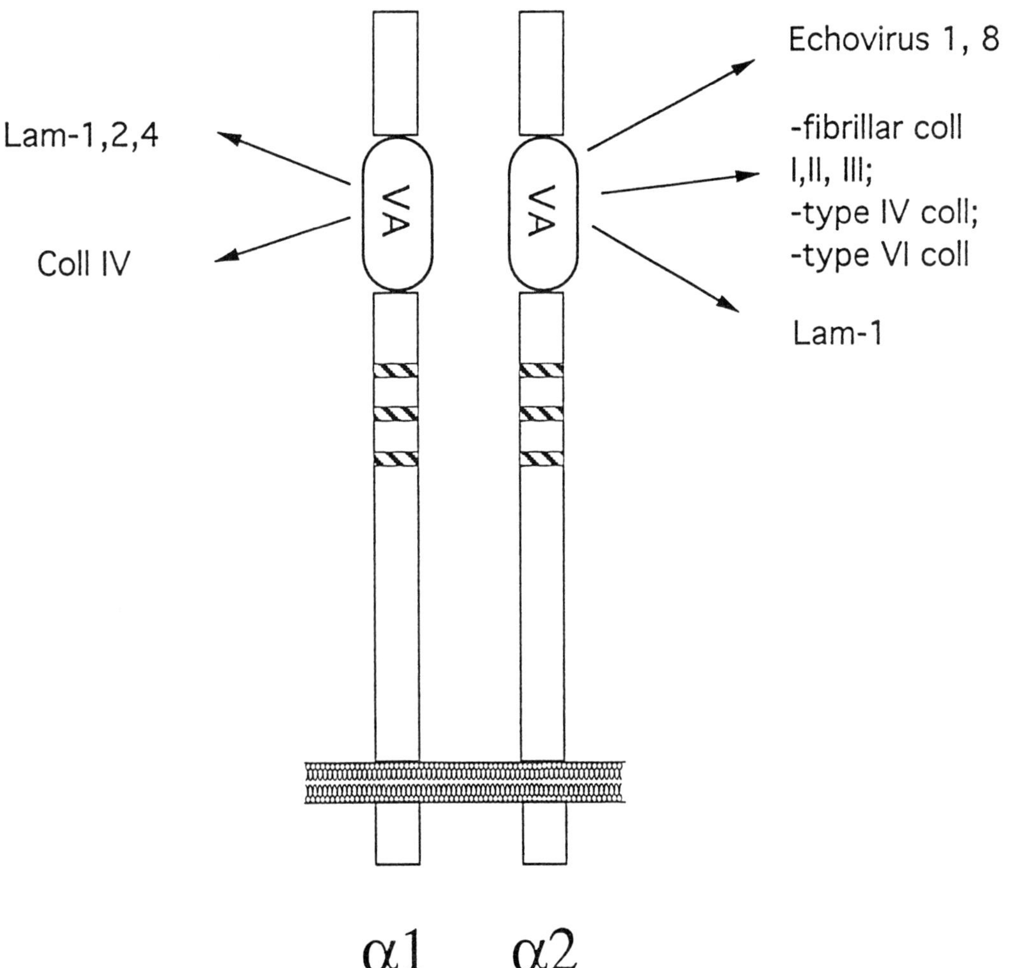

Fig. 3.6. Known ligands of the β1 integrins. Ligands that are recognized through the involvement of the VWFA modules of the β1 integrins are shown.

tion-blocking antibodies, block the attachment of α2-transfected CHO cells to collagen suggesting that these residues are critical for α2β1 binding to collagen.[234] Mutations in the corresponding D140 and D242 residues of the VWFA module of Mac-1 prevent divalent cation binding as well as iC3b ligand binding to Mac-1,[124] suggesting that the equivalent sites in α2β1 also might be involved in divalent cation binding and/or in ligand binding. Mutagenesis studies, performed several years ago in the equivalent residues of the VWFA module of the C2 complement component and that abolished the function of this molecule, concur with the same conclusion.[236] However, the mutations on the α2 VWFA module have no effect (D151A) or only a partial effect (D254A) on collagen binding to the isolated recombinant VWFA module.[237] Binding is inhibited by function-blocking antibodies, suggesting that this mutagenized VWFA module maintains a proper native conformation, and is also divalent cation independent.[237] However, using a nonmutagenized recombinant module other authors did not confirm the cation independent binding to insolubilized collagen.[238] The finding that collagen binding to recombinant α2 VWFA module is not inhibited by up to 5 mM EDTA, while it is well established that platelets[127] and the isolated α2β1 integrin[159] require Mg^{2+} or Mn^{2+} for collagen binding, suggests that cations rather than being directly involved in the actual collagen-VWFA module interaction, maintain an "active" conformation of the α2β1 integrin necessary for the proper α and β chain association or for the formation of a trimolecular complex with the ligand. Thus, residues D151 and D254 apparently are not critical for ligand binding but only as metal ion dependent adhesion sites. Instead, the T221A mutation, and differently from the nearby D219A mutation which is ineffective, fully prevents adhesion of transfected CHO cells to collagen and greatly impairs collagen binding to the recombinant module. Two other mutations, D160A and R242A, also seem critical since

they inhibit binding of function-blocking antibodies. Interestingly, D160 of the α2 subunit corresponds to E146 of the primary sequence of LFA-1, a residue which also is important for binding to ICAM-1.[239] In conclusion, the finding that T221, D160 and R242 are critical for binding to collagen of both α2β1 on CHO cells and of the purified α2 VWFA fusion protein suggests that these residues might be part of the ligand binding interface of the α2β1 integrin VWFA module. D151 and D254, since they coordinate the cation in the MIDAS motif, are important for the function of the α2β1 integrin but not for the isolated VWFA module which appears to be in an "active" conformation by default. How these findings relate to the different conformations determined for the crystal of Mac-1 VWFA module and which depend upon the cation available, remains to be seen.[240]

Analogous to the findings with α2β1, an α1β1 function-blocking antibody also maps to the VWFA module of this latter integrin.[83] While this antibody still binds to a D253A mutant (this mutation corresponding to the D254A mutation of α2β1 and to the D242A mutation of Mac-1), NIH3T3 cells stably transfected with the D253A mutant do not adhere to type IV collagen and the isolated α1β1 mutagenized receptor does not bind to a Sepharose column coupled with the CB3(IV) fragment.[83] Also in the case of the α1β1 integrin, cations are necessary for binding to type IV collagen since cell adhesion is prevented in the presence of EDTA.[83] No data are available yet on the α1β1 isolated VWFA module to show whether removal of the module from its natural environment renders it "active" and fully capable of binding even in the absence of cations as found with α2β1[237] and with Mac-1 in certain cases.[241,242]

INTERACTION OF α2β1 WITH ECHOVIRUS

Binding of Echovirus 1 and 8 serotypes depending on the α2 subunit has been determined by the use of function-blocking antibodies and transfection of α2 cDNA in nonpermissive cells.[243] Furthermore, the mechanisms of α2β1-dependent binding of Echovirus and of collagen or laminin are well distinct in several aspects[244]: (a) in contrast to the findings with ECM molecules that are recognized differentially according to the functional status of the α2 subunit,[177] the virus does not discriminate among α2 forms: it binds equally well to cells transfected with α2 subunits displaying distinct ECM substrate specificities (i.e., cells which adhere to both collagen and laminin, only to collagen, or to neither of the two ligands bind virus to the same extent); (b) neither PMA nor anti–β1 activating antibodies such as TS2/16 stimulate Echovirus binding; (c) in addition, virus binding takes place even in the presence of EDTA and the binding is not influenced by any particular cation; (d) mapping of function-blocking antibodies for virus and ECM proteins indicates that their respective epitopes are only partly overlapping; (e) and finally, chimeric α2 molecules that show altered collagen gel contraction ability and migratory behavior bind virus as the wild type molecules.[244] Similar results are obtained using solubilized α2β1.

That the VWFA module is essential for Echovirus 1 binding was then shown using chimeric α2 constructs. [245] In addition, the virus binds specifically to a fusion protein of the α2β1 VWFA module but not to a similar protein containing the Mac-1 VWFA module,[246] suggesting that all the essential elements for virus binding are contained in the α2β1 module. The binding to this fusion protein is prevented by α2 function-blocking antibodies indicating that the same receptor structures are involved in virus binding to both the isolated VWFA module and to the intact α2β1 receptor expressed at the cell surface. Although mutations D160A and R242A inhibit binding of antibodies that can block cell adhesion to collagen and binding of Echovirus,[237] it seems likely that the α2β1 contact sites for Echovirus are quite distinct from those utilized to recognize

ECM constituents. In fact, at variance with human α2β1, murine α2β1 does not promote binding of Echovirus 1.[85] This species-specific difference is peculiar for Echovirus since both human and murine integrins display a similar capacity to promote cell attachment to type I collagen and Lam-1. A likely explanation is suggested by the comparison of the two sequences: the human and murine sequences are most divergent in the N-terminal two-thirds of the VWFA module and maybe these are important sites for virus binding.

REFERENCES

1. Hynes RO. Integrins: a family of cell surface receptors. Cell 1987; 48:549-554.
2. Ruoslahti E, Pierschbacher MD. New perspectives in cell adhesion: RGD and integrins. Science 1987; 238:491.
3. Hemler ME. VLA proteins in the integrin family: structures, functions, and their role on leukocytes. Annu Rev Immunol 1990; 8:365-400.
4. Hynes RO. Integrins: versatility, modulation, and signaling in cell adhesion. Cell 1992; 69:11-25.
5. Lenter M, Vestweber D. The integrin chains β1 and α6 associate with the chaperone calnexin prior to integrin assembly. J Biol Chem 1994; 269:12263-12268.
6. Busk M, Pytela R, Sheppard D. Characterization of the integrin αVβ6 as a fibronectin-binding protein. J Biol Chem 1992; 267:5790-5796.
7. Smith JW, Cheresh DA. Labelling of integrin αVβ3 with 58Co(III). J Biol Chem 1991; 266:11429-11432.
8. Vogel BE, Tarone G, Giancotti FG et al. A novel fibronectin receptor with an unexpected subunit composition (αVβ1). J Biol Chem 1990; 11:5934-5937.
9. Wayner EA, Garcia-Pardo A, Humphries MJ et al. Identification and characterization of the lymphocyte adhesion receptor for an alternative cell attachment domain in plasma fibronectin. J Cell Biol 1989; 109:1321-1330.
10. Pierschbacher MD, Rouslahti E. Cell attachment activity of fibronectin can be duplicated by small synthetic fragments of the

molecule. Nature 1984; 309:30-33.

11. Carrell NA, Fitzgerald LA, Steiner B et al. Structure of human platelet membrane glycoprotein IIb and IIIa as determined by electron microscopy. J Biol Chem 1985; 260:1743.

12. Nermut MV, Green NM, Eason P et al. Electron microscopy and ultrastructural model of human fibronectin receptor. EMBO J 1988; 7:4093-4099.

13. Weisel JW, Nagaswami C, Vilaire G et al. Examination of the platelet membrane glycoprotein IIB-IIIa comlex and its interaction with fibrinogen and other ligands by electron micoscopy. J Biol Chem 1992; 267:16637-16643.

14. Parise LV, Phillips DR. Platelet membrane glycoprotein IIb/IIIa complex incorporated into phospholipid vescicles. Preparation and morphology. J Biol Chem 1985; 260:1750-1756.

15. Calvete JJ, Mann K, Alvarez MV et al. Proteolytic dissection of the isolated platelet fibrinogen receptor, integrin GPIIb/IIIa. Localization of GPIIb and GPIIIa sequences putatively involved in the subunit interface and in intrasubunit and intrachain contacts. Biochem J 1992; 282:523-532.

16. Calvete JJ, Schaefer W, Mann K et al. Localization of the cross-linking sites of RGD and KQAGDV peptides to the isolated fibrinogen receptor, the human platelet integrin glycoprotein IIb/IIIa-influence of peptide length. Eur J Biochem 1992; 206:759-765.

17. Calvete JJ, Arias J, Alvarez MV et al. Further studies on the topography of the N-terminal region of human platelet glycoprotein IIIa: localization of monoclonal antibody epitopes and the putative fibrinogen-binding sites. Biochem J 1991; 274:457-463.

18. Rocco M, Spotorno B, Hantgan RR. Modeling the αIIbβ3 integrin solution conformation. Prot Sci 1993; 2:2154-2166.

19. Hemler ME, Crouse C, Sonnenberg A. Association of the VLA α6 subunit with a novel protein: a possible alternative to the common VLA β1 subunit on certain cell lines. J Biol Chem 1989; 264:6529-6535.

20. Kajiji S, Tamura RN, Quaranta V. A novel integrin (αEβ4) from human epithelial cells suggests a fourth family of integrin adhesion receptors. EMBO J 1989; 8:673-680.

21. Tuckwell DS, Brass A, Humphries MJ. Homology modelling of integrin EF-hands. Biochem J 1992; 285:325-331.

22. Michishita M, Videm V, Arnaout MA. Anovel divalent cation-binding site in the α domain of the β2 integrin CR3 (CD11b/CD18) is essential for ligand binding. Cell 1993; 72:857-867.

23. Takada Y, Elices MJ, Crouse C et al. The primary structure of α4 subunit of VLA-4: homology to other integrins and possible cell-cell adhesion function. EMBO J 1989; 8:1361-1368.

24. Shaw SK, Cepek KL, Murphy EA et al. Molecular cloning of the human mucosal lymphocyte integrin αE subunit. J Biol Chem 1994; 269:6016-6025.

25. Williams MJ, Hughes PE, Ginsberg MH et al. The inner world of cell adhesion: integrin cytoplasmic domains. Trends Cell Biol 1994; 4:109-112.

26. O'Toole TE, Mandelman D, Forsyth J et al. Modulation of the affinity of integrin αIIbβ3 (GPIIb-IIIa) by the cytoplasmic domain of αIIb. Science 1991; 254:845-847.

27. O'Toole TE, Katagiri Y, Faull RJ et al. Integrin cytoplasmic domains mediate inside-out signal transduction. J Cell Biol 1994; 124:1047-1059.

28. Sastry SK, Horwitz AF. Integrin cytoplasmic domains: mediators of cytoskeletal linkages and extra- and intracellular initiated transmembrane signaling. Curr Opin Cell Biol 1993; 5:819-831.

29. Hemler ME, Weitzman JB, Pasqualini R et al. Structure, biochemical properties, and biological functions of integrin cytoplasmic domains. In: Takada Y, ed. Integrin: The Biological Problem. Ann Arbor, MI: CRC Press, 1994: 1-35.

30. Lee J-O, Rieu P, Amin Arnaout M et al. Crystal structure of the A domain from the α subunit of integrin CR3 (CD11b/CD18). Cell 1995; 80:631-638.

31. D'Souza SE, Haas TA, Piotrowicz RS et al. Ligand and cation binding are dual functions of a discrete segment of the integrin β3 subunit: cation displacement is involved

in ligand binding. Cell 1994; 79:659-667.

32. Huang XZ, Chen A, Agrez M et al. A point mutation in the integrin beta 6 subunit abolishes both alpha v beta 6 binding to fibronectin and receptor localization to focal contacts. Am J Respir Cell Mol Biol 1995; 13:245-251.

33. Smith JW, Cheresh DA. Integrin (αvβ3)-ligand interaction. J Biol Chem 1990; 265:2168-2172.

34. Kamata T, Puzon W, Takada Y. Identification of putative ligand-binding sites of the integrin α4β1 (VLA-4, CD49d/CD29). Biochem J 1995; 305:945-951.

35. Masumoto A, Hemler ME. Mutation of putative divalent cation sites in the α4 subunit of the integrin VLA-4: distinct effects on adhesion to CS1/fibronectin, VCAM-1, and invasin. J Cell Biol 1993; 123:245-253.

36. Loftus JC, Smith JW, Ginsberg MH. Integrin mediated cell adhesion: the extracellular face. J Biol Chem 1994; 269:25235-25238.

37. Loftus JC, O'Toole TE, Plow EF et al. A β3 integrin mutations abolishes ligand binding and alters divalent cation-dependent conformation. Science 1990: 249:915-918.

38. Altruda F, Cervella P, Tarone G et al. A human integrin β1 with an unique cytoplasmic domain generated by alternative mRNA processing. Gene 1990; 95:261-266.

39. Cooper HM, Tamura RN, Quaranta V. The major laminin receptor of mouse embryonic stem cells is a novel isoform of the α6β1 integrin. J Cell Biol 1991; 115:843-850.

40. Languino LR, Ruoslahti E. An alternative form of the integrin beta 1 subunit with a variant cytoplasmic domain. J Biol Chem 1992; 267:7116-7120.

41. Suzuki S, Naitoh Y. Amino acid sequence of a novel integrin β4 subunit and primary expression of the mRNA in epithelial cells.EMBO J 1990; 9:757-763.

42. Hagervost F, Kuikman I, van Kessel AG et al. Molecular cloning of the human alpha 6 integrin subunit. Alternative splicing of alpha 6 integrin subunit. Alternative splicing of alpha 6 mRNA and chromosomal localization of the alpha 6 and beta 4 genes. Eur J Biochem 1991; 199:425-433.

43. Ziober BL, Vu MP, Waleh N et al. Alternative extracellular and cytoplasmic domains of the integrin α7 subunit are differentially expressed during development. J Biol Chem 1993; 268:26773-26783.

44. Van Kuppevelt TH, Languino LR, Gailit JO et al. An alternative cytoplasmic domain of the integrin beta 3 subunit. Proc Natl Acad Sci USA1989; 86:5415-5418.

45. Meredith J Jr, Takada Y, Fornaro M et al. Inhibition of cell cycle progression by the alternatively spliced integrin β1C. Science 1995; 269:1570-1572.

46. Belkin AM, Zhidkova NI, Balzac F et al. β1D integrin displaces the β1A isoform in striated muscles: localization at junctional structures and signaling potential in nonmuscle cells. J Cell Biol 1996; 132:211-226.

47. Brown NH, King DL, Wilcox M et al. Developmentally regulated alternative splicing of *Drosophila* integrin PS2 α transcript. Cell 1989; 59:185-195.

48. Bray PF, Leung CS, Shuman MA et al. Human platelets and megakaryocytes contain alternately spliced glycoprotein IIb mRNAs. J Biol Chem 1990; 265:9587-9590.

49. Bajt ML, Loftus JC. Mutation of a ligand binding domain of beta 3 integrin. J Biol Chem 1994; 269:20913-20919.

50. Takada Y, Ylanne J, Mandelman D et al. A point mutation of integrin β1 subunit blocks binding of α5β1 to fibronectin and invasin but not recruitment to adhesion plaques. J Cell Biol 1992; 119:913-921.

51. Bajt ML, Goodman T, McGuire SL. β2 (CD18) mutations abolish ligand recognition by I domain integrins LFA-1 (αLβ2, CD11a/CD18) and MAC-1 (αMβ2, CD11b/CD18). J Biol Chem 1995; 270:94-98.

52. Berlin C, Berg EL, Briskin MJ et al. α4β7 integrin mediates lymphocyte binding to the mucosal vascular addressin MAdCAM-1. Cell 1993; 74:185-195.

53. Almeida EAC, Huovila APJ, Sutherland AE et al. Mouse egg integrin α6β1 functions as a sperm receptor. Cell 1995; 81:1095-1104.

54. Isberg RR, Leong JM. Multiple β1 chain integrins are receptor for invasin, a protein that promotes bacterial penetration into mammalian cells. Cell 1990; 60:861-871.

55. Ohta H, Tsurudome M, Matsumura H et al. Molecular and biological characterization of fusion regulatory proteins (FRPs): anti-FRP mAbs induced HIV-mediated cell fusion via an integrin system. EMBO J 1994; 13:2044-2055.

56. Relman D, Tuomanen E, Falkow S et al. Recognition of a bacterial adhesin by an integrin: macrophage CR3 (αMβ2, CD11b/CD18) binds filamentous hemagglutinin of *Bordetella pertussis*. Cell 1990; 61:1375-1382.

57. Nemerow GR, Cheresh DA, Wickham TJ. Adenovirus entry into host cells: a role for αV integrins. Trends Cell Biol 1994; 4:52-55.

58. Roivanen M, Hyypiae T, Piirainen L et al. RGD-dependent entry of coxsackievirus A9 into host cells and its bypass after cleavage of VP1 protein by intestinal proteases. J Virol 1991; 65:4735-4740.

59. Bergelson JM, Shepley MP, Chan BMC et al. Identification of the integrin VLA-2 as a receptor for echovirus. Science 1992; 255:1718-1720.

60. Clark EA, Brugge JS. Integrins and signal transduction pathways: the road taken. Science 1995; 268:233-239.

61. Hynes RO. Fibronectin. New York, Springer Verlag 1990.

62. Doliana R, Bonaldo P, Colombatti A. Multiple forms of chicken α3(VI) collagen chain generated by alternative splicing in type A repeat domains. J Cell Biol 1990; 111:2197-2205.

63. Tucker RP, Spring J, Baumgartner S et al. Novel tenascin variants with a distinctive pattern of expression in the avian embryo. Development. 1994; 120:637-647.

64. Koch M, Bohrmann B, Matthison M et al. Large and small splice variants of collagen XII: differential expression and ligand binding. J Cell Biol 1995; 103:1005-1014.

65. Zachary I, Rozengurt E. Focal adhesion kinase (p125FAK): a point of convergence in the action of neuropeptides, integrins, and oncogenes. Cell 1992; 71:891-894.

66. Wang N, Ingber DE. Control of cytoskeletal mechanics by extracellular matrix, cell shape, and mechanical tension. Biophys J 1994; 66:2181-2189.

67. Roskelley CD, Desprez PY, Bissell MJ. Extracellular matrix-dependent tissue-specific gene expression in mammary epithelial cells requires both physical and biochemical signal transduction. Proc Natl Acad Sci USA 1994; 91:12378-12382.

68. Boudreau N, Myers C, Bissell MJ. From laminin to laminin: regulation of tissue-specific gene expression by the ECM. Trends Cell Biol 1995; 5:1-4.

69. Schwartz MA, Ingber DE. Integrating with integrins. Mol Biol Cell 1994; 5:389-393.

70. Kloczewiak M, Timmons S, Lukas TJ et al. Platelet receptor recognition site on human fibrinogen. Synthesis and structure-function relationship of peptides corresponding to the carboxy-terminal segment of the γ chain. Biochemistry 1984; 23:1767-1774.

71. Farrell DH, Thiagarajan P, Chung DW et al. Role of fibrinogen alpha and gamma chain sites in platelet aggregation. Proc Natl Acad Sci USA 1992; 89:10729-10732.

72. Humphries MJ, Komoriya A, Akiyama S.K et al. Identification of two distinct regions of the type III connecting segment of human plasma fibronectin that promote cell type specific adhesion. J Biol Chem 1987; 262:6886-6892.

73. Sanchez-Aparicio P, Dominguez-Jiménez C, Garcia-Pardo A. Activation of the $\alpha_4\beta_1$ integrin through the β1 subunit induces recognition of the RGDS sequence in fibronectin. J Cell Biol 1994; 126:271-279.

74. Jones EY, Harlos K, Bottomley MJ et al. Crystal structure of an integrin-binding fragment of vascular cell adhesion molecule-1 at 1.8A resolution. Nature 1995; 373:539-544.

75. Küehn K, Eble J. The structural basis of integrin-ligand interactions. Trends Cell Biol 1994; 4:256-261.

76. Mercurio AM. Laminin receptors: achieving specificity through cooperation. Trends Biochem Sci 1995; 5:419-423.

77. Bergelson JM, Hemler ME. Do integrins use a 'MIDAS touch' to grasp an Asp? Curr Biol 1995; 5:615-617.

78. Edwards JG, Hameed H, Campbell G. Induction of fibroblast spreading by Mn2+: a possible role for unusual binding sites for divalent cations in receptors for proteins containing Arg-Gly-Asp. J Cell Sci 1988; 89: 507-513.

79. Miyamoto S, Akiyama SK, Yamada KM. Synergistic roles for receptor occupancy and aggregation in integrin transmembrane function. Science 1995; 267:883-885.

80. Zutter MM, Fong AM, Krigman HR et al. Differential regulation of the α2β1 and αIIbβ3 integrin genes during megakaryocytic differentiation of pluripotential K562 cells. J Biol Chem 1992; 28: 20233-20238.

81. Ignatius MJ, Large TH, Houde H et al. Molecular cloning of the rat integrin α1-subunit: a receptor for laminin and collagen. J Cell Biol 1990; 111:709-720.

82. Briesewitz R, Epstein MR, Marcantonio EE. Expression of native and truncated forms of the human integrin α1 subunit. J Biol Chem 1993; 268:2989-2996.

83. Kern A, Briesewitz R, Bank I et al. The role of the I domain in ligand binding of the human integrin α1β1. J Biol Chem 1994; 269:22811-22816.

84. Takada Y, Hemler M. The primary structure of the VLA-2/collagen receptor α2 subunit (platelet GPIa): homology to other integrins and the presence of a possible collagen binding domain. J Cell Biol 1989; 109:397-407.

85. Edelman JM, Chan BMC, Uniyal S et al. The mouse VLA-2 homologue supports collagen and laminin adhesion but not virus binding. Cell Adhes Commun 1994; 2: 131-143.

86. Bahou WF, Potter CL, Mirza H. The VLA-2 (α2β1) I domain functions as a ligand-specific recognition sequence for endothelial cell attachment and spreading: molecular and functional characterization. Blood 1994; 11: 3734-3741.

87. Kamata T, Puzon W, Takada Y. Identification of putative ligand binding sites within I domain of integrin α2β1 (VLA-2, CD49b/CD29). J Biol Chem 1994; 269:9659-9663.

88. Hemler ME, Jacobson JG, Brenner MB et al. VLA-1: a T cell surface antigen which defines a novel late stage of human T cell activation. Eur J Immunol 1985; 15:502-508.

89. Hall DE, Reichardt LF, Crowley E et al. The α1β1 and α6β1 integrin heterodimers mediate cell attachment to distinct sites on laminin. J Cell Biol 1990;110:2175-2184.

90. Ignatius MJ, Reichardt LF. Identification of a neuronal laminin receptor: an Mr 200K/120K integrin heterodimer that binds laminin in a divalent cation-dependent manner. Neuron 1988; 1:713-725.

91. Tawil NJ, Houde M, Blacher R et al. α1β1 integrin heterodimer functions as a dual laminin/collagen receptor in neural cells. Biochemistry 1990; 29:6540-6544.

92. Gullberg D, Turner DC, Borg TK et al. Different β1-integrin collagen receptors on rat hepatocytes and cardiac fibroblasts. Exp Cell Res 1990; 190:254-264.

93. Hemler ME Jacobson JG. Cell matrix adhesion-related proteins VLA-1 and VLA-2: regulation of expression on T cells. J Immunol 1987; 138:2941-2948.

94. Hemler ME, Ware CF, Strominger JL. Characterization of a novel differentiation antigen complex recognized by a monoclonal antibody (A-1A5): unique activation-specific molecular forms on stimulated T cells. J Immunol 1983; 131:334-340.

95. Santoro SA. Identification of a 160,000 dalton platelet membrane protein that mediates the initial divalent cation-dependent adhesion of platelets to collagen. Cell 1986; 46:913-920.

96. Giltay JC, Brinkman HJM, Modderman PW et al. Human vascular endothelial cells express a membrane protein complex immunochemically indistinguishable from the platelet VLA-2 (Glycoprotein Ia-IIa) complex. Blood 1989; 73:1235-1241.

97. O'Connell PJ, Faull R, Russ GR et al. VLA-2 is a collagen receptor on endothelial cells. Immunol Cell Biol 1991; 69:103-110.

98. Albelda SM, Daise M, Levine EM et al. Identification and characterization of cell-substratum adhesion receptors on cultured human endothelial cells. J Clin Invest 1989; 83:1992-202.

99. Hemler ME, Sanchez-Madrid F, Flotte TJ et al. Glycoproteins of 210.000 and 130.000 m.w. on activated T cells: cell distribution and antigenic relations to components on resting cells and T cell lines. J Immunol 1984; 132:3011-3018.

100. Bank I, Book M, Ware R. Functional role of VLA-1 (CD49A) an adhesion, cation-

dependent spreading, and activation of cultured human T lymphocytes. Cell Immunol 1994; 156:424-437.

101. Choy M-Y, Richman PI, Horton MA et al. Expression of the VLA family of integrins in human intestine. J Pathol 1990; 160: 35-40.

102. Saltini C, Hemler ME, Crystal RG. T lymphocytes compartmentalized on the epithelial surface of the lower respiratory tract express the very late activation antigen complex VLA-1. Clin Immunol Immunopathol 1988; 46:221-233.

103. Picker LJ, Treer JR, Nguyen M et al. Coordinate expression of β1 and β2 integrin activation epitopes during T cell responses in secondary lymphoid tissue. Eur J Immunol 1993; 23:2751-2757.

104. Andersson EC, Christensens JP, Marker O et al. Changes in cell adhesion molecule expression on T cells associated with systemic virus infection. J Immunol 1994; 152:1237-1245.

105. Alcocer-Varela J, Aleman-Hoey D, Alarcon-Segovia D. Interleukin-1 and interleukin-6 activities are increased in the cerebrospinal fluid of patients with CNS lupus erythematosus and correlate with local late T-cell activation markers. Lupus 1992; 1:111-117.

106. Hemler ME, Glass D, Coblyn JS et al. Very late activation antigens on rheumatoid synovial fluid T lymphocytes - Association with stages of T cell activation. J Clin Invest 1986; 78:696-702.

107. Miyake S, Sakurai T, Okumura K et al. Identification of collagen and laminin receptor integrins on murine T lymphocytes. Eur J Immunol 1994; 24:2000-2005.

108. Bank I, Roth D, Book M et al. Expression and functions of very late antigen 1 in inflammatory joint diseases. J Clin Immunol 1991; 11:29-38.

109. Shimizu Y, Shaw S. Lymphocyte interactions with extracellular matrix. FASEB J 1991; 5:2292-2299.

110. Pacifici R, Basilico C, Roman J et al. Collagen-induced release interleukin-1 from human blood mononuclear cells. Potentiation by fibronectin binding to the α5β1 integrin. J Clin Invest 1992;

89:61-67.

111. Pacifici R, Roman J, Kimble R et al. Ligand binding to monocyte α5β1 integrin activates the α2β1 receptor via the α5 subunit cytoplasmic domain and protein kinase C. J Immunol 1994; 153:2222-2233.

112. Soligo D, Schiro R, Luksch R et al. Expression of integrins in human bone marrow. Br J Haematol 1990; 76:323-332.

113. van den Berg TK, van der Ende M, Dropp EA et al. Localization of β1 integrins and their extracellular ligands in human lymphoid tissues. Am J Pathol 1993; 143: 1098-1110.

114. Syfrig J, Mann K, Paulsson M. An abundant chick gizzard integrin is the avian α1β1 integrin heterodimer and functions as a divalent cation-dependent collagen IV receptor. Exp Cell Res1991; 194: 165-173.

115. Kelly T, Molony L, Burridge K. Purification of two smooth muscle glycoproteins related to integrin. J Biol Chem 1987; 262: 17189-17198.

116. Belkin VM, Belkin AM, Kotelianski VE. Human smooth muscle VLA-1 integrin: purification, substrate specificity, localization in aorta, and expression during development. J Cell Biol 1990; 111:2159-2170.

117. Lallier T, Bronner-Fraser M. α1β1 integrin on neural crest cells recognizes some laminin substrata in a Ca2+-independent manner. J Cell Biol 1992; 119:1335-1345.

118. Tawil N, Wilson P, Carbonetto S. Integrins in point contacts mediate cell spreading: factors that regulate integrin accumulation in point contacts vs. focal contacts. J Cell Biol 1993; 120:261-271.

119. Grenz H, Carbonetto S, Goodman SL. a3b1 integrin is moved into focal contacts in kidney mesangial cells. J Cell Science 1993; 105:739-751.

120. Cosio FG, Sedmak DD, Nahman NSJ. Cellular receptors for matrix proteins in normal human kidney and human mesangial cells. Kidney Int 1990; 38:886-895.

121. Simon EE and McDonald JA. Extracellular matrix receptors in the kidney cortex. Am J Physiol 1990; 259:F783-F792.

122. Salter DM, Hughes DE, Simpson R et al.

Integrin espression by human articular chondrocytes. Br J Rheum 1992; 31: 231-234.

123. Salter DM, Godolphin JL, Gourlay MS. Chondrocyte heterogeneity: immuno-histologically defined variation of integrin expression at different sites in human fetal knees. J Histochem Cytochem 1995; 43:447-457.

124. Michishita M, Videm V, Arnaout MA. A novel divalent cation-binding site in the a domain of the β2 integrin CR3 (CD11b/CD18) is essential for ligand binding. Cell 1993; 72:857-867.

125. Lallier T, Deutzmann R, Perris R, et al. Neural crest cell interactions with laminin: structural requirements and localization of the α1β1 binding site. Dev Biol 1994; 162: 451-464.

126. Pischel KD, Hemler ME, Huang C et al. Use of the monoclonal antibody 12F1 to characterize the differentiation antigen VLA-2. J Immunol 1987; 138:226-233.

127. Staatz WD, Rajpara SM, Wayner EA et al. The membrane glycoprotein Ia-IIa (VLA-2) complex mediates the Mg++-dependent adhesion of platelets to collagen. J Cell Biol 1989; 108:1917-1924.

128. Kunicki TJ, Nugent D, Staatz S et al. The human fibroblast class II extracellular matrix receptor mediates platelet adhesion to collagen and is identical to the platelet glycoprotein Ia-IIa complex. J Biol Chem 1988; 263:4516-4519.

129. Pischel KD, Bluestein HG, Woods VL Jr. Platelet glycoprotein Ia, Ic and IIa are physycochemically indistinguishable from the very late activation antigens adhesion related proteins of lymphocytes and other cell types. J Clin Invest 1988; 81:505-513.

130. Burger SR, Zutter MM, Sturgill-Koszycki S et al. Induced cell surface expression of functional α2β1 integrin during megakaryocytic differentiation of K562 leukemic cells. Exp Cell Res 1992; 202:28-35.

131. Carter WG, Wayner EA, Bouchard TS et al. The role of α2β1 and α3β1 in cell-cell and cell-substrate adhesion of human epidermal cells. J Cell Biol 1990; 110: 1387-1404.

132. Takada Y, Wayner EA, Carter WG et al. Extracellular matrix receptors ECMR II and ECMR I for collagen and fibronectin correspondence to VLA-2 and VLA-3 in the VLA family of heterodimers. J Cell Biochem 1988; 37:385-393.

133. Wayner EA, Carter WG. Identification of multiple cell adhesion receptors for collagen and fibronectin in human fibrosarcoma cells possessing unique α and β subunits. J Cell Biol 1987; 105:1873-1884.

134. Zutter M, Santoro S. Wide-spread histologic distribution of the α2β1 integrin cell-surface collagen receptor. Am J Pathol 1990; 137:113-120.

135. Gullberg D, Terracio L, Rubin K. Membrane glycoproteins involved in hepatocyte adhesion to collagen type I. Exp Cell Res 1988; 175:388-395.

136. Giltay JC, Brinkman H-JM, Modderman PW et al. Human vascular endothelial cells express a membrane protein complex immunochemically indistinguishable from the platelet VLA-2 (Glycoprotein Ia-IIA) complex. Blood 1989; 73:1235-1241.

137. Lampugnani MG, Resnati M, Dejana E et al. The role of integrins in the maintenance of endothelial monolayer integrity. J Cell Biol 1991; 112:479-490.

138. Leavesley J, Schwartz MA, Rosenfield M, Cheresh DA. Integrin β1-and β3-mediated endothelial cell migration is triggered through distinct signalling mechanisms. J Cell Biol 1993; 121:163-170.

139. Gamble JR, Matthias LJ, Meyer G et al. Regulation of in vitro capillary tube formation by anti-integrin antibodies. J Cell Biol 1993; 121:931-943.

140. Jackson CJ, Knop A, Giles I et al. VLA-2 mediates the interaction of collagen with endothelium during in vitro vascular tube formation. Cell Biol Int 1994; 18:859-867.

141. Defilippi P, van Hinsbergh V, Bertolotto A et al. Differential distribution and modulation of expression of alpha1/beta1 integrin on human endothelial cells. J Cell Biol 1991; 114:855-863.

142. Korhonen M, Ylanne J, Laitinen L et al. The α1-α6 subunits of integrins are characteristically expressed in distinct segments of developing and adult human nephron. J Cell Biol 1990; 111:1245-1254.

143. Gettner SN, Kenyon CJ, Reichardt LF. Characterization of βpat-3 heterodimers, a family of essential integrin receptors in *C. elegans*. J Cell Biol 1995; 129:1127-1141.

144. Rossino P, Defilippi P, Silengo L et al. Up-regulation of the integrin α1β1 in human neuroblastoma cells differentiated by retinoic acid: correlation with increased neurite outgrowth response to laminin. Cell Regul 1991; 2:1021-1033.

145. Fingerman E, Hemler ME. Regulation of proteins in the VLA cell substrate adhesion family: influence of cell growth conditions on VLA-1, VLA-2 and VLA-3 expression. Exp Cell Res 1988; 177:132-142.

146. Santala P, Heino J. Regulation of integrin-type cell adhesion receptors by cytokines. J Biol Chem 1991; 34:23505-23509.

147. Heino J, Ignotz RA, Hemler ME et al. Regulation of cell adhesion receptors by transforming growth factor-β. J Biol Chem 1989; 264:380-388.

148. Kagami S, Border WA, Ruoslahti E et al. Coordinated expression of β1 integrins and transforming growth factor-β-induced matrix proteins in glomerulonephritis. Lab Invest 1993; 69:68-76.

149. Zhang Z, Tarone G, Turner DC. Expression of integrin α1β1 is regulated by nerve growth factor and dexamethasone in PC12 cells. Functional consequences for adhesion and neurite outgrowth. J Biol Chem 1993; 268:5557-5565.

150. Ezoe K, Horikoshi T. Tumor necrosis factor-increased the integrin α2β1 expression and cell attachment to type I collagen in human dermal fibroblast. Biochem Biophys Res Comm 1993; 192:281-287.

151. Heino J, Ignotz RA, Hemler MA et al. Regulation of cell adhesion receptors by transforming growth factor beta. J Biol Chem. 1989; 264:380-388.

152. Heino J, Massagué J. Transforming growth factor-β switches the pattern of integrins expressed in MG-63 human osteosarcoma cells and causes a selective loss of cell adhesion to laminin. J Biol Chem 1989; 264:21806-21811.

153. Turner DC, Flier LA, Carbonetto S. Identification of a cell-surface protein involved in PC12 cell-substratum adhesion and neurite outgrowth on laminin and collagen. J Neurosci 1989; 9:387-3296.

154. Goldman R, Harvey J, Hogg N. VLA-2 is the integrin used as a collagen receptor by leukocytes. Eur J Immunol 1992; 22:1109-1114.

155. Coller BS, Beer JH, Scudder LE et al. Collagen-platelet interactions: evidence for a direct interaction of collagen with platelet GPIa/IIa and an indirect interaction with platelet GPIIb/IIIa mediated by adhesive proteins. Blood 1989; 74:182-192.

156. Kramer RH, Marks N. Identification of integrin collagen receptors on human melanoma cells. J Biol Chem 1989; 264:4684-4688.

157. Eberhard Klein C, Steinmayer T, Kaufmann D et al. Identification of a melanoma progression antigen as integrin VLA-2. J Invest Dermatol 1991; 96:281-284.

158. Wayner EA, Carter WG. Identification of multiple cell adhesion receptors for collagen and fibronectin in human fibrosarcoma cells possessing unique alpha and common beta subunits. J Cell Biol 1987; 105:1873-1884.

159. Kirchhofer D, Languino LR, Ruoslahti E et al. α2β1 integrins from different cell types show different binding specificities. J Biol Chem 1990; 265:615-618.

160. Elices MJ, Hemler ME. The human integrin VLA-2 is a collagen receptor on some cells and a collagen/laminin receptor on others. Proc Natl Acad Sci USA 1989; 86:9906-9910.

161. Hemler ME, Elices MJ, Chan BMC et al. Multiple ligand binding functions for VLA-2 (α2β1) and VLA-3 (α3β1) in the integrin family. Cell Differ Devel 1990; 32:229-238.

162. Toyota B, Carbonetto S, David S. A dual laminin/collagen receptor acts in peripheral nerve regeneration. Proc Natl Acad Sci USA 1990; 87:11319-11322.

163. Languino LR, Gehlsen KR, Wayner E et al. Endothelial cells use α2β1 integrin as a laminin receptor. J Cell Biol 1989; 109:2455-2462.

164. Grzesiak JJ, Davis GE, Kirchhofer D et al. Regulation of α2β1-mediated fibroblast migration on type I collagen by shifts in the concentrations of extracellular Mg2+ and

Ca2+. J Cell Immunol 1992; 5:1109-1117.

165. Grzesiak JJ, Pierschbacher MD. Changes in the concentrations of extracellular Mg++ down-regulate E-cadherin and up-regulate alpha 2 beta 1 integrin function, activating keratinocyte migration on type I collagen. J Invest Dermatol 1995; 104:768-774.

166. Kunicki TJ, Orchelowski R, Annis D et al. Variability of integrin $\alpha2\beta1$ activity on human platelets. Blood 1993; 82:2693-2703.

167. Nieuwenhuis HK, Akkerman J, Houdijk W et al. Human blood platelets showing no response to collagen failed to express surface glycoprotein Ia. Nature 1985; 318:470-472.

168. Nieuwenhuis HK, Sakariassen KS, Houdijk WPM et al. Deficiency of platelet membrane glycoprotein Ia associated with a decreased platelet adhesion to subendothelium. A defect in platelet spreading. Blood 1986; 68:692-695.

169. Deckmyn H, Chew SL, Vermylen J. Lack of platelet response to collagen associated with an autoantibody against glycoprotein Ia: a novel cause of acquired qualitative platelet dysfunction. Thromb Haemost 1990; 63:74-79.

170. Polanowska-Grabowska R, Gear ARL. High-speed platelet adhesion under conditions of rapid flow. Proc Natl Acad Sci USA 1992; 89:5754-5758.

171. Saelman EUM, Horton LF, Barnes MJ. Platelet adhesion to Cyanogen-bromide fragments of collagen $\alpha1(I)$ under flow conditions. Blood 1993; 82:3029-3033.

172. Saelman EUM, Nieuwenhuis HK, Hese KM et al. Platelet adhesion to collagen types I through VIII under conditions of stasis and flow is mediated by GPIa/IIa ($\alpha2\beta1$-integrin). Blood 1994; 83:1244-1250.

173. Polanowska-Grabowska R, Geanacopoulos M, Gear ARL. Platelet adhesion to collagen via the $\alpha2\beta1$ integrin under arterial flow conditions causes rapid tyrosine phosphorylation of pp125[FAK]. Biochem J 1993; 296:543-547.

174. Kiefel V, Santoso S, Katzmann B et al. The Br[a]/Br[b] alloantigen system on human platelets. Blood 1989; 73:2219-2223.

175. Santoso S, Kiefel V, Mueller-Eckhardt C. Human platelet alloantigens Br[a]/Br[b] are expressed on the very late activation antigen 2 (VLA-2) of T lymphocytes. Hum Immunol 1989; 25:237-245.

176. Santoso S, Kalb R, Walka M et al. The human platelet halloantigens Br[a] and Br[b] are associated with a single amino acid polymorphism on glycoprotein Ia (integrin subunit $\alpha2$). J Clin Invest 1993; 92:2427-2432.

177. Chan BMC, Hemler ME. Multiple functional forms of the integrins VLA-2 can be derived from a single $\alpha2$ cDNA clone: interconversion of forms induced by an anti-$\beta1$ antibody. J Cell Biol 1993; 120:537-543.

178. Grinnell F. Fibroblasts, myofibroblasts, and wound mechanisms of disease. J Cell Biol 1994; 124:401-404.

179. Schiro J, Chan B, Roswit W et al. Integrin $\alpha2\beta1$ (VLA-2) mediates reorganization and contraction of collagen matrices by human cells. Cell 1991; 67:403-410.

180. Chan BMC, Matsuura N, Takada Y et al. *In vitro* and *in vivo* consequences of VLA-2 expression on rhabdomyosarcoma cells. Science 1991; 251:1600-1602.

181. Lee RT, Berdichevsky F, Cheng GC et al. Integrin-mediated collagen matrix reorganization by cultured human vascular smooth muscle cells. Circ Res 1995; 76:209-214.

182. Langholz O, Rockel D, Mauch C et al. Collagen and collagenase gene expression in three-dimensional collagen lattices are differentially regulated by $\alpha1\beta1$ and $\alpha2\beta1$ integrins. J Cell Biol 1995; 131:1903-1915.

183. Riikonen T, Koivisto L, Vihinen P et al. Transforming growth factor-β regulates collagen gel contraction by increasing $\alpha2\beta1$ integrin expression in osteogenic cells. J Biol Chem 1995; 270:376-382.

184. Klein EC, Dressel D, Steinmayer T et al. Integrin $\alpha2\beta1$ is upregulated in fibroblasts and highly aggressive melanoma cells in three-dimensional collagen lattices and mediates the reorganization of collagen I fibrils. J Cell Biol 1991; 115:1427-1436.

185. Riikonen T, Westermarck J, Koivisto L et al. Integrin $\alpha2\beta1$ is a positive regulator of collagenase (MMP-1) and collagen $\alpha1(I)$ gene expression. J Biol Chem 1995; 270:13548-13552.

186. Briesewitz R, Kern A, Marcantonio EE.

Ligand-dependent and -independent integrin focal contact localization: the role of the α chain cytoplasmic domain. Mol Biol Cell 1993; 4:593-604.

187. Chan BMC, Kassner PD, Schiro A et al. Distinct cellular functions mediated by different VLA integrins α subunits cytoplasmic domains. Cell 1992; 68:1051-1060.

188. Kassner PD, Alon R, Springer TA et al. Specialized functional properties of the integrin α4 cytoplasmic domain. Mol Biol Cell 1995; 6:661-674.

189. Kawaguchi S, Bergelson JM, Finberg RW et al. Integrin α2 cytoplasmic domain deletion effects: loss of adhesive activity parallels ligand-independent recruitment into focal adhesions. Mol Biol Cell 1994; 5:977-988.

190. Kawaguchi S, Hemler ME. Role of the α subunit cytoplasmic domain in regulation of adhesive activity mediated by the integrin VLA-2. J Biol Chem 1993; 268: 16279-16285.

191. Prockop DJ, Kivirikko KI. Collagens: molecular biology, diseases, and potentials for therapy. Ann Rev Biochem 1995; 64: 403-434.

192. Timpl R, Rohde H, Gehron Robey P et al. Laminin—a glycoprotein from basement membranes. J Biol Chem 1979; 254: 9933-9937.

193. Burgeson RE, Chiquet M, Deutzmann R et al. A new nomenclature for laminins. Matrix Biol 1994; 5: 209-211.

194. Timpl R, Brown JC. The laminins. Matrix Biol 1994; 14:275-281.

195. Engel J. Structure and function of laminin. In: Rohrbach DH, Timpl R, eds. Molecular and Cellular Aspects of Basement Membranes. San Diego, CA: Academic Press, 1993:147-176.

196. Utani A, Nomizu M, Sugiyama S et al. A specific sequence of the laminin α2 chain critical for the initiation of heterotrimer assembly. J Biol Chem 1995; 270: 3292-3298.

197. Antonsson P, Kammeter RA, Schulthess T et al. Stabilization of the α-helical coiled-coil domain in laminin by C-terminal disulfide bonds. J Mol Biol 1995; 250:74-79.

198. Edgar D, Timpl R, Thoenen H. The heparin binding-domain of laminin is responsible for its effects on neurite outgrowth and neuronal survival. EMBO J 1984; 3: 1463-1468.

199. Goodman SL, Deutzmann R, von der Mark K. Two distinct cell binding domains in laminin can independently promote nonneuronal cell adhesion and spreading. J Cell Biol 1987; 105:589-598.

200. Deutzmann R, Aumailley M, Wiedemann H et al. Cell adhesion, spreading and neurite stimulation by laminin fragment E8 depends on maintenance of secondary and tertiary structure in its rod and globular domain. Eur J Biochem 1990; 191:513-522.

201. Sung U, O'Rear JJ, Yurchenco PD. Cell and heparin binding in the distal long arm of laminin: identification of active and cryptic sites with recombinant and hybrid glycoprotein. J Cell Biol 1993; 123:1255-1268.

202. Tomaselli KJ, Hall DE, Reichardt LT et al. A neuronal cell line (PC12) expresses two β1-class integrins -α1β1 and α3β1- that recognize different neurite outgrowth promoting domains in laminin. Neuron 1990; 5:651-662.

203. Aumailley M, Timpl R, Sonnenberg A. Antibody to integrin alpha-6 subunit specifically inhibits cell-binding to laminin fragment 8. Exp Cell Res 1990; 188:55-60.

204. Sonnenberg A, Linders CJT, Modderman PW et al. Integrin recognition of different cell-binding fragments of laminin (P1,E3,E8) and evidence that α6β1 but not α6β4 functions as a major receptor for fragment E8. J Cell Biol 1990; 110:2145-2155.

205. Kramer RH, Vu MP, Cheng Y-F et al. Laminin binding-integrin α7β1: functional characterization and expression in normal and malignant melanocytes. Cell Regul 1991; 2:805-817.

206. Lotz MM, Korzelius CA, Mercurio AM. Human colon carcinoma cells use multiple receptors to adhere to laminin: involvment of α6β4 and α2β1 integrins. Cell Regul 1990; 1:249-257.

207. Aumailley M, Gerl M, Sonnenberg A et al. Identification of the Arg-Gly-Asp sequence in laminin A chain as a latent cell-binding site being exposed in fragment P1. FEBS Lett 1990; 262:82-86.

208. Sonnenberg A, Gehlsen KR, Aumailley M et al. Isolation of α6β1 integrins from platelets and adherent cells by affinity chromatography on mouse laminin fragment E8 and human laminin pepsin fragment. Exp Cell Res 1991; 197:234-244.

209. Pfaff M, Goehring W, Brown JC et al. Binding of purified collagen receptors (α1β1, α2β1) and RGD-dependent integrins to laminins and laminin fragments. Eur J Biochem 1994; 225:975-984.

210. Colognato-Pyke H, O'Rear JJ, Yamada Y et al. Mapping of network-forming, heparin-binding, and α1β1 integrin-recognition sites within the α-chain short arm of laminin-1. J Biol Chem 1995; 270: 9398-9406.

211. Perris R, Brandenberger R, Chiquet M. Differential neural crest cell attachment and migration on avian laminin isoforms. Int J Dev Biol 1996; in press.

212. Goodman SL, Aumailley M, von der Mark H. Multiple cell surface receptors for the short arms of laminin: α1β1 integrin and RGD-dependent proteins mediate cell attachment only to domains III in murine tumor laminin. J Cell Biol 1991; 113:931-941.

213. Delwel GO, Hogervorst F, Kuikman I et al. Expression and function of the cytoplasmic variants of the integrin α6 subunit in transfected K562 cells: activation-dependent adhesion and interaction with isoform of laminin. J Biol Chem 1993; 268:25865-25875.

214. Delwel GO, de Melker AA, Hogervorst F et al. Distinct and overlapping ligand specificities of the α3Aβ1 and α6Aβ1 integrins: recognition of laminin isoforms. Mol Biol Cell 1994; 5:203-215.

215. Underwood PA, Bennet FA, Kirkpatrick A et al. Evidence for the location of a binding sequence for the α2β1 integrin of endothelial cells, in the β1 subunit of laminin. Biochem J 1995; 309:765-771.

216. Vanderberg P, Kern A, Ries A et al. Characterization of a type IV collagen major cell binding site with affinity to the α1β1 and the α2β1 integrins. J Cell Biol 1991; 113:1475-1483.

217. Gullberg D, Gehlsen KR, Turner DC et al. Analysis of α1β1, α2β1 and α3β1 integrins in cell-collagen interactions: identification of conformation dependent α1β1 binding sites in collagen type I. EMBO J 1992; 11:3865-3873.

218. Kern A, Eble J, Goblik R et al. Interaction of type IV collagen with the isolated integrins α1β1 and α2β1. Eur J Biochem 1993; 215:151-159.

219. Aumailley M, Timpl R. Attachment of cells to basement membrane collagen type IV. J Cell Biol 1986; 103:1569-1575.

220. Morton LF, Peachey AR, Barnes MJ. Platelet-reactive sites in collagens type I and type III. Evidence for separate adhesion and aggregatory sites. Biochem J 1989; 258:157-163.

221. Staatz DS, Walsh JJ, Pexton T et al. The α2β1 integrin cell surface collagen receptor binds to the α1(I)-CB3 peptide of collagen. J Biol Chem 1990; 265:4778-4781.

222. Morton LF, Peachey AR, Zijenah LS et al. Conformation-dependent platelet adhesion to collagen involving integrin α2β1-mediated and other mechanisms: multiple α2β1-recognition sites in collagen type I. Biochem J 1994; 299:791-797.

223. Rikonen T, Vihinen P, Potila M et al. Antibody against human alpha 1 beta 1 integrin inhibits HeLa cell adhesion to laminin and to type I, IV and V collagens. Biochem Biophys Res Commun 1995; 209:205-212.

224. Staatz WD, Fok K, Zutter MM et al. Identification of tetrapeptide recognition sequence for the α2β1 integrin in collagen. J Biol Chem 1991; 266:7363-7367.

225. Tuckwell DS, Ayad S, Grant ME et al. Conformation dependence of integrin-type II collagen binding. Inability of collagen peptides to support α2β1 binding, and mediation of adhesion to denatured collagen by a novel α5β1-fibronectin bridge. J Cell Sci 1994; 107:993-1005.

226. Eble JA, Golbik R, Mann K et al. The α1β1 integrin recognition site of the basement membrane collagen molecule (α1(IV)2α2(IV). EMBO J 1993; 12:4795-4802.

227. Pfaff M, Aumailley M, Specks U et al. Integrin and Arg-Gly-Asp dependence of the native and unfolded triple helix of collagen Type VI. Exp Cell Res 1993; 206:167-176.

228. Main AL, Harvey TS, Baron M et al. The three-dimensional structure of the tenth type-III module of fibronectin: an insight into RGD-mediated interactions. Cell 1992; 71:671-678.

229. Cardarelli PM, Yamagata S, Taguchi I et al. The collagen receptors α2β1 from MG-63 and HT1080 cells, interacts with a cyclic RGD peptide. J Biol Chem 1992; 267: 23159-23164.

230. Winterbottom N, Tondravi MM, Harrington TL et al. Cartilage matrix protein is a component of the collagen fibril of cartilage. Dev Dyn 1992; 193:266-276.

231. Tondravi MM, Winterbottom N, Haudenschild DR et al. Cartilage matrix protein binds to collagen and plays a role in collagen fibrillogenesis. In: Fallon JF, Goetinck PF, Kelly RO Stocum DL, eds. Limb Development and Regeneration. New York, NY, Wiley-Liss, 1993: 515-522.

232. Roth GL, Titani K, Hoyer LW et al. Localization of binding sites within human von Willebrand factor for monomeric type III collagen. Biochemistry 1986; 25:8357-8361.

233. Pareti FI, Niiya K, McPherson JM et al. Isolation and characterization of two domains of human von Willebrand factor that interact with fibrillar collagen types I and III. J Biol Chem 1987; 262:13835-13841.

234. Kamata T, Puzon W, Takada Y. Identification of putative ligand binding sites within I domain of integrin α2β1 (VLA-2, CD49b/CD29). J Biol Chem 1994; 269:9659-9663.

235. Bahou WF, Potter CL, Mirza H. The VLA-2 (α2β1) I domain functions as a ligand-specific recognition sequence for endothelial cell attachment and spreading: molecular and functional characterization. Blood 1994; 11:3734-3741.

236. Horiuchi T, Macon KJ, Engler JA et al. Site-directed mutagenesis of the region around Cys-241 of complement component C2: evidence for a C4b binding site. J Immunol 1991; 147:584-589.

237. Kamata T, Takada Y. Direct binding of collagen to the I domain of integrin α2β1 (VLA-2, CD49b/CD29). J Biol Chem 1994; 269:26006-26010.

238. Tuckwell D, Calderwood D, Green L et al. Integrin α2 I-domain is a binding site for collagens. J Cell Sci 1995; 108:1629-1637

239. Huang C, Springer TA. A binding interface on the I domain of lymphocyte function-associated antigen-1 (LFA-1) required for specific interaction with intercellular adhesion molecule 1 (ICAM-1). J Biol Chem 1995; 270:19008-19016.

240. Lee J-O, Bankston LA, Arnaout MA et al. Two conformations of the integrin A-domain (I-domain): a pathway for activation? Structure 1995; 3:1333-1340.

241. Rieu P, Ueda T, Haruta I et al. The A-domain of β2 integrin CR3 (CD11b/CD18) is a receptor for the hookworm-derived neutrophil adhesion inhibitor NIF. J Cell Biol 1994; 127:2081-2091.

242. Moyle M, Foster DL, McGrath DE et al. A hookworm glycoprotein that inhibits neutrophil functions is a ligand of the integrin CD11b/CD18. J Biol Chem 1994; 269:10008-10015.

243. Bergelson JM, St John N, Kawaguchi S et al. Infection by Echovirus 1 and 8 depends on the α2 subunit of human VLA-2. J Virol 1993; 67:6847-6852.

244. Bergelson JM, Chan BMC, Finberg RW et al. The integrin VLA-2 binds Echovirus 1 and extracellular matrix ligands by different mechanisms. J Clin Invest 1993; 92:232-239.

245. Bergelson JM, St. John N, Kawaguchi S et al. The I domain is essential for Echovirus 1 interaction with VLA-2. Cell Adhes Commun 1994; 2:455-464.

246. King SL, Cunnigham JA, Finberg RW et al. Echovirus 1 interaction with the isolated VLA-2 I domain. J Virol 1995; 69: 3237-3239.

247. Bork P, Bairoch A. Extracellular protein modules. Trends Biochem Sci 1995; 3.

β2 Integrins

The β2 integrin subfamily is composed of four distinct heterodimers expressed exclusively on leukocytes that mediate static and dynamic adhesive functions in a large variety of homotypic and heterotypic cellular events. They include interaction of immature thymocytes with thymic epithelium, firm adhesion to and transmigration through endothelium during the process of leukocytes recirculation, and chemotaxis and phagocytosis of granulocytes and monocytes.[1] Both historical and practical aspects still determine the multiple denominations of the β2 integrins, but we will refer to the most common LFA-1, Mac-1 and p150,95, throughout this chapter. LFA-1 (αLβ2) is an acronym for lymphocyte function associated antigen-1; Mac-1 (αMβ2) is an abbreviated name for macrophage antigen-1 and it embodies the complement receptor type-3 (CR-3); p150,95 (αXβ2) is the complement receptor type-4 (CR-4); the α subunits of LFA-1, Mac-1 and p150,95 also are designated CD11a, CD11b and CD11c. The common β2 subunit is designated CD18 in accord with the Human Leukocyte Differentiation Antigen Workshops. The recently identified fourth member of the β2 integrin subfamily, is designated αDβ2. In vitro assays; monoclonal antibodies that inhibit β2 integrin-mediated processes; natural genetic diseases affecting the β2 subunit, such as those of patients suffering from the leukocyte adhesion deficiency (LAD-1); and finally, recombinant subunits and their fragments, have all contributed to the understanding of the properties of the β2 integrins.

MOLECULAR STRUCTURE

All four β2 integrins consist of a common β2 subunit which migrates in SDS-PAGE with an apparent molecular mass of about 95 kD, and of α subunits with apparent molecular masses of 150 kD (p150,95),[2] 155 kD (αDβ2),[3] 170 kD (Mac-1)[4] and 180 kD (LFA-1).[2]

The human β2 gene contains 16 exons and spans a region of approximately 40 kb.[5] The human gene is localized to chromosome 21p22 close to the common breakpoint of chromosomal translocations in chronic myeloid leukemia.[6] Five exons (from exon 5 through exon 9) encode the conserved region of about 200 amino acid residues containing a MIDAS like cation-binding motif.[7] The identity with other β subunits approaches 60% to 89% in some subsegments of this region.

The Superfamily with von Willebrand Factor VA Domains, edited by
Alfonso Colombatti and Roberto Doliana. © 1996 R.G. Landes Company.

The entire human Mac-1[8] and p150,95[9] α subunit genes have been characterized and a partial description of the human LFA-1 α subunit gene also has been reported.[10] Both the Mac-1 and p150,95 a subunit genes contain 31 exons arranged in seven clusters and spanning a region of about 55 and 25 kb, respectively.[8,9] Structural comparison of the genomic organization of Mac-1 and p150,95 α subunit genes indicates that they are highly homologous and suggests that these two genes arose by a recent duplication event. Both the number of exons and the phases of intron/exon junctions are identical. Each of the seven EF hand-like repeats is located in a separate exon[8,9] and the VWFA module is coded for by four exons. The genes encoding the α chains of LFA-1, Mac-1, and p150,95 are clustered between bands p11-p13.1 on chromosome 16.[6]

The amino acid sequence deduced from the cDNA of the β2 subunit consists of a 701 residues long extracellular domain, a 23 amino acids transmembrane sequence, and a 45 amino acid long cytoplasmic tail.[11,12] The 200 residue long N-terminal part of the β2 subunit is highly conserved among different β subunits[13,14] as well as is involved in α/β subunits association and/or ligand binding. The ligand-binding motifs of the β3 and of other β subunits[14] and several artificially induced[15] and naturally occurring[16] mutations of the β2 subunit, that impair heterodimer formation and cell surface expression, occur in this same region. In analogy with all integrin β subunits, in the C-terminal part of the extracellular domain there are four consecutive repeats of 40 amino acid residues containing eight cysteines each. The murine[17] and the chicken[18] β2 subunits are highly homologous to the human molecule with an 81% and a 65% identity, respectively.

The α subunits of the β2 integrins are highly homologous: Mac-1 and p150,95 are more related at the deduced amino acid level to each other (63% identity) than to LFA-1 (36% identity). This structural similarity is paralleled at the functional level, inasmuch as both Mac-1 and p150,95

can bind iC3b[19,20] and both are active in granulocyte and monocyte homotypic/heterotypic adhesion phenomena. The α subunits consist of an extracellular domain ranging from 1,063 for LFA-1 to 1,077 for Mac-1, a 29 residue similar transmembrane sequence, and a cytoplasmic tail ranging from 53 residues for LFA-1 to 57 residues for p150,95.[21-24] The extracellular domains contain a VWFA module of 194 amino acid residues, and seven 50-60 residues repeats the last three of which, domains V-VII, are related to the EF hand motif present in calcium binding proteins[25,26] (Fig. 4.1). These repeats also are conserved in the α subunits of other integrin subfamilies. The leukocyte integrins require divalent cations for ligand binding and these ions, by stabilizing the subunits, have been conveniently used for the affinity purification of functional heterodimers.[10] All α subunits of the β2 subfamily present the conserved GFFKR sequence at the junction between the transmembrane and cytoplasmic domains. While not strictly required to mediate integrin/cytoskeleton interactions this sequence seems particularly important for the regulation of integrin affinity.[27]

TISSUE EXPRESSION

Mac-1 was the first member to be identified among the β2 integrins as a marker of myeloid cells in the mouse[4] and later in the human.[19,28] LFA-1 was discovered using a different approach, i.e., screening for antibodies able to inhibit T cytotoxic cell mediated killing of tumor cell targets.[29-31] The third member of this subfamily, p150,95, was identified in human cells by immunoprecipitation with β2 subunit antibodies.[2,32,33] Very recently, αDβ2 was recognized as a unique and distinct entity expressed in selected tissue macrophages[3,34] and constitutively active for ICAM-3.[3] β2 integrins are restricted to cells of the immune system and their expression is controlled both by rapid cell surface transport of preformed receptors and by de novo biosynthesis. Mobilization of integrins stored in intracellular pools re-

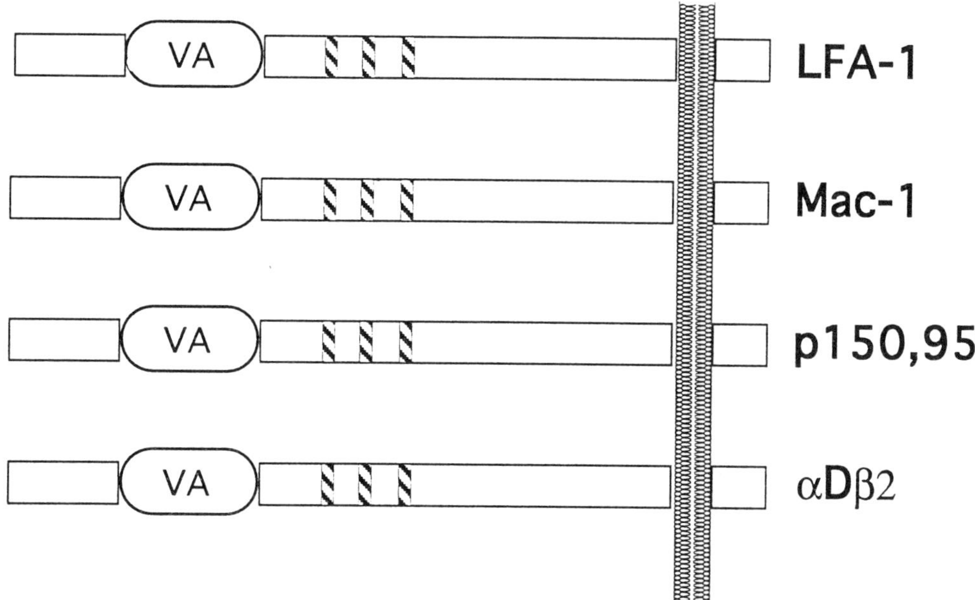

Fig 4.1. Schematic diagram of the structural features of the α chains of β2 integrins. The new designation (proposed by Bork and Bairoch)[271] of the VWFA/I modules (VA) is followed. The stripped boxes correspond to the EF hand-like cation binding sites.

sults in a dramatic up-regulated expression in a matter of minutes. This rapid mobilization subserves a fundamental function in responding to changes in the local environment and these changes also contribute greatly to the accumulation of monocytes and neutrophils at sites of acute inflammation. Most Mac-1 and p150,95 molecules are in fact stored in neutrophil and monocyte granules and secretory vescicles.[35-38] In contrast to the fast up-regulation from intracellular storage pools, de novo synthesis is relatively slow and depends on the presence of physiological differentiation stimuli.

LFA-1 is expressed on all leukocytes and also on early progenitors of burst and erythroid colony-forming units (CFUs), granulocyte/macrophage (GM)-CFUs, and monocyte (M)-CFUs.[39] During B cell development, the levels of LFA-1 increase coincidentally with the maturation of the cells in the bone marrow.[40,41] Mac-1 is detected primarily on terminally differentiated myeloid cells including monocytes, granulocytes, macrophages and large granular lymphocytes[42,43] and also can be found on small subsets of CD8[+44] and CD4[+] T cells[45] and on a few CD5[+] B cells.[46] Macrophages, monocytes, granulocytes, activated B cells, and some T cell subpopulations express p150,95.[47-49] Both Mac-1 and p150,95 are absent from erythroid and GM-CFU and are instead first detected on committed precursors at the myelocytic and monoblastic stages, respectively.[39] Further differentiation of monocytes upon extravasation and maturation into resident macrophages is followed by a drop in cell surface levels of LFA-1.[50] In contrast, the relative abundance of Mac-1 and p150,95 is reversed: while monocytes express more Mac-1 than p150,95, in macrophages p150,95 is by far the most representative β2 integrin.[51] Mac-1 is rarely present in the large majority of B cells and p150,95 is transiently expressed at higher levels following activation of mature B cells.[49] αDβ2 was initially identified on the basis of its restricted topographic distribution pattern: its absence from monocytes and granulocytes in peripheral blood and its predominant expression on macrophages in specialized tissue compartments such as spleen red pulp, on certain peripheral blood CD8[+] T cells and on spleen CD4[-]CD8[-] lymphocytes presumably expressing the T cell receptor (TCR) γδ.[3]

At the level of resolution of a low-voltage field emission scanning electron microscopy (EM), it appears that in unactivated neutrophils and in contrast to L-selectin, which is clustered at the tip of microvilli and membrane ruffles, Mac-1 is localized primarily at the cell body.[52] When cells are activated, Mac-1 expression is up-regulated and it also can be found at the microvilli level organized in microclusters.

BIOSYNTHESIS

The β2 subunit precursor is synthesized in larger excess compared to the α subunit precursors. α and β subunits then associate noncovalently in a 1:1 stoichiometric ratio in the endoplasmic reticulum, a stage followed by carbohydrate processing in the Golgi apparatus.[53,54] Finally, the mature heterodimer is either transported to the cell surface or stored (except LFA-1) in intracellular granules. The association of the subunit precursors is necessary for further processing and transport. If association does not take place, as in LAD patients,[16] the heterodimer is absent from the cell surface. In addition to the different number of potential glycosylation sites among the α and β subunits, there is great variation in the level of glycosylation and of sialylation in different cell types.[55-57] At present, the functional significance of this variation is unknown, but some of the potential glycosylation/sialylation sites are localized to ligand binding regions in both α and β subunits and may be implicated in the regulation of the receptor-ligand interaction.

Expression of the genes encoding CD11/CD18 is tightly regulated during differentiation of leukocyte subpopulations.[58] Studies on the cell lines HL60 and U973, which can be induced to differentiate by retinoic acid and phorbol esters[59,60] have suggested that the coordinate expression of the CD11/CD18 genes might depend on common genetic elements. Both transcriptional[61,62] and post-transcriptional[59] mechanisms have been proposed as responsible for regulating mRNA levels of the α and β subunit genes during late myeloid differentiation. In addition, several analogies in these genes are found: lack of TATA and CAAT boxes, multiple transcription start sites and the presence of common putative regulatory sequences in the promoter regions.[63-69] Reporter gene constructs have been used to characterize the baseline expression and the phorbol ester inducibility of the LFA-1 and Mac-1 promoters. Using this approach it was found that the different extracellular signals available during differentiation induce responses of equivalent intensity suggesting that similar transcription factors may act to coordinately regulate the expression of the α and β subunits.[70,71] In particular, the binding of nuclear factor PU.1 to both αM and β2 genes has shown that PU.1 is critical for the activity of both genes. PU.1, the product of the protooncogene Sp-1, a member of the Ets family of transcription factors and a "master switch" gene in hematopoietic differentiation, regulates not only Mac-1 α and β2 genes but also the tissue specific expression of other myeloid genes such as the macrophage colony-stimulating factor[70] On the other hand, lymphocytes which express both PU.1 and β2 but not the Mac-1 α subunit, probably have other factors that may specifically repress Mac-1 expression. Finally, in line with this suggestion are the results obtained in transgenic mice in which a human CD4 reporter gene driven by a Mac-1 α subunit promoter construct was introduced:[72] as expected from the constitutive pattern of Mac-1 expression, the transgene was expressed in granulocytes and peritoneal macrophages. However, expression also was detected in lymphocytes in two founder lines, suggesting that in addition to the proximal PU.1 sites other regulatory sequences, excluded from the 1.5 kb promoter constructs used in those experiments, are necessary for the specific Mac-1 expression.

FUNCTION

The β2 integrins expressed on leukocytes undergo activation phenomena strikingly similar to those shown by β1 and β3 integrins such that leukocyte activation is in general a required prerequisite for ligand binding.[73] Consequently, the ligand affinity of leukocyte integrins is not constitutive, rather, these adhesion receptors fluctuate between low and high avidity states for their ligands and these shifts depend on triggering events mediated by intracellular signals generated from other cell surface receptors and from the extracellular environment. The ability of leukocyte integrin receptors to switch rapidly from a low- to a high-avidity state allows cells to circulate freely and then stick firmly at required sites where local conditions contribute to the up-regulation of integrin activity. The increase in average binding affinity, which can be as high as 200-fold between the resting and the activated cells,[74] is correlated with augmented ligand binding. An alternative model suggests that integrin receptor activation does not result from a reversible increase in affinity between the inactive and the active receptors, since the two types of receptors are isoenergetic, but from lowering the activation energy necessary to shift the receptor from an inactive to an active state.[75]

A discussion on the intracellular mechanisms that direct, regulate, and modulate LFA-1 (but also Mac-1 and p150,95) adhesion is beyond the scope of the present chapter. A number of recent reviews have dealt with both "outside in" and "inside out" mechanisms of activation[73,76-79] and with the role played by the α and β subunit cytoplasmic domains and to those reviews the reader is referred for more detailed informations.

LEUKOCYTE ADHESION

LFA-1, which is expressed on all leukocytes, is required during both the afferent and efferent arms of the immune response. Using function-blocking antibodies it turned out that LFA-1 represents one of the major adhesion receptors during immune responses.[80] For instance, during T cell priming by antigen presenting cells (APCs), LFA-1 provides the necessary adhesive strength with ICAM-1,[81-85] ICAM-2,[86,87] and ICAM-3[87-91] counter-receptors involved. While ICAM-2 and ICAM-3, which are expressed at higher levels on resting T cells, seem the major counterreceptors during early stages of primary antigenic responses,[88,89,92] ICAM-1 is the principal counter-receptor on memory T cells.[93] T cells typically express more than 10^5 LFA-1 molecules per cell, but they do not display any adherence for cells expressing ICAM-1 or for surfaces coated with solubilized ICAM-1. TCR engagement is sufficient to convert a fraction of LFA-1 molecules to high affinity binding[94] and T cell activation is necessary to induce a rapid and transient increase in binding to ICAM-1. This also is achieved by cross-linking of relevant cell surface receptors such as CD2,[94] CD7,[95] CD28,[95] CD43,[96] CD62L[97] or MHC class II molecules,[98] or by exposure to phorbol esters.[99,100] LFA-1 also plays an important role in B cell activation.[105-108] The LFA-1/ICAM-1 adhesion pair is certainly involved in the processes leading to the killing of various types of target cells by effector T cells.[105,106] However, inhibition studies with LFA-1 function-blocking antibodies have clearly suggested that rather than interfering with the killing event they function by preventing the formation of the initial cell-cell conjugate.[47,107,108]

LFA-1 does not only function to promote cell-cell contact during the various activation steps, but it also performs a distinct role as a signal transducer molecule.[109,110] In fact, adhesion and signal transduction are essential elements of a cascade of events leading to antigen-specific activation of T-lymphocytes. LFA-1 also supports antigen presentation by monocytes[111] and B cells.[112-114]

Adhesion through LFA-1 is a complex process, as suggested by its sensitivity to low temperature, metabolic energy inhibitors and cytoskeleton disrupting drugs. Hence it seems likely that adhesion is regulated by several negative and positive factors such as kinases, phosphatases and phospholipases that result in changes in intracellular calcium,[115-118] in phosphorylation,[119-123] in elevation of cyclic AMP[115,124,125] and of the hydrolysis of inositol phospholipids.[126,127] Cross-linking of TCR induces actin polymerization and rearrangement of the cytoskeleton: a fraction of LFA-1 molecules associate with the cytoskeleton after PMA activation,[128,129] although not all the data have been consistent with this conclusion.[130] The importance of the cell environment also is underscored by the finding that LFA-1 transfected in nonhematopoietic cells is constitutively active.[131]

A small number of antibodies raised against LFA-1 bind to epitopes expressed under conditions promoting ligand binding.[132,133] These antibodies define a change of LFA-1 upon activation resulting in enhanced adhesion. They poorly recognize LFA-1 on resting T lymphocytes but show high reactivity against T lymphocytes activated by various means.[134-136] This change is detected for instance by the L16 antibody[135] which recognizes only a fraction of LFA-1 molecules expressed by resting lymphocytes, a fraction that is dramatically augmented upon in vitro cell activation.[74,116,135] These two states may correspond to different conformations of the integrin, as defined by antibody L16[135] or by antibody 24, the latter of which binds to a Mg^{2+}-induced epitope.[136] However, these types of reporter antibodies might bind to epitopes induced by an aggregated versus a non-aggregated integrin form as found for Mac-1.[137] In fact, membrane distribution analysis indicates that a high expression of the L16 epitope corresponds to a distribution of LFA-1 in macroclusters on the cell surface and it is well known that Ca^{2+}-induced clustering is a prerequisite for acquisition of adhesive function.[116] Furthermore, in both a T cell line and in LFA-1 transfected T cells the membrane distribution of high avidity LFA-1 is highly localized in macroclusters while non-activated LFA-1 is evenly distributed

on the cell surface.[138] Cation-dependent epitopes of antibodies recognizing conformational states in LFA-1 do not necessarily interact with the integrin cation binding domains but may recognize epitopes on both α and β subunits that appear on the receptor upon cation or ligand binding.[133,135-139] Therefore, LFA-1 can be present on cell surfaces in several activation states: inactive LFA-1 lacking L16 epitopes; inactive LFA-1 with low L16 expression and low Ca^{2+} binding; potentially active LFA-1 with a high affinity Ca^{2+} binding and hence with clustered receptors but not sufficient for LFA-1 mediated cell aggregation; active LFA-1 with Mg^{2+} bound substituting for Ca^{2+}; and finally, ligand bound LFA-1 with an altered conformation and high epitope 24 expression.[140] Other antibodies against the β2 subunit were described that can by themselves stimulate "conformational changes" or macroaggregations and generate different ligand binding states in LFA-1 such that it can bind to ICAM-1 and ICAM-3 but not to ICAM-2.[141] What is the meaning of these distinct functional forms of LFA-1? Given the transitory nature of lymphocyte function it would appear advantageous if LFA-1 interaction could be modified quickly in order to regulate adhesion and facilitate de-adhesion, for instance by changing or removing the cation available as suggested recently.[75]

Mac-1 and p150,95 play a minor role in leukocyte-leukocyte interactions, but activated neutrophils form homotypic aggregates in vitro[142] and p150,95 specific antibodies can inhibit conjugate formation between target cells and cytotoxic T lymphocytes.[47] Furthermore, while a quantitative rise in LFA-1 is not required for T and B cell adhesion responses, quantitative changes through a rapid degranulation and transport of intracellular pools to the cell membrane occur for Mac-1 and p150,95 in granulocytes and monocytes both in vitro and in vivo.[35-37,143,144] However, since the magnitude of increased adhesion cannot be explained solely by the augmented expression, several Mac-1 mediated functions occur despite no measurable increase in cell surface expression,[145,146] and thus also Mac-1 undergoes activation via conformational changes[147,148] and/or clustering[149] as suggested for LFA-1.[140]

As observed with LFA-1,[140] activation[150] prompts acquisition by a subset of Mac-1 molecules on neutrophils, monocytes and CHO transfected cells of a competent conformation which facilitates binding to both ICAM-1 and fibrinogen.[151] Activated cells concurrently express the CBRM1/5 epitope whose presence is strictly dependent upon divalent cations and correlates with highly avid forms of Mac-1 molecules. This reporter antibody binds to neutrophils and monocytes activated with chemoattractants, cytokines or phorbol esters and recognizes only a fraction of Mac-1 molecules. CBRM1/5 completely abolish adhesion to both ICAM-1 and fibrinogen[151] suggesting that only a fraction of cell surface integrins are engaged at any given time in ligand binding.

LEUKOCYTE-ENDOTHELIUM INTERACTION

The migration of leukocytes through different body compartments subserves a primary immune surveillance function. Lymphocytes constantly recirculate from the blood into lymphoid tissues ("homing") and this ensues that antigens are more easily encountered by antigen specific cells. Similarly, localization of lymphocytes, granulocytes, and monocytes at sites of inflammation is dependent upon specific adhesion to the vascular endothelium through interaction with specific adhesive ligands. This process is regulated by the constitutive and/or induced expression and activation of several cell surface receptors recognizing ligands on endothelial cells and within the ECM and by an array of chemotactic cytokines.[152] Expression of adhesive ligands vary in endothelial cells of different sites: for instance, the endothelial cells of the high endothelial venules of peripheral lymph nodes are different from those of mucosal lymphoid tissues and from the flat endothelium lining non-lymphoid tissues

in both normal and inflamed conditions. Further, the combined action of cytokines may result in antagonistic, additive, or synergistic consequences suggesting that the expression of adhesive molecules is finely regulated. The various signals act on leukocytes in a distinct manner and give reason for the selective localization of leukocyte subsets.

The processes leading to leukocytes binding to endothelium and entry into inflamed tissues are well described and can be summarized as follows:[1,153-155] the first step is mediated by binding of selectins to carbohydrate ligands. This has been conclusively demonstrated for neutrophils by means of function-blocking antibodies and purified proteins[156-161] and more recently by gene knock-out mice.[162] Selectins have fast on/off rates for binding to their ligands,[163] hence, they are optimal players for mediating the initial labile attachment with a high tensile strength. Initial contact with the vessel wall (tethering) seems to be a random event, perhaps stimulated by local alterations in flow characteristics and generation of tissue mediators. Tethering is followed by rolling, which represents a compromise of adhesive interactions between leukocytes and endothelial cells on one side and shear forces on individual leukocytes on the other side. This step is facilitated by continuous release by the activated endothelium of cytokines, chemokines and chemoattractants which bind to their receptors and transduce signals for the activation of integrins. As mentioned above, local stimuli may be specific for certain cell subtypes and thus promote selective cell recruitment or may influence the function of several adhesive proteins and/or leukocyte subtypes. Rolling is then followed by firm sticking through activation of β2 integrins. Mediators generated during the strengthening phase of leukocyte recruitment can function by enhancing[164-166] but also by reducing[167-169] leukocyte-endothelial interactions. If adhesion promoting factors predominate then shear resistant cell adhesion via activated β2 integrins with endothelial ligands will follow. This adhesive process is very fast: as shown by intravital microscopy, within 1 to 3 seconds, shear-sensitive rolling is replaced by shear-resistant leukocyte adhesion.[170] Hemodynamic flow conditions, by directly upregulating ICAM-1 expressed on endothelial cells,[171] also play a major role on the process of β2 integrin-dependent leukocyte adhesion. Finally, firm adhesion is followed by transendothelial migration involving PECAM-1, ICAM-1 and VCAM-1 on endothelium and β2 integrins on leukocytes which accumulate then at sites of immune reaction or inflammation.[172] The subsequent migration of cells depends on the transient nature of adhesiveness i.e. attachment to and detachment from the ECM ligand(s) by rapidly activated and deactivated β1 and β3 integrins localized at the leading and trailing edges of migrating leukocytes. A role of β2 integrins in this step is suggested by recent data, since activated monocytes appear to utilize β2 rather than β1 integrins to attach to heparin[173] and to migrate on laminin and fibronectin.[174]

In lymphocytes, in particular memory lymphocytes which lack expression of both L-selectin and the ligand for E-selectin, tethering and rolling on VCAM-1 can be mediated by the α4β1 integrin which recognizes both fibronectin and VCAM-1.[175,176] This function precedes the activation events necessary for the LFA-1- and Mac-1-mediated firm adhesion, spreading and transmigration.[172,177] The α4β1-dependent mechanism also is used for migration of monocytes into inflamed joints in arthritis.[178] It is likely that the α4β1/VCAM-1 interaction has a high dissociation kinetics, similar to that observed between selectins and their counter-receptors and differing from the firm interaction between LFA-1/Mac-1 and ICAM-1. An important aspect of this multiple cell-adhesion model is that by providing combinatorial flexibility it allows specificity of control in leukocyte migration.[1,153,155,179]

ASSOCIATION WITH OTHER CELL SURFACE RECEPTORS

There is increasing evidence that integrins can physically associate with other receptors or cell-membrane molecules. For instance, a significant percentage of CD2, which contributes to T cell activation and consequently activates LFA-1-mediated functions,[94] is associated with LFA-1 in thymocytes and spleen T cells.[180] Although the structural elements of LFA-1 participating in this interaction and the functional role of this interaction have not yet been clarified, the possibility exists that this close association provides a mechanism for fine-tuning the activation events immediately following the initial TCR engagement to the antigenic peptide.

During the process of phagocytosis Fc and complement receptors CR1, Mac-1 (CR3) and p150,95 (CR4) activate signaling cascades involved in tyrosine phosphorylation of paxillin and activation of the fgr tyrosine kinase,[119-123] actin polymerization,[127] enhanced respiratory burst[117,122] and transient increase in intracellular calcium.[117] The glycosylphosphatidylinositol (GPI)-linked FcγRIII (CD16) receptor is not only functionally linked[181,182] but also cocaps and is physically associated with Mac-1.[184,185] This association is N-acetyl-D-glucosamine dependent and the sugar can inhibit the formation of the complex between the two receptors. Binding of antibody VIM12 to its epitope at the C-terminus of the extracellular Mac-1 domain activates granulocytes, upregulates Mac-1 expression and induces actin polymerization.[186] This region of Mac-1 is very rich in N-linked sugars and N-acetyl-D-glucosamine can inhibit VIM12 binding to its epitope. Since the same sugar inhibits the formation of a cell membrane complex between FcγRIII and Mac-1[183] it could be assumed that the C-terminus of the extracellular Mac-1 domain is involved in the formation of this and other multi-receptor complexes on the neutrophil cell membrane.[181,182,184] LFA-1-dependent adhesion induced by PMA is inhibited by treatment with okadaic acid[187] which is a potent serine/threonine protein phosphatase inhibitor[188] as is the LFA-1-dependent homotypic T-cell aggregation following treatment with an ICAM-2 peptide.[189] Consistent with the above observations on LFA-1 is the finding that Mac-1 α subunit is constitutively phosphorylated on serine residues and a potential involvement of serine/threonine phosphatases in the regulation of the activation-dependent Mac-1-stimulated cell adhesion is likely. The evidence that deletion of the α subunit cytoplasmic tail leads to a significant increase in ligand binding suggests the possibility that not only the β2 but also the Mac-1 α subunit negatively regulates receptor avidity[190] through phosphorylation/dephosphorylation events. The consequences of VIM12 binding to Mac-1 on neutrophils also can be inhibited by okadaic acid.[186] Therefore, if VIM12 binding mimics the naturally occurring cooperation between Mac-1 and FcγRIII, the epitope recognized by the VIM2 antibody might be directly involved in the interaction prompted by this antibody. Alternatively, VIM12 might act indirectly via changes in the conformation of distant interacting sites (i.e., within the VWFA module) of the Mac-1 α subunit. Recently, also the FcγRIIA receptor was found to be associated with Mac-1.[191]

Another receptor identified in a membrane complex together with Mac-1 as well as LFA-1 is the plasminogen activator receptor.[184,192] The finding of a close physical association of these components implies that β2 integrin-mediated functions might involve localized proteolysis.

Interaction with Soluble Ligands

Neutrophil extravasation into tissues and phagocytosis of iC3b-coated particles are essential steps in host defense against infections and Mac-1 (CR3) is a major component used by circulating cells not only to migrate into inflamed sites but also to phagocytize opsonized particles.[193] The first evidence that p150,95 also has iC3b-binding capability was provided when p150,95 from extracts of solubilized cells was successfully purified on iC3b-Sepharose columns.[194,195] That p150,95 functions as a fully active complement receptor (CR4) and does not need to work in concert with

other β2 integrins was then demonstrated by cotransfecting both α and β subunits of p150,95 in cells lacking complement receptors.[196]

Additional β2 integrin-dependent mechanisms contributing to the general leukocyte adhesion to endothelium also have been described. This indirect form of cell-cell adhesion is dependent upon the bridging function of soluble ligands for vascular receptors. Thus, fibrinogen[197-199] and factor X[199] can potentiate adhesion of activated myeloid and lymphoid cells to resting endothelium be 2- to 5-fold. This increased adhesion depends on the interaction between soluble fibrinogen and/or factor X and ICAM-1 expressed on the endothelial site and between fibrinogen and/or factor X and activated Mac-1 on leukocytes (Fig. 4.2). Similarly, rapid adhesion of neutrophils to endothelium can be mediated by binding of iC3b to Mac-1 and to complement receptors on endothelial cells.[200,201]

The hemostatic system is finely regulated to keep blood in a fluid state until normal hemostasis or pathologic thrombosis are activated. Inflammation with its sequela of leukocyte activation and adhesion and early vascular injury is strictly associated with initiation of platelet adhesion and fibrin deposition and these events depend on the nature of the vascular bed and on the extent of shear forces. Leukocytes and in particular neutrophils can interact with activated and adherent platelets under appropriate shear conditions and upregulate Mac-1 expression.[202] Both Mac-1[203-207] and p150,95[208,209] function as fibrinogen receptors, although their binding activity is modulated by different agonists, TPA for Mac-1 and TNF for p150,95. In addition, monocytes can directly activate the zymogen factor X to Xa[210] through a function that monocytes share with herpes simplex infected endothelium.[211] As with the majority of other ligands, leukocytes recognize factor X as a consequence of a transient high avidity state, for instance through an ADP-dependent process.[150] This alternative extrinsic pro-coagulant response[210] can potentially contribute to vascular injury and tissue damage.[212]

Finally, Mac-1 has been shown to bind to several other soluble ligands including NIF[213] (see below), C3dg,[214] LPS,[215] lipophosphoglycan,[216] glycoprotein 63 from leishmania,[217,218] filamentous hemagglutinin of *Bordetella pertussis*,[219] fimbriated *E. coli*,[220] and yeast cell wall antigens.[221,222] Rather unusual is the recognition mechanism of the filamentous hemagglutinin. This ligand, by binding simultaneously to Mac-1 and to the LRI integrin-CD47 signaling complex,[223,224]

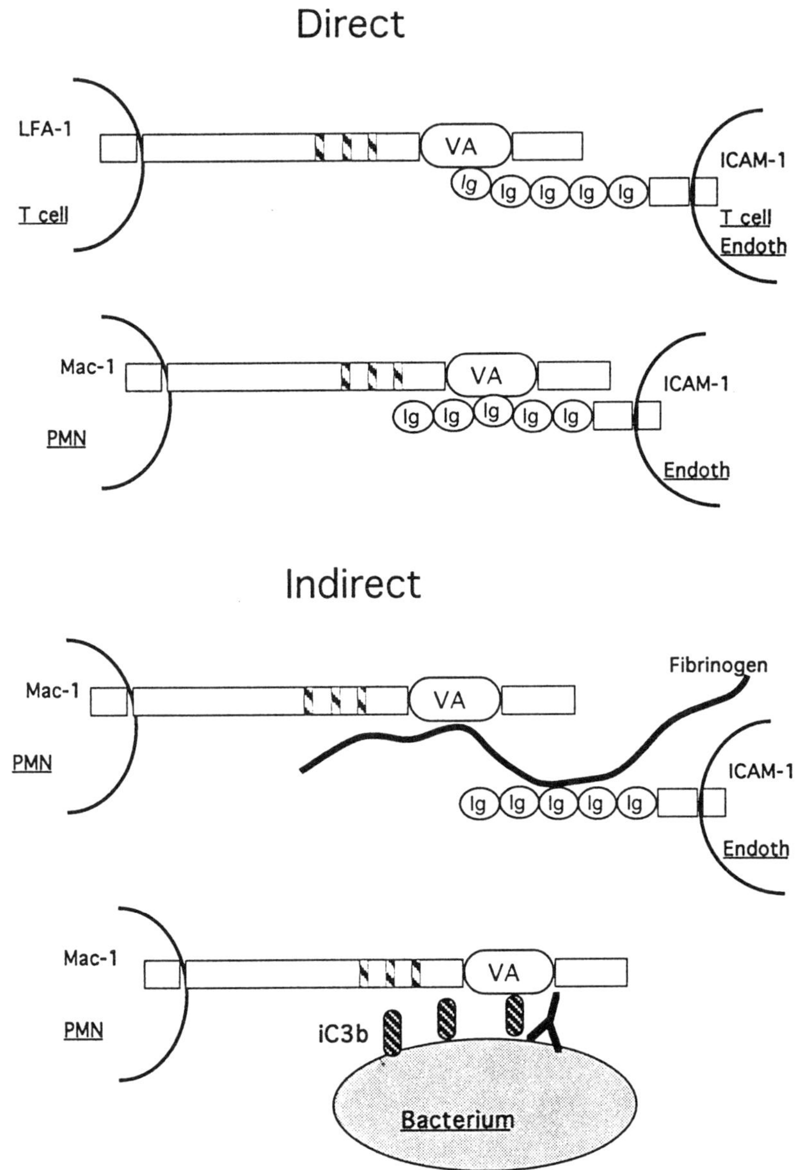

Fig 4.2. Schematic representation of the cell-cell interactions mediated by β2 integrins through their VWFA/I (VA) modules. Direct cell-cell adhesion involves LFA-1 and Mac-1 VWFA modules and the first or third Ig module of ICAM-1, respectively. Indirect cell-cell adhesion between Mac-1 and endothelial cells or a bacterium is mediated by fibrinogen and iC3b, respectively.

leads to an enhanced Mac-1 binding and by this manner the bacterium up-regulates its own attachment to host cells.

STRUCTURE-FUNCTION RELATIONSHIPS

MAPPING OF FUNCTIONAL EPITOPES TO VWFA MODULES (I MODULES)

There is ample evidence that LFA-1 on resting cells does not bind spontaneously to its ligands ICAM-1, -2 and -3, but needs to be activated by a number of stimuli, suggesting that a change in the molecule may render the ligand binding sites accessible.[79,93,99,128,140] Studies of human-mouse hybrids have shown that the ICAM-1 binding site on LFA-1 is located on the α subunit;[225] as the majority of the function-blocking antibodies against the α subunit recognize the isolated VWFA module expressed in an eukaryotic system it might be hypothesized that the isolated fragment retains a conformation similar to that displayed when expressed on the whole α subunit.[132,226] Similarly, most epitopes recognized by function-blocking anti Mac-1 and anti p150,95 antibodies map to the respective VWFA modules of the integrin.[227] The presence of the ICAM-1 and ICAM-3 binding site(s) on the VWFA module of LFA-1 is supported by functional assays:[228] while most antibodies block T cell adhesion to both ICAM-1 and ICAM-3, there are few antibodies that are selective for ICAM-1: one of these antibodies is inducing a high avidity state of LFA-1 for iCAM-1 but is not able to stimulate binding of T cells to ICAM-3, whereas two other antibodies inhibit binding of activated T cells only to ICAM-1. That the binding sites for these two ligands are distinct also is confirmed in an independent assay with COS cells transfected with LFA-1.[226]

Antibodies raised against the human LFA-1 α subunit do not cross-react with the murine counterpart. Based on this observation, amino acid sequences that are important for antibody binding were localized in the VWFA module by chimeras between the human and the murine α subunits.[229,230] Next, a series of replacement mutants were prepared in which murine-specific residues were substituted with the corresponding human residues. This approach indicated that the VWFA module contains three[229] or four[230] distinct regions recognized by antibodies that block LFA-1 function. In one study the regions were identified as IdeA (for I domain epitope A) (residues I126-N129), IdeB (Q143-K149), and IdeC (K197-L203). In a second study the highest level of blocking was obtained with antibodies recognizing epitopes localized between residues M154-L359. Although most antibodies mapped within the VWFA module, also antibodies mapping between the VWFA module and the EF hand-like motifs gave good inhibition (Fig. 4.3).[230] The fact that the residues important for antibody binding are located in sequences that vary the most among the α subunits of β2 integrins accounts for their specificity for LFA-1. Except for a disagreement on the localization of few antibodies, the two studies concur with the same conclusion that residues located on the ligand binding interface and surrounding the residues that directly or indirectly coordinate Mg^{2+} in the MIDAS motif are important for antibody binding. The blocking antibodies may inhibit LFA-1 binding by disrupting the function of multiple structural elements important for ligand binding. Alternatively, the antibodies may inhibit the activity of LFA-1 by affecting the conformation or the activity of the cation-binding MIDAS motif.[7,231]

Activated Mac-1 plays an essential role in immune clearance by facilitating neutrophil adhesion to endothelium, transendothelial migration and phagocytosis of opsonized particles. Several antibodies able to block four Mac-1 ligands including iC3b, ICAM-1, fibrinogen and a still undefined counter-receptor for neutrophil aggregation map in the VWFA module.[227] However, and as also determined with LFA-1,[230] few function-blocking antibodies map outside the VWFA module. In particular, OKM10 maps to an epitope

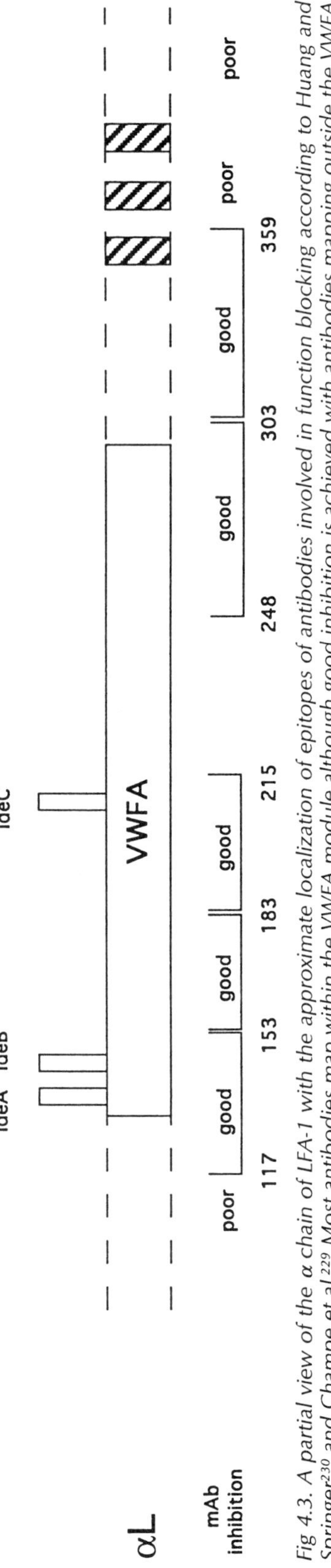

Fig 4.3. A partial view of the α chain of LFA-1 with the approximate localization of epitopes of antibodies involved in function blocking according to Huang and Springer[230] and Champe et al.[229] Most antibodies map within the VWFA module although good inhibition is achieved with antibodies mapping outside the VWFA module. Numbers refer to the amino acid residues of the human Mac-1.

shared by regions that are N- and C-terminal of the VWFA module,[227] suggesting that while physically separated, the N-terminal and the EF hand-like regions are closely associated and structurally apposed. It is interesting that, while the majority of antibodies are strongly inhibitory in at least one functional assay, not all antibodies are able to block the interaction of Mac-1 with its multiple ligands. The different patterns of inhibition suggest the existence of distinct immunoreactive and may be functional subdomains. A likely possibility is that for each ligand some or all of these subdomains may contribute to the overall architecture of the binding site. Alternatively, the VWFA module may contain a core region that facilitates recognition of all ligands with few spatially close sequences contributing instead to the ligand specificity. The use of human/murine chimeric Mac-1/p150,95 constructs and VWFA module deletions indicates that many function-blocking antibodies bind to the C-terminal half of the module.[232] In addition, several antibodies require an intact module for binding to occur suggesting that they recognize conformational epitopes. The epitopes of Mac-1 function-blocking antibodies may not correspond to the genuine ligand-interacting sequence(s). This is exemplified by the OKM1 antibody: although this antibody inhibits the leukocyte-fibrinogen interaction of Mac-1 that is mediated by the VWFA module,[198,233] the epitope recognize by the OKM1 antibody is located outside the VWFA module.[227,233] Therefore, in this case it could be envisioned that engagement of distant epitope(s) induces a significant rearrangement in the spatial configuration of the α subunit or in the Mac-1 heterodimer as a whole, making the VWFA module or the ligand interacting site(s) sterically inaccessible to macromolecular ligands such as fibrinogen. Alternatively, and as mentioned in the case of LFA-1[230] the possibility that epitopes outside the VWFA module contain additional recognition sequences for both LFA-1 and Mac-1 should be considered.

The study of p150,95 function has been hampered by the overlapping binding properties of Mac-1 that is often expressed at higher densities on the same type of cells. Since iC3b binds to p150,95 expressed on cells and to purified p150,95 and this interaction is specifically abolished by function-blocking antibodies that localize to the VWFA module, it can be concluded that, in analogy with Mac-1,[227] the VWFA module of p150,95 also is an important ligand recognition site for iC3b.

In summary, the antibodies inhibiting functional responses in vitro have different mechanisms of action : they compete for the ligand binding site;[74] they stabilize the "activated" or the "unactivated" conformation; they decrease the activation energy for the shift from an inactive to an active state; and they can alter the interactions with divalent cations which mediate the transition between activated and unactivated integrin conformation.[74,75,135,232-236] Finally, that activation-dependent epitopes on stimulated leukocytes also localize to the VWFA module[226,227,232] suggests that this domain, in addition to the ligand binding function, participates in qualitative mechanisms and exerts a regulatory role in receptor activation in both Mac-1 and LFA-1.

THE VWFA MODULES (I MODULES) OF β2 INTEGRINS MEDIATE THEIR FUNCTIONS

LFA-1 binds to the first (N-terminal) immunoglobulin domain of ICAM-1,[84,85,237,238] ICAM-2,[86,87] and possibly also that of ICAM-3[89-91,239] and ICAM-4.[240] On the contrary, Mac-1 recognizes the third immunoglobulin domain of ICAM-1[241,242] (Fig. 4.2). The binding of LFA-1 to ICAM-1 is particularly avid if the latter is dimeric since binding to the monomeric form of ICAM-1 is negligible.[243] A 22-amino acid long peptide derived from the first domain of ICAM-2 behaves as a specific agonist for LFA-1 function:[244] it stimulates T cell aggregation and NK cell activity and it inhibits cell attachment to purified LFA-1.[245] The peptide also binds to Mac-1 but not to p150,95 and this in-

teraction is prevented only by the function-blocking OKM10 antibody, whose epitope is formed by both N-terminal and EF hand-like regions of the Mac-1 α subunit.[244] This latter finding suggests that ICAM-2 and OKM10 binding sites might be very close or overlapping. Although no evidence had been found previously for an interaction between Mac-1 and ICAM-2, the peptide stimulates Mac-1 attachment to fibrinogen very efficiently and iC3b as well as monocytic[244] and NK cell[245] aggregation without inducing the expression of activation dependent epitopes. That a high avidity state can be induced by a peptide agonist which can distinguish between two highly homologous receptors such as Mac-1 and p150,95 suggests that this type of approach might be useful in pharmacological attempts to alter integrin specific functions.

Data demonstrating that the VWFA module of LFA-1 contains the ligand binding site were initially provided in studies utilizing a chimeric protein consisting of the VWFA module joined to the Fc fragment of IgG.[228] In those studies no indication as to which part or residues of the module might actually be involved in ligand binding was provided. In other studies[246] the ligand binding properties of two sets of LFA-1 variants transfected in 293 cells were analyzed: one set, in which the human VWFA module variable sequences of the IdeA, IdeB and IdeC epitopes were replaced by murine sequences, indicated that the binding site for ICAM-1 is not contained in epitopes recognized by LFA-1 function-blocking antibodies.[246] A second set, in which residues conserved throughout the VWFA modules of the β2 integrins were mutagenized, identified residues D137 and D239, which are part of the cation binding MIDAS site[231] as important for binding of LFA-1 to ICAM-1.[246] With these latter mutants no difference is detected between mutated and wild type molecules in binding of function-blocking antibodies. Mutations of the P192 residue also abrogates adhesion, but since antibody binding also is strongly reduced, it is likely that P192 plays a structural role. In this case the lack of adhesion might be the consequence of conformational changes induced by the substitutions. Using in vitro translated LFA-1 protein fragments Hogg and collaborators mapped the LFA-1 binding sites for ICAM-1 outside of the VWFA module to the EF hand-like cation binding motifs V and VI.[247] While the binding is insensitive to EDTA these fragments apparently possess a native folding since they react with function-blocking antibodies raised against the intact LFA-1 molecule. Fine mapping of these sites by blocking experiments with short peptides show that two discontinuous regions (P458-L477 and G497-V516) contribute to the binding site,[247] but compared to the nearly complete inhibition achieved with antibodies, these peptides inhibit only about 40% of T cell binding to ICAM-1. A more detailed investigation of the effects of amino acid replacements, epitope mapping and functional binding studies using transfected COS cells identified four residues (M140, E146, T243 and S245) in two noncontiguous regions of the VWFA module as crucial for species-specific binding of LFA-1 to ICAM-1 (Fig. 4.4).[230] Whether a two step sequential model such that initial cation dependent binding through the VWFA module might induce a change in the area comprising the V and VI motifs leading to a more stable binding is still hypothetical.

Initial data supporting a direct role of Mac-1 VWFA module in ligand binding were provided by studying the binding properties of intermolecular chimeras between Mac-1 and p150,95.[227] Later on it was found that in contrast to the temperature dependency of cell-bound Mac-1/ligand interaction, iC3b binds to the recombinant VWFA module of Mac-1 in a temperature-independent fashion.[248] This finding indicates that the isolated module assumes a functionally active conformation which is lacking in the native Mac-1 molecule, unless the latter is activated by agonists. Furthermore, it suggests that the conformational or clustered condition of the

intact receptor may be mimicked by using immobilized recombinant VWFA modules. The iC3b binding site on Mac-1 localizes to a short linear peptide (peptide A7, residues N232-K245) which also binds iC3b directly and inhibits iC3b binding to the VWFA module as well as to Mac-1 present on neutrophils.[248] However, while the mutation of T209 of Mac-1 blocks adhesion to ICAM-1,[249] peptide A5 (R196-I215) that contains the T209 residue has no inhibitory effect. The apparent contradiction of these results (peptide A5 with T209 is ineffective and peptide A7 without T209 is functional) could be explained by two possibilities: there is more than one potential binding site involved in the iC3b-VWFA module interaction, or the linear peptide(s) do not necessarily assume the proper spatial conformation.

Mutations affecting the conserved amino acid residues D140 and D242 impair iC3b binding to Mac-1 indicating that binding requires an intact MIDAS metal binding site in the Mac-1 module.[7,231,248,249] Similarly, mutations introduced in the conserved residues of the VWFA modules of LFA-1[249] and of $\alpha2\beta1$,[250] and the complement component C2[251] that are part of the primary or secondary coordination shell with the cation in the MIDAS motif, are crucial for a proper function of the module, irrespective of the structurally different ligands recognized (Fig. 4.4). Mutations in the above residues seem critical for cation binding and consequently for binding to ligands when cells with the intact $\beta2$ integrins and recombinant VWFA modules are used.[7,231,248,249] This suggests that the residues coordinating the ion might be involved in actual binding to the ligand. Such regulation could occur through effects on accessibility of ligands to the real binding sites and is likely mediated by binding of divalent cations to the MIDAS cation binding motif.[7] The cations would play a direct or an indirect role in ligand binding perhaps by stabilizing a specific permissive conformation, or by interacting or competing with the ligand. It is worth pointing out that the

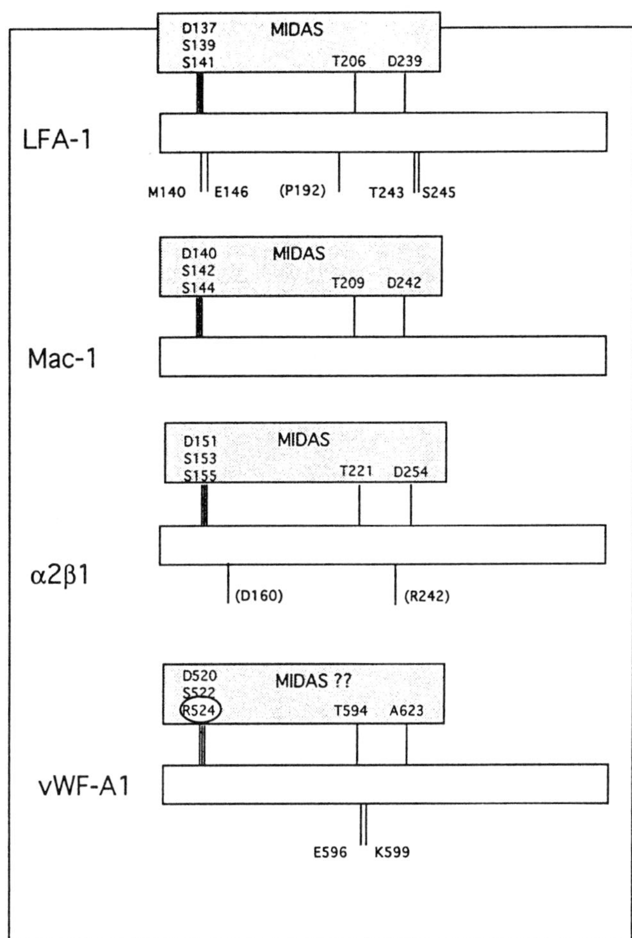

Fig 4.4. Schematic diagram of the VWFA modules of the α chains of LFA-1, Mac-1 and α2β1 integrins and of the A1 module of vWF. The conserved residues of the cation binding MIDAS motif are shown along with the residues (bolded) very likely involved in direct interaction between LFA-1,[230,249] α2β1[250] and vWF[269] with their respective ligands ICAM-1, collagen and GPIb. The R524 residue in the vWF A1 module is encircled since this last one might represent a variant MIDAS motif. Although the interaction of vWF A1 module and platelet GPIb is not known to be dependent upon divalent cations and some of the residues coordinating metal ions are not at all conserved in A1, the MIDAS motif was tentatively included also for this module.

affinity of the ion for the MIDAS motif is one order of magnitude higher than the affinity of the ion for the EF hand-like motifs. Taken together, these results suggest that by isolating all or parts of the VWFA modules it would be possible to promote receptor-ligand interactions in the absence of cations.

The hookworm *Ancylostoma caninum* produces a 41 kD protein called NIF, which binds specifically to Mac-1 and inhibits activated neutrophil-mediated functions.[213] By locally producing a factor able to selectively block adhesion to and spreading on endothelial cell monolayers as well as peroxide release, hookworms may be able to prevent Mac-1-mediated neutrophil extravasation into infected sites and the consequent destruc-

tion of parasites. The binding of NIF to neutrophils is selective and of high affinity, it is equally effective to the inactive as well as the active forms of Mac-1 and it is inhibited by a function-blocking antibody and by a soluble recombinant VWFA module of Mac-1.[252] This inhibition is specific since the VWFA module of LFA-1 is unable to inhibit even at high molar concentrations.[252] The recognition site in the VWFA module of Mac-1 is comprised of non-contiguous sequences, one of which (A7) also serves as the major iC3b binding site.[248] The peptides are centrally located in the VWFA module and overlapping (A6 and A7) with two other peptides contributing to the recognition site that are located at the N-(A1) and C-terminus (A12) of the module.

The peptides are spatially close in the three-dimensional structure of the module[7] and this may explain the finding that NIF inhibits recognition of several Mac-1 ligands: ICAM-1 and iC3b are completely inhibited, while binding to fibrinogen is inhibited only partially. NIF might directly block interaction between Mac-1 and one or more of its ligands, or it may antagonize conformational changes in Mac-1 that are required for ligand recognition. However, peptide inhibition studies should be cautiously considered since several other shorter peptides spanning this region are unable to inhibit integrin ligand interaction.[252]

NIF is an example of a selective natural antagonist for Mac-1 since it does not inhibit the closely related p150,95 integrin. That the interactive region between the VWFA module and NIF is ample (four sequences are involved) may account for the high selectivity of this protein for Mac-1 but not for p150,95 (which also is capable to bind iC3b). In fact, while the A7 region is highly conserved in both α subunits, the regions encoding A1, A6 and A12 are less conserved. The binding of NIF is cation-dependent also when the recombinant VWFA module is used and this is at variance with the findings with other VWFA modules that recognize their respective ligands in the absence of cations or even in the presence of EDTA.[250,253,254] Consequently, NIF does not bind to isolated VWFA modules mutagenized in the D140 or D242 residues,[7] indicating that binding requires an intact MIDAS motif. However, while binding of NIF to neutrophils is completely abolished by EDTA, binding to the recombinant module is only partially decreased in the presence of EDTA.[255] Finally, since the recombinant VWFA module of Mac-1 inhibits NIF in the nanomolar range, whereas it inhibits iC3b binding at micromolar concentrations, it might be used to treat hookworm infections without unwanted negative consequences for other Mac-1 dependent functions.

A 30 kD fragment of fibrinogen, lacking the C-terminus of the γ chain, which is a ligand binding site for the αIIbβ3 integrin,[256] recapitulates the specific fibrinogen binding to Mac-1 and can fully inhibit the binding of intact fibrinogen to Mac-1.[207] While factor X needs a sequential order of addition of three spatially distant surface loops present in the catalytic domain,[211] one single peptide sequence of fibrinogen (G190-V202) is sufficient for bridging through with Mac-1.[257] However, synthetic peptides derived from the three loops can each inhibit factor X binding to Mac-1 and prevent thrombin generation. Fibrinogen and factor X are likely to bind to spatially separated sites of Mac-1 as evidenced by the differential ability of function-blocking antibodies to inhibit either ligand[150] and by the lack of competitive cross inhibition by unlabeled factor X.[233] Furthermore, the recombinant VWFA module of Mac-1 binds fibrinogen with high efficiency and encompasses all the biochemical criteria of specificity and saturability expected for a genuine receptor-mediated interaction.[256] This suggests that the VWFA module is only minimally involved in recognition of factor X, although activation of Mac-1 is associated with the appearance of an activation dependent epitope identified by a reporter antibody,[257] which can block the binding of both factor X and fibrinogen to Mac-1.

It is known that neutrophil chemotaxis within the subendothelial ECM requires the presence of Mac-1 and several reports have indicated that activated neutrophils attach to heparin, but not to chondroitin sulfate A, B, or C.[173] Furthermore, Mac-1 might recognize polysaccharides and it has been shown that heparan sulfate can mediate, at least in part, the Mac-1 mediated adhesion of stromal cells to fibroblasts.[258] The adhesion of neutrophils and of Mac-1 transfected CHO cells to heparin is almost completely inhibited by some function-blocking antibodies that map to the VWFA module, while antibodies that map in the C-terminal part of the extracellular domain of Mac-1 are ineffective.[173] While fewer antibodies block adhesion to heparin than to iC3b, there is one antibody that abolishes binding to heparin but not to ICAM-1 and iC3b. In addition, since heparin does not competitively inhibit neutrophil adhesion to fibrinogen,[173] it is likely that its binding site on the VWFA module is distinct or only partially overlapping with those for the other Mac-1 ligands. Heparin and heparan sulfate proteoglycans also can present chemokines to leukocytes and induce adhesion to endothelium;[259] thus they might subserve a double function as direct ligands for Mac-1 and as molecules that present factors necessary for further activation. The recent report that β2 integrins are required for migration of activated monocytes on laminin and fibronectin[174] expands the ligand specificity and suggests that the VWFA module of β2 integrins also can interact with ECM constituents, thus endowing these integrins with a very broad spectrum of ligands (Fig. 4.5).

DISEASE ASSOCIATION

LAD is an autosomal recessive disorder of human,[15,16] dog[260] and cattle[261] where diverse functional impairments in leukocyte functions are related to their inability to adhere particularly to other leukocytes and to endothelium. Patients with LAD deficiencies affecting different cell adhesion molecules have been described[16,262] but only in LAD-1 patients does the defect concern the β2 integrin subunit. A β2 knock out mouse model also is available to study the functional defects in vivo.[263] The disease is dependent upon the defective expression or complete absence of β2 integrins from the cell surface. As a consequence of this, most patients suffer from severe recurrent bacterial infections often culminating in septicemia in the presence of a prominent leukocytosis. Consistent with our understanding of the process of leukocyte-endothelium interaction, leukocytes from LAD-1 patients exhibit normal selectin-dependent tethering and rolling, but are deficient in β2 integrin-dependent firm attachment and endothelium transmigration. While lymphocytes can overcome the β2 deficiency by usage of the α4β1 mediated adhesion pathway, neutrophils are more severely affected and are not found at sites of inflammation.

The majority of cases in which the β2 subunit fails to associate with the α subunit are of moderate severity and the molecular defects are point mutations or small insertions and deletions[264] that occur in two segments of the β2 chain: one spanning the region conserved among all the β subunits, the other in exon 13 coding for the fourth cysteine-rich segment close to the cell membrane insertion. The single residue substitutions in the conserved region impair either partially[265] or completely[266] the non-covalent association of the α and β subunits. Mutations in residues highly conserved in all β integrin subunits (D106G,G147R,P156L and N329S) and comprised in the region important for cation and ligand binding abolish expression at the cell surface.[265] Some of the mutations in exon 13 (G548D and R571C) impair integrin expression[265,266] suggesting that also changes in the rigid cysteine-rich stalk can affect the conformation of the distantly located contact area between the α and β subunits. The functional defect can be easily rescued in vitro if cells from LAD-1 patients are transfected with the β2 cDNA.[267]

CONCLUSIONS

The crystal structures of the VWFA module of Mac-1 differ considerably depending upon whether the crystal is grown in the presence of Mg^{2+} or Mn^{2+} (see chapter 1).[268] The results of the structural analysis indicate that in the case of Mg^{2+}, one coordination bond might come from the ligand, whereas in the case of Mn^{2+}, being the thermodynamically favored form, there is no need for an external coordination bond. These findings suggest that the VWFA module exists in at least two discrete conformations representing the active and inactive functional states. This is consistent with the reactivities of certain

Fig 4.5. Ligands of the β2 integrins. Known ligands that are recognized through the involvement of the VWFA modules of β2 integrins are shown. In two instances the counter-receptors (endothelium counter-receptor interacting with p150,95 and neutrophil homotypic adhesion receptor have not yet been molecularly identified. Other ligands such as laminin and fibronectin[174] and heparin[173] are not included since the role of the VWFA module in this interaction is not formally proven yet.

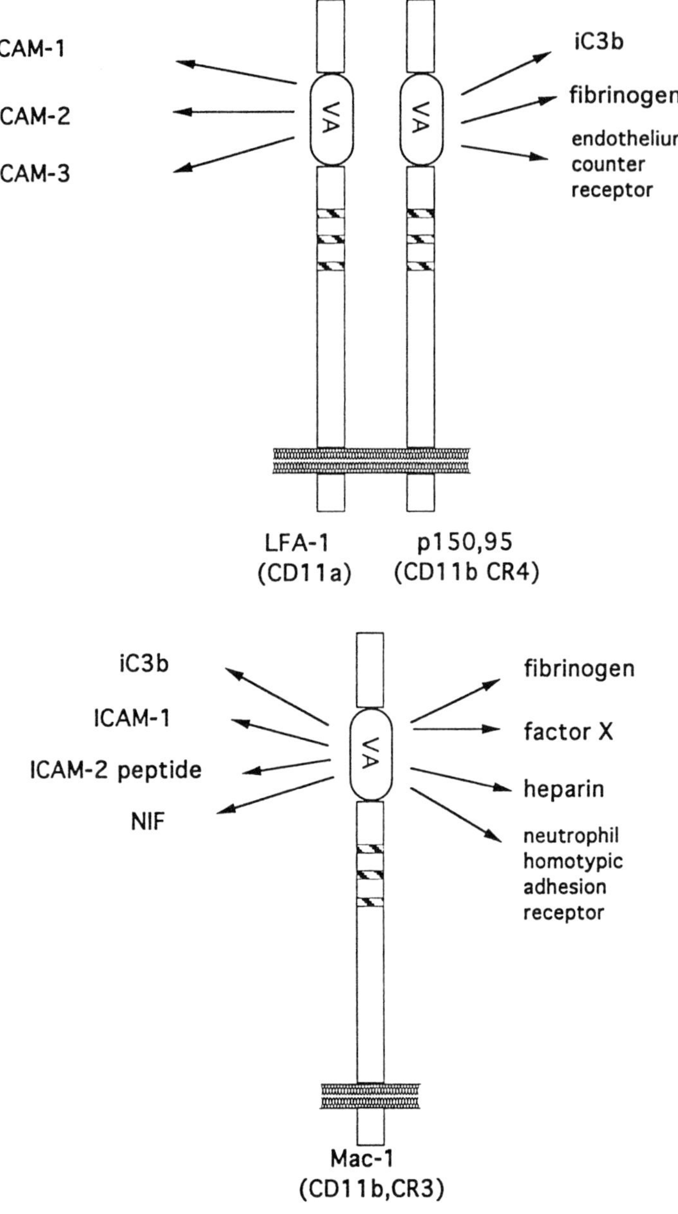

antibodies against the VWFA modules of α chains that can discriminate between the active and inactive states of β2 integrins,[132,151,257] and with analogous findings in the hemostatic system where vWF is present in at least two conformational states.[269,270] Thus, the VWFA modules of β2 integrins participate in receptor function by providing direct interaction with the ligand via contact sites with some residues and via interaction via the divalent cation and/or by providing structural elements necessary to maintain the conformation of a ligand binding site in a remote part of the chain. An interesting possibility is that this module represents an ion-sensitive regulatory domain that governs the transition between activated and unactivated conformation.

REFERENCES

1. Springer TA. Traffic signals for lymphocyte recirculation and leukocyte emigration: the multi-step paradigm. Cell 1994; 76: 301-314.
2. Sanchez-Madrid F, Nagy J, Robbins E et al. A human leukocyte differentiation antigen family with distinct alpha subunits and a common beta subunit: the lymphocyte function-associated antigen (LFA-1), the C3bi complement receptor (OKM1/Mac-1), and the p150,95 molecule. J Exp Med 1983; 158: 1785-1803.
3. Danilenko DM, Rossitto PV, Van der Vieren M et al. A novel canine leukointegrin $\alpha_d\beta_2$ is expressed by specific macrophage subpopulations in tissue and a minor CD8⁺ lymphocyte subpopulation in peripheral blood. J Immunol 1995; 155:35-44.
4. Springer T, Galfre G, Secher DS et al. Mac-1: a macrophage differentiation antigen identified by monoclonal antibody. Eur J Immunol 1979; 9:301-306.
5. Weizmann JB, Wells CE, Wright AH et al. The gene organization of the human beta 2 integrin subunit (CD18). FEBS 1992; 294:97-103.
6. Corbi AL, Larson RS, Kishimoto TK et al. Chromosomal location of the genes encoding the leukocyte adhesion receptors LFA-1, Mac-1 and p150,95. Identification of a gene cluster involved in cell adhesion. J Exp Med 1988; 167:1597-1607.
7. Lee J-O, Rieu P, Arnaout MA et al. Crystal structure of the A domain from the α subunit of integrin CR3 (CD11b/CD18). Cell 1995; 80:631-638.
8. Fleming JC, Pahl HL, Gonzales DA et al. Structural analysis of the CD11b gene and phylogenetic analysis of the α-integrin gene family demonstrate remarkable conservation of genomic organization and suggest early diversification during evolution. J Immunol 1993; 150:480-490.
9. Corbi AL, Garcia-Aguilar J, Springer TA. Genomic structure of an integrin α subunit, the leukocyte p150,95 molecule. J Biol Chem 1990; 265:2782-2788.
10. Larson RS, Springer TA. Structure and function of leukocyte integrins. Immunol Rev 1990; 114:181-217.
11. Law SKA, Gagnon J, Hildreth JEK et al. The primary structure of the β-subunit of the cell surface adhesion glycoproteins LFA-1, CR3 and p150,95 and relationship to the fibronectin receptor. EMBO J 1987; 6:915-919.
12. Kishimoto TK, O'Connor K, Lee A et al. Cloning of the β subunit of the leukocyte adhesion proteins: homology to an extracellular matrix receptors defines a novel supergene family. Cell 1987; 48:681-690.
13. Bajt ML, Loftus JC. Mutation of a ligand binding domain of beta 3 integrin. J Biol Chem 1994; 269:20913-20919.
14. Loftus JC, Smith JW, Ginsberg MH. Integrin-mediated cell adhesion: the extracellular face. J Biol Chem 1994; 269: 25235-25238.
15. Bait ML, Goodman T, McGuire SL. β2 (CD18) mutations abolish ligand recognition by I domain integrins LFA-1 (αLβ2, CD11a/CD18) and MAC-1 (αMβ2, CD11b/CD18). J Biol Chem 1995; 270:94-98.
16. Arnaout MA, Michishita M. Genetic abnormalities in leukocyte adhesion molecule deficiency. In : Gupta S, Griscelli C, eds. New Concepts in Immunodeficiency Diseases. John Wiley & Sons, 1993:191-202.
17. Zeger DL, Osman N, Hennings M et al. Mouse macrophage β subunit (CD11b) cDNA for the CR3 complement receptor/Mac-1 antigen. Immunogenetics 1990; 31:191-197.
18. Bilsland CAG, Springer TA. Cloning and expression of the chicken CD18 cDNA. J Leuk Biol 1994; 55:501-506.
19. Wright SD, Rao PE, Van Voorhis WC et al. Identification of the C3bi receptor of human monocytes and macrophages by using monoclonal antibodies. Proc Natl Acad Sci USA 1983; 80:5699-5703.
20. Micklem KJ, Sim RB. Isolation of complement-fragment-iC3b-binding proteins by affinity chromatography. Biochem J 1985; 231:233-236.
21. Larson RS, Corbi AL, Berman L et al. Primary structure of the leukocyte function-associated molecule-1 α subunit: an integrin with an embedded domain defining a protein superfamily. J Cell Biol 1989; 108:703-712.

22. Pytela R. Amino acid sequence of the murine Mac-1 α chain reveals homologuous with the integrin family and an additional domain related to von Willebrand factor. EMBO J 1988; 7:1371-1378.

23. Corbi AL, Miller LJ, O'Connor K et al. cDNA cloning and complete primary structure of the α subunit of a leukocyte adhesion glycoprotein, p150,95. EMBO J 1987; 6:4023-4028.

24. Corbi AL, Kishimoto TK, Miller LJ et al. The human leukocyte adhesion glycoprotein Mac-1 (complement receptor type 3, CD11b) α subunit. J Biol Chem 1988; 263:12403-12411.

25. Strynadka NCJ, James MNG. Crystal structures of the helix-loop-helix calcium-binding proteins. Ann Rev Biochem 1989; 58:951-998.

26. Tuckwell DS, Brass A, Humphries MJ. Homology modelling of integrin EF-hands. Biochem J 1992; 285:325-331.

27. Williams MJ, Hughes PE, O'Toole TE et al. The inner world of cell adhesion: integrin cytoplasmic domains. Trends Biochem Sci 1994; 4:109-112.

28. Dana N, Styrt B, Griffin J et al. Two functional domains in the phagocyte membrane glycoprotein Mo1 identified with monoclonal antibodies. J Immunol 1986; 137:3259-3263.

29. Kuerzinger K, Reynolds T, Germain RN et al. A novel lymphocyte function-associated antigen (LFA-1): cellular distribution, quantitative expression and structure. J Immunol 1981; 127:596-602.

30. Sanchez-Madrid F, Krensky AM, Ware CF et al. Three distinct antigens associated with human T lymphocyte-mediated cytolysis: LFA-1, LFA-2 and LFA-3. Proc Natl Acad Sci USA 1982; 79:7489-7493.

31. Hildreth JEK, Gotch FM, Hildreth PDK et al. A human lymphocyte-associated antigen involved in cell-mediated lympholysis. Eur J Immunol 1983; 13:202-208.

32. Springer TA, Miller LJ, Anderson DC. p150,95, the third member of the Mac-1, LFA-1 human leukocyte adhesion glycoprotein family. J Immunol 1986; 136:240-245.

33. Lanier LL, Arnaout MA, Schwarting R et al. p150,95, third member of the LFA-1/ CR3 polypeptide family identified by anti-Leu M5 monoclonal antibody. Eur J Immunol 1985; 15:713-718.

34. Cobbold S, Holmes M, Willet B. The immunology of companion animals: reagents and therapeutic strategies with potential veterinary and human clinical applications. Immunol Today 1994; 15:347-352.

35. Todd RF III, Arnaout MA, Rosin RE et al. Subcellular localization of the large subunit of Mo1 (Mo1 alpha; formerly gp110), a surface glycoprotein associated with neutrophil adhesion. J Clin Invest 1984; 74: 1280-1290.

36. Bainton DF, Miller LJ, Kishimoto TK et al. Leukocyte adhesion receptors are stored in peroxidase-negative granules of human neutrophils. J Exp Med 1987; 166: 1641-1653.

37. Miller LJ, Bainton DF, Borregaard N et al. Stimulated mobilization of monocyte Mac-1 and p150,95 adhesion proteins from an intracellular vesicular compartment to the cell surface. J Clin Invest 1987; 80:535-544.

38. Sengelov H, Kjedelsen L, Kroeze W et al. Secretory vesicles are the intracellular reservoir of complement receptor 1 in human neutrophils. J Immunol 1994; 153:804-810.

39. Miller BA, Antognetti G, Springer TA. Identification of cell surface antigens present on murine hematopoietic stem cells. J Immunol 1985; 134:3286-3290.

40. Kansas GS, Dailey MO. Expression of adhesion structures during B cell development in man. J Immunol 1989; 142:3058-3062.

41. Desroches CV, Andreoni C, Rigal D. Differential expression of the LFA-1 molecule on the human peripheral blood mononuclear cell subpopulations. Immunol Lett 1990; 24:13-20.

42. Hickstein DD, Hickey MJ, Collins SJ. Transcriptional regulation of the leukocyte adherence protein β subunit during human myeloid cell differentiation. J Biol Chem 1988; 263:13863-13867.

43. Miller JM, Schwarting R, Springer TA. Regulated expression of the Mac-1, LFA-1, p150,95 glycoprotein family during leukocyte differentiation. J Immunol 1986; 137:2891-2900.

44. Posnett DN, Sinha R, Kabak S et al. Clonal

populations of T cells in normal elderly humans: the T cell equivalent to "benign monoclonal gammopathy". J Exp Med 1994; 179: 609-618.

45. Hoshino T, Yamada A, Honda J et al. Tissue-specific distribution and age-dependent increase of human CD11b⁺ T cells. J Immunol 1993; 151:2237-2246.

46. Kasaian MT, Ikematsu H, Casali P. Identification and analysis of a novel human surface CD5-B lymphocyte subset producing natural antibodies. J Immunol 1992; 148:2690-2702.

47. Keizer GD, Borst J, Visser W et al. Membrane glycoprotein p150,95 of human cytotoxic T cell clones is involved in conjugate formation with target cells. J Immunol 1987; 138:3130-3136.

48. Schwarting R, Stein H, Wang CY. The mAbs anti S-HCL 1 (anti Leu14) and anti S-HCL 3 (anti Leu M5) allow the diagnosis of hairy cell leukemia. Blood 1985; 65:974-983.

49. Postigo A, Corbi AL, Sanchez-Madrid F et al. Regulated expression and function of CD11c/CD18 integrin on human B lymphocytes. Relation between attachment to fibrinogen and triggering of proliferation through CD11c/CD18. J Exp Med 1991; 174:1313-1322.

50. Strasmann G, Springer TA, Haskill SJ et al. Antigens associated with the activation of murine mononuclear phagocytes in vivo: differential expression of lyphocyte function-associated antigen in the several stages of development. Cell Immunol 1985; 94: 265-275.

51. Martz E, LFA-1 and other accessory molecules functioning in adhesions of T and B lymphocytes. Hun Immunol 1987; 18:3-37.

52. Erlandsen SL, Hasslen SR, Nelson RD. Detection and spatial distribution of the β2 integrin (Mac-1) and L-selectin (LECAM-1) adherence receptors on human neutrophils by high-resolution field emission SEM. J Histochem Cytochem 1993; 41:327-333.

53. Ho M-K, Springer TA. Biosynthesis and assembly of the alpha and beta subunits of Mac-1, a macrophage glycoprotein associated with complement receptor function. J Biol Chem 1983; 258:2766-2769.

54. Springer TA, Thompson WS, Miller LJ et al. Inherited deficiency of the Mac-1, LFA-1, p150,95 glycoprotein family and its molecular basis. J Exp Med 1984; 160: 1901-1918.

55. Dahms NM, Hart GW. Lymphocyte function-associated antigen 1 (LFA-1) contains sulfated N-linked oligosaccharides. J Immunol 1985; 134:3978-3986.

56. Takeda A. Sialyation patterns of lymphocyte function-associated antigen 1 (LFA-1) differ between T and B lymphocytes. Eur J Immunol 1987; 17:281-286.

57. Skubitz KM, Snook RW. II. Monoclonal antibodies that recognize lacto-N-fucopentaose III (CD15) react with the adhesion-promoting glycoprotein family (LFA-1/HMAC-1/GP 150,95) and CR1 on human neutrophils. J Immunol 1987; 139:1631-1639.

58. Miller JM, Schwarting R, Springer TA. Regulated expression of the Mac-1, LFA-1, p150,95 glycoprotein family during leukocyte differentiation. J Immunol 1986; 137:2891-2900.

59. Hickstein DD, Rack AL, Collins SJ. Regulation of expression of the CD11b and CD18 subunits of the neutrophil adherence receptor during human myeloid differentiation. J Biol Chem 1989; 264:21812-21817.

60. Rosmarin AG, Weil S, Law SK et al. Differential expression of Mo1 and myeloperoxidase genes during myeloid differentiation. Blood 1988; 73:131-136.

61. Pahl HL, Rosmarin AG, Tenen DG. Characterization of the myeloid-specific CD11b promoter. Blood 1992; 79:865-870.

62. Bellon T, Lopez-Rodriguez C, Rubio MA et al. Regulated expression of p150,95 (CD11c/CD18; αX/β2) and VLA-4 (CD49d/CD29; α4/β1) integrins during myeloid cell differentiation. Eur J Immunol 1994; 24:41-47.

63. Rosmarin AG, Levy R, Tenen DG. Cloning and analysis of the CD18 promoter. Blood 1992; 79:2598-2604.

64. Agura ED, Howard M, Collins SJ. Identification and sequence analysis of the promoter for the leukocyte integrin β-subunit (CD18): a retinoic acid-inducible gene. Blood 1992; 79:602-609.

65. Cornwell RD, Gollahon KA, Hickstein DD. Description of the leukocyte function-associated-antigen-1 (LFA-1 or CD11a) promoter. Proc Natl Acad Sci USA 1993; 90:4221-4225.

66. Chen H-M, Pahl HL, Scheibe RJ et al. The Sp1 transcription factor binds the CD11b promoter specifically in myeloid cells in vivo and is essential for myeloid-specific promoter activity. J Biol Chem 1993; 268:8230-8239.

67. Lopez-Cabrera M, Nueda A, Vara A et al. characterization of the p150,95 leukocyte integrin α subunit (CD11c) gene promoter: identification of cis-acting elements. J Biol Chem 1993; 268:1187-1193.

68. Boettinger EP, Shelley CS, Farokhzad OC et al. The human β2 integrin CD18 promoter consists of two inverted ets cis elements. Mol Cell Biol 1994; 14:2604-2615.

69. Voso MT, Burn TC, Wulf G et al. Inhibition of hematopoiesis by competitive binding of transcription factor PU.1. Proc Natl Acad Sci USA 1994; 91:7932-7936.

70. Pahl HL, Scheibe RJ, Zhang D-E et al. The photo-oncogene PU.1 regulates expression of the myeloid-specific CD11b promoter. J Biol Chem 1993; 268:5014-5020.

71. Rosmarin AG, Caprio D, Levy R et al. CD18 (β2 leukocyte integrin) promoter requires PU.1 transcription factor for myeloid activity. Proc Natl Acad Sci USA 1995; 92:801-805.

72. Back A, East K, Hickstein D. Leukocyte integrin CD11b promoter directs expression in lymphocytes and granulocytes in transgenic mice. Blood 1995; 85:1017-1024.

73. Stuiver I, O'Toole TE. Regulation of integrin function and cellular adhesion. Stem Cells 1995; 13:250-262.

74. Lollo BA, Chan KWH, Hanson EM et al. Direct evidence for two affinity states for lymphocyte function-associated antigen 1 on activated T cells. J Biol Chem 1993; 268:21693-21700.

75. Cai T-Q, Wright SD. Energetics of leukocyte integrin activation. J Biol Chem 1995; 270:14358-14365.

76. Pardi R, Inverardi L, Bender JR. Regulatory mechanisms in leukocyte adhesion: flexible receptors for sophisticated travelers.

Immunol Today 1992; 13:224-230.

77. Edwards SW. Cell signalling by integrins and immunoglobulin receptors in primed neutrophils. Trends Biol Sci 1995; 20:362-367.

78. Yamada KM, Miyamoto S. Integrin transmembrane signaling and cytoskeletal control. Curr Opin Cell Biol 1995; 7:681-389.

79. Lub M, van Kooyk Y, Figdor CG. Ins and outs of LFA-1. Immunol Today 1995; 16:479-483.

80. van Seventer GA, Shimizu Y, Horgan KJ et al. Remote T-cell costimulation via LFA-1/ICAM-1 and CD2/LFA-3: demonstration with immobilized ligand/mAb and implication in monocyte-mediated costimulation. Eur J Immunol 1991; 21:1711-1718.

81. Rothlein R, Dustin ML, Marlin SD et al. A human intercellular adhesion molecule (ICAM-1) distinct from LFA-1. J Immunol 1986; 137:1270-1274.

82. Marlin SD, Springer TA. Purified intercellular adhesion molecule-1 (ICAM-1) is a ligand for lymphocyte function-associated antigen 1 (LFA-1). Cell 1987; 51:813-819.

83. Staunton DE, Marlin SD, Stratowa C et al. Primary structure of ICAM-1 demonstrates interaction between members of the immunoglobulin and integrin supergene families. Cell 1988; 52:925-933.

84. Makgoba M, Sanders M, Luce GEG et al. ICAM-1 a ligand for LFA-1 dependent adhesion of B, T, and myeloid cells. Nature 1988; 331:86-88.

85. Mazerolles F, Lumbroso C, Lecomte O et al. The role of lymphocyte function-associated antigen 1 (LFA-1) in the adherence of T lymphocyte to B lymphocytes. Eur J Immunol 1988; 18:1229-1234.

86. Staunton DE, Dustin ML, Springer TA. Functional cloning of ICAM-2, a cell adhesion ligand for LFA-1 homologous to ICAM-1. Nature 1989; 339: 61-64.

87. de Fougerolles AR, Stacker SA, Schwarting R et al. Characterization of ICAM-2 and evidence for a third counter-receptor for LFA-1. J Exp Med 1991; 174:253-267.

88. de Fougerolles AR, Springer TA. Intercellular adhesion molecule 3, a third adhesion counter-receptor for lymphocyte function-associated molecule 1 on resting lympho-

cytes. J Exp Med 1992; 175:185-190.

89. Vazeux R, Hoffman PA, Tomita JK et al. Cloning and characterization of a new intercellular adhesion molecule ICAM-R. Nature 1993; 360:485-488.

90. Juan M, Vilella R, Mila J et al. CDw50 and ICAM-3: two names for the same molecule. Eur J Immunol 1993; 23:1508-1512.

91. Fawcett J, Holness CLL, Nedham LA et al. Molecular cloning of ICAM-3, a third ligand for LFA-1, constitutively expressed on resting leukocytes. Nature 1992; 360:481-484.

92. Damle NK, Klussman K, Aruffo A. Intercellular adhesion molecule-2, a second counter-receptor for CD11a/CD18 (leukocyte function-associated antigen-1), provides a costimulatory signal for T-cell receptor-initiated activation of human T cells. J Immunol 1992; 148: 665-671.

93. Cabanas C, Hogg N. Ligand ICAM-1 has a necessary role in the activation of integrin LFA-1. Proc Natl Acad Sci USA 1993: 90:5838-5842.

94. van Kooyk Y, van de Wiel van Kemenade P, Weder P et al. Enhancement of LFA-1-mediated cell adhesion by triggering through CD2 or CD3 on T Lymphocytes. Nature 1989; 342:811-813.

95. Shimizu Y, van Seventer GA, Ennis E et al. Crosslinking of the T cell-specific accessory molecules CD7 and CD28 modulates T cell adhesion. J Exp Med 1992; 175:577-582.

96. Cyster JG, Williams AF. The importance of cross-linking in the homotypic aggregation of lymphocytes induced by anti-leukosialin (CD43) antibodies. Eur J Immunol 1992; 22:2565-2572.

97. Simon SI, Burns AR, Taylor AD et al. L-selectin (CD62L) cross-linking signals neutrophil adhesive functions via the Mac-1 (CD11b/CD18) β2-integrin. J Immunol 1995; 155:1502-1514.

98. Mourad W, Geha RS, Chatila T. Engagement of major histocompatibility complex class II molecules induces sustained, lymphocyte function-associated molecule 1-dependent cell adhesion. J Exp Med 1990; 172:1513-1516.

99. Rothlein R, Springer TA. The requirement for lymphocyte function-associated antigen 1 in homotypic leukocyte adhesion stimulated by phorbol ester. J Exp Med 1986; 163:1132-1149.

100. Dustin ML, Springer TA. T-cell receptor cross-linking transiently stimulates adhesiveness through LFA-1. Nature 1989; 341: 619-624.

101. Mentzer SJ, Gromkowski SH, Krenski AM et al. LFA-1 membrane molecule in the regulation of homotypic adhesions of human B lymphocytes. J Immunol 1985; 135:9-11.

102. Tedder TF, Schmidt R, Rudd CE et al. Function of the LFA-1 and T4 molecules in the direct activation of resting human B lymphocytes by T lymphocytes. Eur J Immunol 1986; 16:1539-1543.

103. Howard DR, Eaves AC, Takei F. Lymphocyte function-associated antigen (LFA-1) is involved in B cell activation. J Immunol 1986; 136:4013-4018.

104. Barret TB, Shu G, Clark EA. CD40 signaling activates CD11a/CD18 (LFA-1)-mediated adhesion in B cells. J Immunol 1991; 146:1722-1729.

105. Hildreth JEK, Gotch FM, Hildreth PDK et al. A human lymphocyte-associated antigen involved in cell-mediated lympholysis. Eur J Immunol 1983; 13:202-208.

106. Malefyt RD, Verma S, Bejarano MT et al. CD2/LFA-3 or LFA-1/ICAM-1 but not CD28/B7 interactions can augment cytotoxicity by virus specific CD8[+] cytotoxic-lymphocytes. Eur J Immunol 1993; 23:418-424.

107. Davignon D, Martz E, Reynolds T et al. Lymphocyte-function associated antigen 1 (LFA-1): a surface antigen distinct from Lyt-2,3 that participates in T lymphocyte-mediated killing. Proc Natl Acad Sci USA 1981; 78:4535-4539.

108. Krensky AM, Sanchez-Madrid F, Robbins E et al. The functional significance, distribution and structure of LFA-1, LFA-2 and LFA-3: cell surface antigens associated with CTL-target interactions. J Immunol 1983; 131:611-616.

109. van Noesel C, Miedema F, Brouwer M et al. Regulatory properties of LFA-1 α and β chains in human lymphocyte activation. Nature 1988; 333:850-852.

110. Wacholtz MC, Patel SS, Lipsky PE. Leukocyte function-associated antigen 1 is an ac-

tivation molecule for human T cells. J Exp Med 1989; 170:431-448.

111. Dougherty GJ, Hogg N. The role of monocyte lymphocyte function-associated antigen 1 (LFA-1) in accessory cell function. Eur J Immunol 1987; 17:943-947.

112. Moy VT, Brian AA. Signaling by lymphocyte function-associated antigen 1 (LFA-1) in B cells: enhanced antigen presentation after stimulation through LFA-1. J Exp Med 1992; 175: 1-7.

113. Tohma S, Hirohata S, Lipsky PE. The role of CD11a/CD18-CD54 interaction in human T cell-dependent B cell activation. J Immunol 1991; 146:492-499.

114. Sanders VM, Vitetta ES. B cell-associated LFA-1 and T cell-associated ICAM-1 transiently cluster in the area of contact between interacting cells. Cell Immunol 1991; 132:45-55.

115. van Kooyk Y. Weder P, Heije K et al. Role of intracellular Ca^{2+} levels in the regulation of CD11a/CD18 mediated cell adhesion. Cell Adhes Commun 1993; 1:21-32.

116. Cabanas C, Hogg N. Ligand intercellular adhesion molecule 1 has a necessary role in activation of integrin lymphocyte function-associated molecule 1. Proc Natl Acad Sci USA 1993; 90:5838-5842.

117. Sehgal G, Zhang K, Todd F et al. Lectin-like inhibition of immune complex receptor-mediated stimulation of neutrophils: effects on cytosolic calcium release and superoxide production. J Immunol 1993; 150:4571-4580.

118. Wacholtz MC, Patel SS, Lipsky PE. Leukocyte function-associated antigen 1 is an activation molecule for human T cell. J Exp Med 1989; 170:431-448.

119. Chatila TA, Geha RS, Arnaout MA. Constitutive and stimulus-induced phosphorylation of CD11b/CD18 leukocyte adhesion molecules. J Cell Biol 1989; 109: 3435-3444.

120. Buyon JP, Slade SG, Reibman J et al. Constitutive and induced phosphorylation of the α-and β-chains of the CD11b/CD18 leukocyte integrin family. J Immunol 1990; 144:191-197.

121. Berton G, Fumagalli L, Laudanna C et al. β2 integrin-dependent protein tyrosine phosphorylation and activation of the FGR protein tyrosine kinase in human neutrophils. J Cell Biol 1994; 126:1111-1121.

122. Zhou M, Brown EJ. CR3 (Mac-1, αMβ2, CD11b/CD18) and FcγRIII cooperate in generation of a neutrophil respiratory burst: requirement for FcγRIII and tyrosine phosphorylation. J Cell Biol 1994; 125: 1407-1416.

123. Graham IL, Anderson DC, Holers VM et al. Complement receptor 3 (CR3, Mac-1, integrin αMβ2, CD11b/CD18) is required for tyrosine phosphorylation of paxillin in adherent and nonadherent neutrophils. J Cell Biol 1994; 127:1139-1147.

124. Haverstick DM, Gray LS. Lymphocyte adhesion mediated by lymphocyte function-associated antigen-1. I. Long term augmentation by transient increases in intracellular cAMP. J Immunol 1992; 149:389-396.

125. Haverstick DM, Gray LS. Lymphocyte adhesion mediated by lymphocyte function-associated antigen-1. II. Interaction between phorbol ester- and cAMP sensitive pathways. J Immunol 1992; 149:397-402.

126. van Seventer GA, Bonvini E, Yamada H et al. Costimulation of TCR/CD3-mediated activation of resting of human CD4+ T-cells by LFA-1 ligand ICAM-1 involves prolonged inositol phospholipid hydrolysis and sustained increase of intracellular Ca++ levels. J Immunol 1992; 149:3872-3880.

127. Loefgren RJ, Ng-Sikorski J, Sioelander A et al. β2 integrin engagement triggers actin polymerization and phosphatidylinositol trisphosphate formation in non-adherent human neutrophils. J Cell Biol 1993; 123:1597-1605.

128. Pardi R, Inverardi L, Rugarli C et al. Antigen-receptor complex stimulation triggers protein kinase C-dependent CD11a/CD18-cytoskeleton association in T lymphocytes. J Cell Biol 1992; 116:1211-1220.

129. Karlheinz P, O'Toole TE. Modulation of cell adhesion by changes in αLβ2 (LFA-1, CD11a/CD18) cytoplasmic domain/ cytoskeleton interaction. J Exp Med 1995; 181:315-326.

130. Dustin ML, Carpen O, Springer TA. Regulation of locomotion and cell-cell contact

area by the LFA-1 and ICAM-1 adhesion receptors. J Immunol 1992; 148:2654-2663.

131. Larson RS, Hibbs ML, Springer TA. The leukocyte integrin LFA-1 reconstituted by cDNA transfection in an nonhematopoietic cell line is functionally active and not transiently regulated. Cell Regul 1990; 1: 359-367.

132. Landis RC, Bennett RI, Hogg N. A novel LFA-1 activation epitope maps to the I domain. J Cell Biol 1993; 120: 1519-1527.

133. Dransfield I, Cabanas C, Craig A et al. Divalent cation regulation of the function of the leukocyte integrin LFA-1. J Cell Biol 1992; 116:219-226.

134. Keizer GD, Visser W, Vliem M et al A monoclonal antibody (NKI-L16) directed against a unique epitope on the α-chain of human leukocyte function-associated antigen 1 induces homotypic cell-cell interactions. J Immunol 1988; 140:1393-1400.

135. van Kooyk Y, Weder P, Hogervorst F et al. Activation of LFA-1 through Ca^{2+}-dependent epitope stimulates leukocyte adhesion. J Cell Biol 1991; 112:345-354.

136. Dransfield I, Hogg N. Regulated expression of Mg^{2+} binding epitope on leukocyte integrin α subunit. EMBO J 1989; 8: 3759-3765.

137. Detmers PA, Wright SD, Olsen E et al. Aggregation of complement receptors on human neutrophils in the absence of ligand. J Cell Biol 1987; 105:1137-1145.

138. Pyszniak AM, Welder CA, Takei F. Cell surface distribution of high-avidity LFA-1 detected by soluble ICAM-1-coated midrospheres. J Immunol 1994; 152:5241-5249.

139. Robinson MK, Andrew D, Rosen H et al. Antibody against the Leu-CAM β-chain (CD18) promotes both LFA-1 and CR3-dependent adhesion events. J Immunol 1992; 148:1080-1085.

140. van Kooyk Y, Figdor CG. Integrins and integrin regulation. In: Shimizu Y, ed. Lymphocyte Adhesion Molecules. Austin: RG Landes, 1993:1-25.

141. Ortlepp S, Stephens PE, Hogg N et al. Antibodies that activate β2 integrins can generate different ligand binding sites. Eur J Immunol 1995; 25:637-643.

142. Anderson DC, Miller LJ, Schmalstieg FC et al. Contributions of the Mac-1 glycoprotein family to adherence-dependent granulocyte functions: structure-function assessments employing subunit-specific monoclonal antibodies. J Immunol 1986; 137:15-27.

143. Myones BL, Dalzell JG, Hogg N et al. Neutrophil and monocyte cell surface p150,95 has iC3b-receptor (CR4) activity resembling CR3. J Clin Invest 1988; 82:640-651.

144. Keizer GD, te Velde AA, Schwarting R et al. Role of p150,95 in adhesion, migration, chemotaxis and phagocytosis of human monocytes. Eur J Immunol 1987; 17: 1317-1322.

145. Buyon JP, Abramson SP, Philips MR et al. Dissociation between increased expression of Gp165/95 and homotypic neutrophil aggregation. J Immunol 1988; 140:3156-3160.

146. Vedder NB, Harlan JM. Increased surface expression of CD11b/CD18 (Mac-1) is not required for stimulated neutrophils adherence to cultured endothelium. J Clin Invest 1988; 81:676-682.

147. Philips MR, Buyon JP, Winchester R et al. Up-regulation of the iC3b receptor (CR3) is neither necessary nor sufficient to promote neutrophil aggregation. J Clin Invest 1988; 82:495-501.

148. Vedder NB, Harlan JM. Increased surface expression of CD11b/CD18 (Mac-1) is not required for stimulated neutrophil adherence to cultured endothelium. J Clin Invest 1988; 81:676-682.

149. Detmers PA, Wright SD, Olsen E et al. Aggregation of complement receptors on human neutrophils in the absence of ligand. J Cell Biol 1987; 105:1137-1145.

150. Altieri DC, Edgington TS. The saturable high affinity association of coagulation factor X to ADP stimulated human monocytes defines a novel function of the Mac-1 receptor. J Biol Chem 1988; 263: 7007-7015.

151. Diamond MS, Springer TA. A subpopulation of Mac-1 (CD11b/CD18) molecules mediated neurophil adhesion to ICAM-1 and fibrinogen. J Cell Biol 1993; 120:545-556.

152. Murphy PM. The molecular biology of leukocyte chemoattractant receptors. Annu Rev

Immunol 1994; 12:593-633.

153. Carlos TM, Harlan JM. Leukocytes-endothelial adhesion molecules. Blood. 1994; 84:2068-2101.

154. Butcher EC. Leukocyte-endothelial cell recognition: three (or more) steps to specificity and diversity. Cell 1991; 64:1033-1036.

155. Lasky LA. Selectins: Interpreters of cell-specific carbohydrate information during inflammation. Science 1992; 258:964-969.

156. Ley K, Gaehtgens P, Fennie C et al. Lectin-like cell adhesion molecule 1 mediates leukocyte rolling in mesenteric venules in vivo. Blood 1991; 77:2553-2555.

157. von Andrian UH, Chambers JD, McEvoy LM et al. Two-step mode of leukocyte-endothelial cell interaction in inflammation: distinct role for LECAM-1 and the leukocyte β2 integrins in vivo. Proc Natl Acad Sci USA 1991; 88:7538-7542.

158. Lawrence MB, Springer TA. Leukocytes roll on a selectin at physiologic flow rates: Distinction from and prerequisite for adhesion though integrins. Cell 1991; 65:859-873.

159. Abbassi O, Kishimoto TK, McIntire LV et al. E-selectin supports neutrophil rolling in vitro under conditions of flow. J Clin Invest 1993; 92:2719-2730.

160. Jones DA, Abbassi O, McIntire LV et al. P-selected mediates neutrophil rolling on histamine-stimulated endothelial cells. Biophys J 1993; 65:1560-1569.

161. Lawrence MB, Bainton DF, Springer TA. Neutrophil tethering to and rolling on E-selectin are separable by requirement for L-selectin. Immunity 1994; 1:137-145.

162. Mayadas TN, Johnson RC, Rayburn H et al. Leukocyte rolling and extravasation are severely compromised in P-selectin-deficient mice. Cell 1993; 74:541-554.

163. Alon R, Hammer DA, Springer TA. Lifetime of the P-selectin-carbohydrate bond and its response to tensile force in hydrodynamic flow. Nature 1995; 374:539-542.

164. Lorant DE, Patel KD, McIntyre TM et al. Coexpression of GMP-140 and PAF by endothelium stimulated by histamine or thrombin: a juxtacrine system for adhesion and activation of neutrophils. J Cell Biol 1991; 115:223-234.

165. Huber AR, Kunkel SL, Todd RF III et al. Regulation of transendothelial migration by endogenous interleukin-8. Science 1991; 254:99-102.

166. Tanaka Y, Adams DH, Hubscher S et al. T-cell adhesion induced by proteoglycan-immobilized cytokine MIP-1β. Nature 1993; 361:79-82.

167. Hetchman DH, Cylbusky MI, Fuchs HJ et al. Intravascular IL-8: inhibitor of polymorphonuclear leukocyte accumulation at sites of acute inflammation. J Immunol 1991; 147:883-892.

168. Kubes P, Suzuki M, Granger DN. Nitric oxide: an endogenous modulator of leukocyte adhesion. Proc Natl Acad Sci USA 1991; 88:4651-4655.

169. Gamble JR, Khew-Goodall Y, Vadas MA. Transforming growth factor-β inhibits E-selectin expression on human endothelial cells. J Immunol 1993; 150:4494-4503.

170. Bargatze RF, Butcher EC. Rapid G protein-regulated activation event involved in lymphocyte binding to high endothelial venules. J Exp Med 1993; 178: 367-372.

171. Morigi M, Zoja C, Figliuzzi M et al. Fluid shear stress modulates expression of adhesion molecules by endothelial cells. Blood 1995; 85:1696-1703.

172. Kavanaugh AF, Lightfoot E, Lipsky PE et al. Role of CD11/CD18 in adhesion and transendothelial migration of T cells. Analysing utilizing CD18-deficient T cell clones. J Immunol 1991; 146:4149-4156.

173. Diamond MS, Alon R, Parkos CA et al. Heparin is an adhesive ligand for the leukocyte integrin Mac-1 (CD11b/CD18). J Cell Biol 1995; 130:1473-1482.

174. Penberthy TW, Jiang Y, Luscinskas FW et al. MCP-1-stimulated monocytes preferentially utilize beta 2-integrins to migrate on laminin and fibronectin. Am J Physiol 1995; 269:C60-68.

175. Alon R, Kassner PD, Woldemar Carr M et al. The integrin VLA-4 supports tethering and rolling in flow on VCAM-1. J Cell Biol 1995; 128:1243-1253.

176. Berlin C, Bargatze RF, von Andrian UH et al. α4 integrins mediate lymphocyte attachment and rolling under physiologic flow. Cell 1995; 80:413-422.

177. Luscinskas FW, Ding H, Lichtman AH. P-selectin and vascular cell adhesion molecule 1 mediate rolling and arrest, respectively, of CD4+ T lymphocyte on tumor necrosis factor α-activated vascular endothelium under flow. J Exp Med 1995; 181:1179-1186.

178. Issekutz AC, Issekutz TB. Monocyte migration to arthritis in the rat utilizes both CD11/CD18 and very late activation antigen 4 integrin mechanisms. J Exp Med 1995; 181:1197-1203.

179. Schweighoffer T, Shaw S. Adhesion cascades: diversity through combinatorial strategies. Curr Opin Cell Biol 1992; 4:824-829.

180. Altin JG, Pagler EB, Parish CR. Evidence for cell surface association of CD2 and LFA-1 (CD11a/CD18) on T lymphocytes. Eur J Immunol 1994; 24:450-457.

181. Kew RR, Grimaldi CM, Furie MB et al. Human neutrophil FcγRIII and formyl peptide receptors are functionally linked during formyl-methionyl-leucyl-phenylalanine-induced chemotaxis. J Immunol 1992; 149:989-997.

182. Petty HR, Todd RF III. Receptor-receptor interactions of complement receptor type 3 in neutrophil membranes. J Leuk Biol 1993; 54:492.

183. Zhou M, Todd RF III, van de Winkel JGJ et al. Cocapping of the leukoadhesin molecules complement receptor type 3 and lymphocyte function-associated antigen-1 with Fcγ receptor III on human neutrophils. J Immunol 1993; 150:3030-3041.

184. Xue W, Kindzelskii AL, Todd RF III et al. Physical association of complement receptor type 3 and urokinase-type plasminogen activator receptor in neutrophils membranes. J Immunol 1994 152:4630-4640.

185. Poo H, Krauss JC, Mayo-Bond L et al. Interaction of the Fcγ receptor Type IIIB with complement receptor type 3 in fibroblasts transfectants: evidence from lateral diffusion and resonance energy transfer studies. J Mol Biol 1995; 247:597-603. J Mol Biol 1994;247:597

186. Stockl J, Majdic O, Pickl WF et al. Granulocyte activation via a binding site near the C-terminal region of complement receptor type 3 α-chain (CD11b) potentially involved in intramembrane complex formation with glycosylphosphatidylinositol-anchored FcγRIIIB (CD16) molecules. J Immunol 1995;154:5452-5463.

187. Hedman H, Lundgren E. Regulation of LFA-1 avidity in human B cells: requirement for dephosphorylation events for high avidity ICAM-1 binding. J Immunol 1992; 149:2290-2295.

188. Cohen P, Holmes CFB, Tsukitani Y. Okadaic acid: a new probe for the study of cellular regulation. Trends Biochem Sci 1990; 15:98-102.

189. Li R, Nortamo P, Kantor C et al. A leukocyte integrin binding peptide from intracellular adhesion molecule-2 stimulates T cells adhesion and natural killer cell activity. J Biol Chem 1993; 268:21474-21477.

190. Rabb H, Michishita M, Sharma CP et al. Cytoplasmatic tail of human complement receptor type 3 (CR3, CD11b/CD18) regulates ligand avidity and the internalization of occupied receptors. J Immunol 1993; 151:990-1002.

191. Annenkov A, Ortlepp S, Hogg N. The β2 integrin Mac-1 but not p150,95 associates with FcγRIIA. Eur J Immunol 1996; 26: 207-212.

192. Bohuslav J, Horejsi AL, Hansmann C et al. Urokinase plasminogen activator receptor, β2-integrins, and src-kinases within a single receptor complex of human monocytes. J Exp Med 1995; 181:1381-1390.

193. Arnaout MA. Structure and function of the leukocyte adhesion molecules CD11/CD18. Blood 1990; 75:1037-1050.

194. Malhotra V, Hogg N, Sim RB. Ligand binding by the p150,95 Ag of U937 monocytic cells: properties in common with complement receptors type 3 (CR3). Eur J Immunol 1986; 16:1117-1123.

195. Myones BL, Daizell JG, Hogg N et al. Neutrophil and monocyte cell surface p150,95 has iC3b-receptors (CR4) activity resembling CR3. J Clin Invest 1988; 82:640-651.

196. Bilsland CAG, Diamond MS, Sim RB. The leukocyte integrin p150,95 (CD11c/CD18) as a receptor for iC3b. J Immunol 1994; 152:4582-4589.

197. Languino LR, Plescia J, Duperray A et al.

Fibrinogen mediates leukocyte adhesion to vascular endothelium through an ICAM-1-dependent pathway. Cell 1993; 73: 1423-1434.

198. Altieri DC, Plescia J, Plow EF. The structural motif glycine-190-valine 202 of the fibrinogen γ chain interacts with CD11b/CD18 integrin (αMβ2, Mac-1) and promotes leukocyte adhesion. J Biol Chem 1993; 268:1847-1853.

199. Elmer GS, Edgington TS. Monoclonal antibody to an activation neoepitope of αMβ2 inhibits multiple αMβ2 functions. J Immunol 1994; 152:5836-5844.

200. Marks RM, Todd RF III, Ward PA. Rapid induction of neutrophil-endothelial adhesion by endothelial complement fixation. Nature 1989; 339:314-317.

201. Vercellotti GM, Platt JL, Bach FH et al. Neutrophil adhesion to xenogeneic endothelium via iC3b. J Immunol 1991; 146:730-734.

202. Yeo EL, Sheppard JI, Fuerstein IA. Role of P-selectin and leukocyte activation in polymorphonuclear cell adhesion to surface adherent activated platelets under physiologic shear conditions (an injury vessel wall model). Blood 1994; 83:2498-2507.

203. Altieri DC, Bader R, Mannucci PM et al. Oligospecificity of the cellular adhesion receptor Mac-1 encompasses an inducible recognition specificity for fibrinogen. J Cell Biol 1988; 107:1893-1900.

204. Wright SD, Weitz JI, Huang AJ et al. Complement receptor type 3 (CD11b/CD18) of human polymorphonuclear leukocytes recognizes fibrinogen. Proc Natl Acad Sci USA 1988; 85:7734-7738.

205. Trezzini C, Jungi TW, Kuhnert P et al. Fibrinogen association with human monocytes: evidence for constitutive expression of fibrinogen receptors and for involvement of Mac-1 (CD18, CR3) in the binding. Biochem Biophys Res Commun 1988; 156:477-484.

206. Gustafson EJ, Lukasiewicz H, Wachtfogel YT et al. High molecular weight kininogen inhibits fibrinogen binding to cytoadhesins of neutrophils and platelets. J Cell Biol 1989; 109:377-387.

207. Altieri DC, Agbanyo FR, Plescia J et al. A unique recognition site mediates the interaction of fibrinogen with leukocyte integrin Mac-1 (CD11b/CD18). J Biol Chem 1990; 265:12119-12122.

208. Loike JD, Sodeik B, Cao L et al. CD11c/CD18 on neutrophils recognizes a domain at the N terminus of the Aα chain of fibrinogen. Proc Natl Acad Sci USA 1991; 88:1044-1048.

209. Postigo AA, Corbi AL, Sanchez-Madrid F et al. Regulated expression and function of CD11c/CD18 integrin on human B lymphocytes. Relation between attachment to fibrinogen and triggering of proliferation through CD11c/CD18). J Exp Med 1991; 174:1313-1321.

210. Altieri DC, Morissey JH, Edgington TS. Adhesive receptor Mac-1 coordinates the activation of factor X on stimulated cells of monocyte and myeloid differentiation: an alternative initiation of the coagulation protease cascade. Proc Natl Acad Sci USA 1988; 85:7462-7468.

211. Altieri DC, Etingin OR, Fair DS et al. Structurally homologous ligand binding of integrin Mac-1 and viral glycoprotein C receptors. Science 1991; 254:1200-1202.

212. Hoffman M, Monroe DM, Roberts HR et al. Human monocytes support factor X activation by factor VIIa, independent of tissue factor: implications for the therapeutic machanism of high dose factor VIIa in hemophilia. Blood 1994; 83:38-42.

213. Moyle M, Foster DL, McGrath DE et al. A hookworm glycoprotein that inhibits neutrophil functions is a ligand of the integrin CD11b/CD18. J Biol Chem 1994; 269:10008-10015.

214. Ross GD, Reed W. The leukocyte integrin and complement receptor CR3 (CD11b/CD18) has specificity for C3dg, as well as for iC3b. FASEB J 1992; 6:A2013.

215. Wright SD, Jong MTC. Adhesion-promoting receptors on human macrophages recognize *Escherichia coli* by binding to lipopolysaccharide. J Exp Med 1986; 164:1876-1888.

216. Talamas-Rohana P, Wright SD, Lennartz MR et al. Lipophosphoglycan from *Leishmania mexicana* promastigotes binds to members of the CR3, p150,95 and LFA-1 fam-

ily of leukocyte integrins. J Immunol 1990; 144:4817-4824.

217. Russel DG, Wright SD. Complement receptor type 3 (CR3) binds to an Arg-Gly-Asp-containing region on the major surface glycoprotein, gp63, of *Leishmania* promastigotes. J Exp Med 1988; 168: 279-292.

218. Mosser DM, Springer TA, Diamond MS. *Leishmania* promastigotes require opsonic complement to bind to the human leukocyte integrin Mac-1 (CD11b/CD18). J Cell Biol 1992; 116:511-520.

219. Relman D, Tuomanen E, Falkow S et al. Recognition of a bacterial adhesin by an integrin: macrophage CR3 (αMβ2, CD11b/CD18) binds filamentous hemagglutinin of *Bordella pertussis*. Cell 1990; 61:1375-1382.

220. Gbarah A, Gahmberg CG, Ofek I et al. Identification of the leukocyte adhesion molecules CD11 and CD18 as receptors for type 1-fimbriated (mannose-specific) *Escherichia coli*. Infect Immun 1991; 59:4524-4530.

221. Ross GD, Cain JA, Myones BL et al. Specificity of membrane complement receptor type three (CR3) for β-glucans. Complement 1987; 4:61-74.

222. Newman SL, Chaturvedi S, Klain BS. The WI-1 antigen of *Blastomyces dermatitidis* yeasts mediates binding to human macrophage CD11b/CD18 (CR3) and CD14. J Immunol 1995; 154: 753-761.

223. Gresham HD, Adams SP, Brown EJ. Ligand binding specificity of the leukocyte response integrin expressed by human neutrophils. J Biol Chem 1992; 267:13895-13902.

224. Ishibashi Y, Claus S, Relman DA. *Bordetella pertussis* filamentous hemagglutin interacts with a leukocyte signal transduction complex and stimulates bacterial adherence to monocyte CR3 (CD11b/CD18). J Exp Med 1994; 180:1225-1233.

225. Claiborne Johnston S, Dustin ML, Hibbs ML et al. On the species specificity of the interaction of LFA-1 with intercellular adhesion molecules. J Immunol 1990; 145:1181-1187.

226. Randi AM, Hogg N. I domain of β2 integrin lymphocyte function-associated antigen-1 contains a binding site for ligand

intercellular adhesion molecule-1. J Biol Chem 1994; 269:12395-12398.

227. Diamond MS, Garcia-Aguilar J, Bickford JK et al. The I domain is a major recognition site on the leukocyte integrin Mac-1 (CD11b/CD18) for four distinct adhesion ligands. J Cell Biol 1993; 120:1031-1043.

228. Landis RC, McDowall A, Holness CLL et al. Involvement of the "I" domain of LFA-1 in selective binding to ligands ICAM-1 and ICAM-3. J Cell Biol 1994; 126: 529-537.

229. Champe M, McIntyre W, Berman PW. Monoclonal antibodies that block the activity of leukocyte function-associated antigen 1 recognize three discrete epitopes in the inserted domain of CD11a. J Biol Chem 1995; 270:1388-1394.

230. Huang C, Springer TA. A binding interface on the I domain of Lymphocyte function-associated antigen-1 (LFA-1) required for specific interaction with intercellular adhesion molecule 1 (ICAM-1). J Biol Chem 1995; 270:19008-19016.

231. Michishita M, Videm V, Arnaout MA. A novel divalent cation-binding site in the α domain of the β2 integrin CR3 (CD11b/CD18) is essential for ligand binding. Cell 1993; 72:857-867.

232. Violette SM, Rusche JR, Purdy SR et al. Differences in the binding of blocking anti-CD11b monoclonal antibodies to the A-domain of CD11b. J Immunol 1995; 155:3092-3101.

233. Zhou L, Lee DHS, Plescia J et al. Differential ligand binding specificities of recombinant CD11b/CD18 integrin I-domain. J Biol Chem 1994; 269:17075-17079.

234. Dransfield I, Cabanas C, Barrett J et al. Interaction of leukocyte integrins with ligand is necessary but not sufficient for function. J Cell Biol 1992; 116:1527-1535.

235. Kuijpers KC, Kuijpers TW, Zeijlemaker WP et al. Analysis of the role of leukocyte function-associated antigen-1 in activation of human influenza virus-specific T cell clones. J Immunol 1990; 144:3281-3287.

236. Altieri DC, Edgington TS. A monoclonal antibody reacting with distinct adhesion molecules defines a transition in the functional state of the receptor CD11b/CD18

(Mac-1). J Immunol 1988; 141:2656-2660.

237. Staunton DE, Dustin ML, Erickson HP et al. The arrangement of the immunoglobulin-like domains of ICAM-1 and the binding sites for LFA-1 and rhinovirus. Cell 1990; 61:243-254.

238. Berendt AR, McDowall A, Craig AG et al. The binding site on ICAM-1 for *Plasmodium falciparum*-infected erytrocytes overlaps, but is distinct from the LFA-1 binding site. Cell 1992; 68:71-81.

239. Sadhu C, Lipsky B, Erickson HP et al. LFA-1 binding site in ICAM-3 contains a conserved motif and non-contiguous amino acids. Cell Adhes Commun 1994; 2: 429-440.

240. Bailly P, Tontti E, Hermand P et al. The red cell LW blood group protein is an intercellular adhesion molecule which binds to CD11/CD18 leukocyte integrins. Eur J Immunol 1995; 25: 3316-3320.

241. Diamond MS, Staunton DE, de Fougerolles AR et al. ICAM-1 (CD54): a counter-receptor for Mac-1 (CD11b/CD18). J Cell Biol 1990; 111:3129-3139.

242. Diamond MS, Staunton DE, Marlin SD et al. Binding of the integrin Mac-1 (CD11b/CD18) to the third immunoglobulin-like domain of ICAM-1 (CD54) and its regulation by glycosylation. Cell 1991; 65:961-971.

243. Miller J, Knorr R, Ferrone M et al. Intercellular adhesion molecule-1 dimerization and its consequences for adhesion mediated by lymphocyte function associated-1. J Exp Med 1995; 182:1231-1241.

244. Li R, Xie J, Kantor C et al. A peptide derived from the intercellular adhesion molecule-2 regulates the avidity of the leukocyte integrins CD11b/CD18 and CD11c/CD18. J Cell Biol 1995; 129:1143-1153.

245. Somersalo K, Carpén O, Saksela E et al. Activation of NK cell migration by leukocyte integrin binding peptide from ICAM-2. J Biol Chem 1995; 270:8629-8636.

246. Edwards CP, Champe M, Gonzalzs T et al. Identification of amino acids in the CD11a I-domain important for binding of the leukocyte function-associated antigen-1 (LFA-1) to intercellular adhesion molecule-1 (ICAM-1). J Biol Chem 1995; 270:12635-12640.

247. Stanley P, Bates PA, Harvey J et al. Integrin LFA-1 α subunit contains an ICAM-1 binding site in domains V and VI. EMBO J 1994; 13:1790-1798.

248. Ueda T, Rieu P, Brayer J et al. Identification of the complement iC3b binding site in the β2 integrin CR3 (CD11b/CD18). Proc Natl Acad Sci USA 1994; 91:10680-10684.

249. Kamata T, Wright R, Takada Y. Critical threonine and aspartic acid residues within the I domains of β2 integrins for interactions with intercellular adhesion molecule 1 (ICAM-1) and C3bi. J Biol Chem 1995; 270:12531-12535.

250. Kamata T, Takada Y. Direct binding of collagen to the I domain of integrin α2β1 (VLA-2, CD49b/CD29) in a divalent cation-independent manner. J Biol Chem 1994; 269:26006-26010.

251. Horiuchi T, Macon KJ, Engler JA et al. Site-directed mutagenesis of the region around Cys-241 of complement component C2: evidence for a C4b binding site. J Immunol 1991; 147:584-589.

252. Rieu P, Ueda T, Haruta I et al. The A-domain of β2 integrin CR3 (CD11b/CD18) is a receptor for the hookworm-derived neutrophil adhesion inhibitor NIF. J Cell Biol 1994; 127:2081-2091.

253. Bergelson JM, Chan BMC, Finberg RW et al. The integrin VLA-2 binds Echovirus 1 and extracellular matrix ligands by different mechanisms. J Clin Invest 1993; 92:232-239.

254. Ikeda Y, Handa M, Kawano K et al. The role of von Willebrand factor and fibrinogen in platelet aggregation under varying shear stress. J Clin Invest 1991; 87: 1234-1240.

255. Muchowski PJ, Zhang L, Chang ER et al. Functional interaction between the integrin antagonist neutrophil inhibitory factor and the I domain of CD11b/CD18. J Biol Chem 1994; 42:26419-26423.

256. Farrell DH, Thiagarajan P, Chung DW et al. Role of fibrinogen α and γ chain sites in platelet aggregation. Proc Natl Acad Sci USA 1992; 89: 10729-10732.

257. Elmer GS, Edgington TS. Monoclonal antibody to an activation neoepitope of αMβ2

inhibits multiple αMβ2 functions. J Immunol 1994; 152:5836-5844.

258. Coombe DR, Watt SM, Parish CR. Mac-1 (CD11b/CD18) and CD45 mediate the adhesion of hematopoietic progenitor cells to stromal cell elements via recognition of stromal heparan sulfate. Blood 1994; 84: 739-752.

259. Webb LMC, Ehrengruber MU, Clark-Lewis I et al. Binding to heparan sulfate or heparin enhances neutrophil responses to interleukin 8. Proc Natl Acad Sci USA 1993; 90:7158-7162.

260. Giger U, Boxer LA, Simpson PJ et al. Deficiency of leukocyte surface glycoproteins Mo1, LFA-1 and Leu M5 in a dog with recurrent bacterial infections: an animal model. Blood 1987; 69:1622-1630.

261. Kehrli ME, Ackermann MR, Shuster DE et al. Animal model of human disease. Bovine leukocyte adhesion deficiency. β2 integrin deficiency in young Holstein cattle. Am J Pathol 1992; 140:1489-1492.

262. Etzioni A, Frydman M, Pollack S et al. Recurrent severe infections caused by a novel leukocyte adhesion deficiency. New Engl J Med 1992; 327:1789-1792.

263. Wilson RW, Ballantyne CM, Smith CW et al. Gene targeting yields a CD18-mutant mouse for study of inflammation. J Immunol 1993; 151:1571-1578.

264. Kishimoto TK, Hollander N, Roberts TM et al. Heterogeneous mutations in the β subunit common to the LFA-1, Mac-1, and p150,95 glycoproteins cause leukocyte adhesion deficiency. Cell 1987; 50:193-202.

265. Arnaout MA, Dana N, Gupta SK et al. Point mutations impairing cell surface expression of the common β subunit (CD18) in a patient with leukocyte adhesion molecule (LeuCAM) deficiency. J Clin Invest 1990; 85:977-981.

266. Nelson C, Rabb H, Arnaout MA. Generic cause of leukocyte adhesion molecule deficiency. Abnormal splicing and a missense mutation in a conserved region of CD18 impair cell surface expression of β2 integrins. J Biol Chem 1992; 267:3351-3357.

267. Hibbs ML, Wardlaw AJ, Stacker SA et al. Transfection of cells from patients with leukocyte adhesion deficiency with an integrin β subunit (CD18) restores lymphocyte function-associated antigen-1 expression and function. J Clin Invest 1990; 85:674-681.

268. Lee J-O, Bankston LA, Arnaout MA et al. Two conformations of the integrin A-domain (I-domain): a pathway for activation? Structure 1995; 3:1333-1340.

269. Matsushita T, Sadler JE. Identification of amino acid residues essential for von Willebrand factor binding to platelet glycoprotein Ib. J Biol Chem 1995; 270: 13406-13414.

270. Cooney KA, Ginsburg D. Comparative analysis of type 2b von Willebrand disease mutations: implications for the mechanism of von Willebrand factor binding to platelets. Blood 1996; 87:2322-2328.

271. Bork P, Bairoch A. Extracellular protein modules. Trends Biochem Sci 1995; 3.

C2 and Factor B

INTRODUCTION TO THE COMPLEMENT CASCADE

Complement, which derives its name from the old observation that one or more serum heat-labile component(s) help or "complement" the lytic function of antibodies, is the major humoral effector system of defense.[1] Complement mediates osmotic lysis of target cells, facilitates phagocytosis by binding (= opsonization) to foreign organisms, activates inflammatory processes through its chemotactic and granule releasing (anaphylotoxic) function, solubilizes potentially tissue-damaging immune complexes and, finally, regulates immune responses.

This system comprises more than 30 different constituent proteins that function as proenzymes, enzymes, enzyme cofactors and cell surface receptors for biologically active fragments of complement proteins.[2] This complex array of proteins exhibits a limited number of conserved and often repeated modules suggesting that during evolution multiple gene duplication and exon shuffling events took place to obtain the present day members.[3]

Two-thirds of the proteins are soluble in plasma and about one-third are membrane-associated, integral or PI-linked. Fifteen different components participate in the complement activation pathway through a process of sequential proenzyme activation consisting of cleavage of one or two peptide bonds. Most of them are designated by the letter C and a number from 1 to 9, C1 being a complex of three distinct proteins, C1q, C1r and C1s. Four additional members of this group are designated factor B, factor D, MBP (membrane-binding protein) and MASP (membrane-binding protein associated serine protease) (Table 5.1).

The process of complement activation is strictly and efficiently controlled by a large group of membrane-associated or soluble proteins. The function of these regulatory proteins is to provide proportionality between the extent of the activation signal and the level of complement activation, thus protecting the host from potentially destructive consequences. The main function of the membrane-associated regulatory proteins is to inactivate the enzymatic system at the level of the host cells to allow focusing of complement on foreign targets, i.e., microbial cell

Table 5.1. Proteins of the complement cascade

Localization	Function		
	Involved in activation	**Receptor**	**Regulatory**
Plasma	C1q, C1r, C1s D, MBP, MASP, C4, C3, **<u>C2</u>**, **<u>B</u>** C5, C6, C7, C8, C9		C1 INH, C4BP, C3a/C5a INA, H, I, P, S
Cell membrane		C1qr, C5aR, CR1, CR2 **<u>Mac-1/CR3, p150, 95/CR4</u>**	CR1, DAF, MCP, HRF, CD59

The components encompassing a VWFA module are underlined and in bold.

membranes. Finally, a number of cell-surface components function as receptors for biologically active fragments of complement proteins, including CR3 (CD11b/Mac-1) and CR4 (CD11c/p150,95) that are described in the chapter on VWFA-containing β2 integrins (see chapter 4).

It has been established that the enzymatically active forms of a complement protein or protein complex are indicated by an overbar, as in $\overline{C3bBb}$, which indicates the complex between C3b and Bb components. Proteolytic cleavage fragments of complement proteins generated during the complement cascade are symbolized by lower-case letters, as in C4a and C4b where, *a* indicates the smaller fragment. The only exception is C2 in which the smaller fragment is indicated by *b*.

Complement can be activated by distinct pathways, the classical, which is the major effector mechanism for antibody-mediated immune response, the alternative, which is activated by charged regions on the surface of pathogens and foreign cells and the lectin pathway, which is triggered by carbohydrates on the surface of pathogens. The major complement component C3 is common to all pathways.[4] There are two key steps in the activation of the complement system and these are the formation of the bi-molecular complexes designated C3 ($\overline{C4b2a}$ for the classical and $\overline{C3bBb}$ for the alternative pathway) and C5

($\overline{C4b2a3b}$ for the classical and $\overline{C3bBb3b}$ for the alternative pathway) convertases. These multiprotein complexes are capable of splitting the α chain of C3 (and C5), thereby initiating the numerous biological activities that depend upon complement activation. In the classical pathway, complement is activated most frequently by the interaction of the C1 complex with immune complexes or aggregates containing immunoglobulins (Ig). In the alternative pathway, complement is activated by the interaction of several non-Ig activators such as bacteria, LPS, fungi, yeast etc. with C3b (on cell surface) or with a C3b-like form of C3, $C3(H_2O)$ in the fluid phase (Fig. 5.1).

The C1 of the classical pathway is a large multimeric molecular complex composed of 22 polypeptides 18 of which (six A, six B and six C polypeptide chains) of about 25kD each form the Ig-binding C1q subunit. Each type of polypeptide contains an N-terminal region of 81 residues of collagen-like sequences (Gly-Xaa-Yaa)[5] and three different polypeptides interact in a 1:1:1 ratio to form a heterotrimeric triple helix with one interruption located at approximately the middle of the collagen rod. Thus, one C1q component is composed of six triple helices aligned in parallel for half of their length and then the remainder of each rod bends outwards to end in a noncollagenous globular domain. Two com-

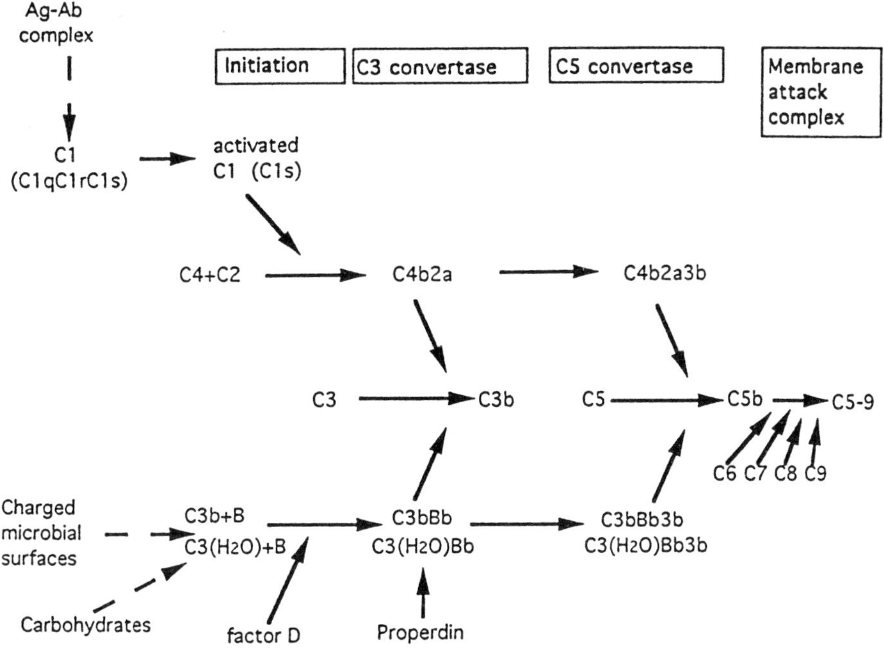

Fig. 5.1. *Major activation steps in the complement pathways are shown.*

plexes of C1r - C1s proenzymes of about 85 kD form a flexible linear tetramer and then associate with C1q. When C1q interacts with an activator (i.e. Ig-Ag complex) a conformational change ensues allowing autoactivation of C1r to yield $\overline{\text{C1r}}$, which is followed by the activation of C1s to $\overline{\text{C1s}}$. Both C1r and C1s are serine proteases.

The C1 complex generates from C4 both C4a (one of the three anaphylotoxins, the others being C3a and C5a) and C4b from C4, thus allowing interaction of the latter polypeptide with the proenzyme C2. This bimolecular complex is activated by $\overline{\text{C1s}}$, which removes C2b (in this case the smaller fragment) from the $\overline{\text{C4b2}}$ complex, leading to the formation of the active $\overline{\text{C4b2a}}$ C3 convertase.[6] Activation of the C1 complex is under the control of the C1-inhibitor (C1-INH), which prevents spontaneous activation of C1, and rapidly forms a proteolytically inactive 1:1 covalent complex with C1r and C1s, thus preventing overactivation of the system. The C4b binding protein (C4bp) regulates the C4b2a C3 convertase by inhibiting its formation and by accelerating its decay via

the displacement of C2a from C4b or acting as cofactor for factor I. Visualized by electron microscopy, the molecule has a spider like structure consisting of seven thin, elongated, and flexible subunits, to which C4b binds.[7,8]

The serine protease factor I also can cause rapid loss of the biological activity associated with C4b by cleaving it into two fragments. The membrane-associated regulatory protein complement receptor type 1 (CR1), a high affinity C4b and C3b receptor,[9,10] displays cofactor activity for the factor I leading to permanent inactivation,[11] processing and clearing of immune complexes. The membrane cofactor protein (MCP)[12,13] also binds to C4b and C3b and is the most efficient cofactor for the I-mediated cleavage of C3b. The decay accelerating factor (DAF/CD55)[14] does not exhibit cofactor activity in the presence of factor I but instead it reversibly prevents assembly of the C3 convertases by competing with C2 for the binding to C4b.[15-17]

In the alternative pathway there is an amplification loop whereby C3 is cleaved by preformed $\overline{\text{C3bBb}}$ or by $\overline{\text{C3(H}_2\text{O)Bb}}$

into C3a and C3b. The latter polypeptide binds the inactive proenzyme B[18] from which the Ba fragment is removed by the active factor D in a similar way to the cleavage of C4b2 by C1s,[19] one major difference being that factor D does not require enzymatic cleavage to be activated.[20] The resulting active $\overline{C3bBb}$ or $\overline{C3(H_2O)Bb}$ is the alternative pathway C3 convertase. The difference between $\overline{C3bBb}$ and $\overline{C3(H_2O)Bb}$ is that the former is particle-bound and the latter is in the fluid phase. The alternative pathway C3 convertase is unstable unless it is stabilized by properdin.

Factor H, in an analogous manner to the C4bp-C4b interaction in the classical pathway, regulates the C3 convertase $\overline{C3bBb}$ by competing for factor B binding to C3b and by accelerating the decay of the $\overline{C3bBb}$ complexes. In the presence of factor H, CR1 and MCP factor I cleaves C3b leaving an inactive iC3b and later even smaller fragments. The microenvironment of particle-bound C3b determines whether C3b will bind to factor B, which causes activation in the pathway, or to factor H, which will abrogate the activation. The conservation of the binding sites of C3 for the different constituents[21,22] is pronounced as C3 from several species contain highly homologous residues in these sites.[23] Both Mac-1(CR3/CD11b)[24] and p150,95 (CR4/CD11c)[25] bind iC3b and mediate phagocytosis of iC3b-coated microbial particles.

Finally, the C3 convertases ($\overline{C4b2a}$ and $\overline{C3bBb}$) split C3 in C3a and C3b, and the latter participates in the formation of the C5 convertases $\overline{C4b2a3b}$ and $\overline{C3bBb3b}$. The C5 convertases split C5 in $\overline{C5a}$ and in the larger fragment $\overline{C5b}$ which, without further proteolysis, initiates the self-assembly of the C(5b-8)C9n complex involved in membrane lysis.

MOLECULAR STRUCTURE

C2 and factor B are very similar in structure, both consisting of three globular domains of approximately similar size as evidenced by electron microscopy.[26] The 2a and Bb components consist of two globular domains and in heterocomplexes

of factor B and monoclonal antibodies against Ba and Bb, the individual domains of factor B are clearly distinguished:[18] furthermore, in the assembled convertases only one of the two domains is seen in close apposition with C3b.[18] Both components have a mosaic structure constituted by three distinct portions, each conveying unique functional properties, and each being encoded by genes derived from different superfamilies.[27,28]

Both C2 and factor B genes reside, together with the duplicated C4 genes and several other unrelated genes, within the class III region of the human,[29-32] mouse,[29,31,33,34] and *Xenopus* MHC.[35,36] C2 and factor B are extremely closely linked in the MHC region and in man they are present between the HLA class II DRα and the HLA class I B loci. In fact, the initiation site for factor B is only 421 bp from the poly(A) site of C2.[37] However, although the two genes lie very closely there is a 10-15-fold difference in their amounts suggesting that their regulation is distinct. There is no doubt that C2 and Factor B have arisen by duplication of an ancestral gene and this was followed later by structural and functional diversification. In fact, despite the overall similarity at the protein and mRNA levels the two genes differ considerably in size. The C2 gene is much larger, about 18 kb versus 6 kb of factor B, but it contains the same number of exons organized in similar fashion as factor B. The only major difference is the length of the introns.[27,38,39] The C2b and the Ba fragments are encoded by four exons and each of the three internal repeats, defined short consensus repeats (SCR) or complement control proteins (CCP), is encoded by one exon. The VWFA module present in the C2a and Bb fragments is encoded by five exons. The serine protease module is encoded by eight exons (11 to 18) and each of the active sites is contained in a separate exon. This region shows a close correlation to the exon organization of the classical serine proteases,[40] except for the presence of an additional exon (No. 15), which is inserted in the middle of the protease domain.[41]

This exon encodes for a region of the C2a and Bb fragments lying between two active sites, D551 and S674. The function of this additional exon might be to confer cleavage specificity by C2a and Bb only for their respective C4 and C3 substrates.

C2 has at least two alternative transcriptional initiation sites that are utilized in a tissue-specific manner and with differential translational efficiency.[42] Both distant (-240 and -180) and proximal (-27) sites are used by hepatocyte, whereas U937 monoblastic cells used only the proximal site. Deletion of the long 5'-untranslated region results in a strong increase in translational efficiency. These observations suggest that the tissue-specific alternative promoters may differentially regulate C2 expression. The C2 promoter is TATA-less since a TATA-like and a CCAAT box are not located at typical distances from the putative transcription initiation site.[27] Alternative initiation of transcription also has been reported for human and mouse factor B:S1 nuclease protection and primer extension assays localized the transcription initiation site of the human factor B to position -175[37] and in the mouse to positions -302 and -106,[43] relative to the translation initiation site. In the mouse the shorter mRNA is preferentially (95%) utilized in the liver while in both kidney and small intestine the two transcripts are expressed in equal amounts.[44] Thus, enhanced gene expression may be contributed also by preferential utilization of transcriptional initiation sites. Differently from C2, both human and murine factor B possess a typical TATA box.[37,45] In addition, the close proximity of the C2 and factor B genes requires some mechanisms for terminating transcription of the C2 upstream gene otherwise the polymerase II transcribing the C2 gene could read through the factor B promoter. A termination or pause sequence for polymerase II has been located downstream from the C2 poly(A) site by footprinting[46,47] and by poly(A) site competition assays.[48]

The cDNA of the human[28,39,49-52] murine[53,54] and *Xenopus*[35] factor B is known.

The human[49,55-58] and murine[59] cDNAs of C2 also have been characterized. As mentioned above the N-terminal domains of both factor B[28,50] and C2[57] contain the three repeated SCR/CCP sequences of 60 residues, homologous to those present in variable numbers in many regulatory and receptor proteins of the complement system (Fig. 5.2). The middle domain is contributed by a VWFA module and the C-terminal domain is homologous to members of the serine protease gene superfamily. Overall conservation of the position of most cysteines and of the catalytically important residues indicate a clear structural and evolutionary relationship between the active sites of C2 and factor B and the classical serine proteases. A partial protein sequence of the chicken factor B also has been obtained[60] and shown to be highly homologous to both human and murine factor B. This partial sequence comprises the Ba fragment that is 42% and 49% identical to C2b and Ba, respectively. This chicken complement component most likely represents the common protease at work in both classical and alternative activation pathways of the chicken complement since there is no evidence for the presence of a C2-like component in chicken serum. Furthermore, as electrophoretic polymorphism showed independent segregation[61] between MHC and chicken factor B, it can be concluded that, at variance with mammals and *Xenopus*, chicken factor B does not map within the MHC complex. In *Xenopus* a second gene has recently been identified,[36] but it seems unlikely that this second gene is the frog counterpart of the mammalian C2 gene although it also maps within the MHC region. The two *Xenopus* genes have a much higher similarity (82%) among themselves and the similarity between both *Xenopus* genes is higher for the mammalian factor B (40%) than for C2 (30%).

Recently, a homologue of factor B has been cloned in a cyclostome, the lamprey;[62] which is one of the most primitive vertebrates and which possesses a functional complement system with C3/C4-like

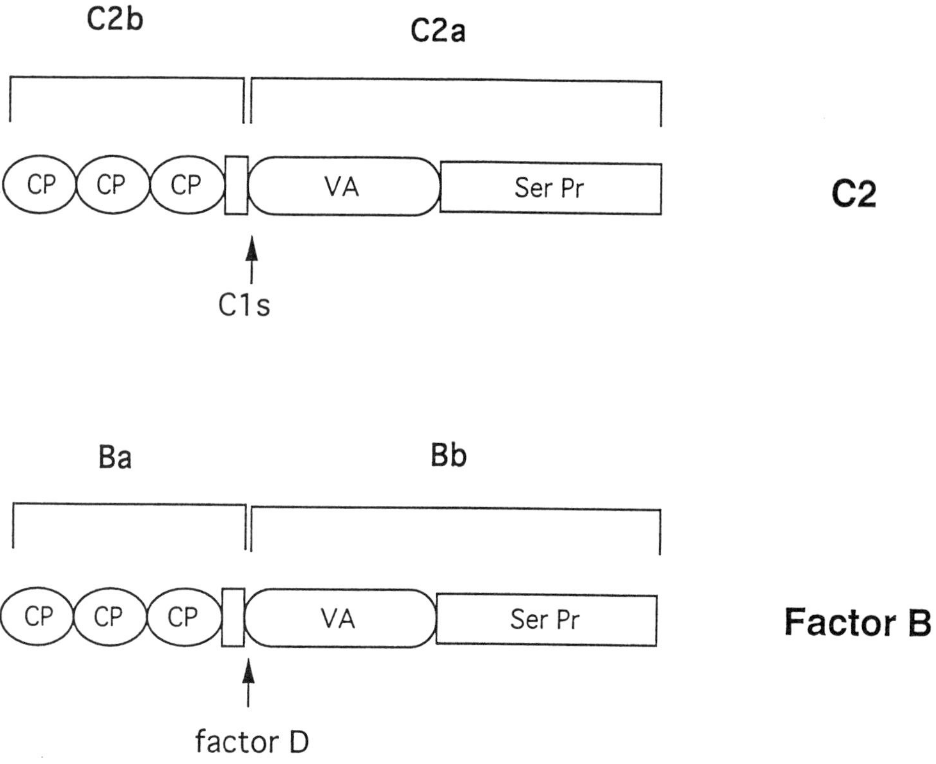

Fig. 5.2. Schematic diagram of C2 and factor B components of the complement pathways. The different modules are designated according to the proposed nomenclature of Bork and Bairoch.[155] The C1s and factor D cleavage sites originating the different fragments (C2b and C2a, and Ba and Bb, respectively) also are indicated.

components. However, this complement system is organized only in the alternative pathway consisting of fewer components than the mammalian system and functions as an opsonic system devoid of lytic activity. The overall sequence identity of the lamprey factor B with mouse C2 and factor B is 29% and 33% respectively, the SCR/CCP modules showing the highest conservation. Thus, the three SCR/CCP modules have 12 cysteines residues at the exact corresponding positions in the other species. Furthermore, in the serine protease domain, nine out of ten cysteines are in identical position as in mouse C2 and factor B. It appears that the lamprey complement system represents a stage in evolution preceding the events that led to C2/ factor B gene duplication. While phylogenetic studies have identified MHC class I and II homologous genes in cartilaginous fish,[63,64] there are no reports on the identification of MHC class I and II genes in cyclostomes. Since Igs are not present either in cyclostomes, the lack of both Igs and MHC class I and II molecules could indicate that these genes were generated between the divergence of cyclostomes and cartilaginous fish and suggests that the complement system consisting of the alternative pathway originated earlier than Igs, MHC, and the classical and lytic complement pathways.

In both cell culture and in vivo the single-copy C2 gene generates mRNAs differing in size due to extensive alternative splicing.[65-67] Biosynthetic studies using U105-MG astroglioma cells,[68] hepatocytes and Hep62 hepatoma cells[70] have shown variant mRNAs and cell-associated C2 polypeptides of a size smaller than the secreted functional C2 polypeptide. Shorter mRNA variants can be generated in the mouse by utilization of an alternative 5' donor site in exon 14.[69] More recently, using liver mRNA and several in vitro cell lines, evidence was provided for several C2 mRNA species since there might be splicing out of a) exons 2 and 3; b) exon 3; c) exon 6; d) exon 17; or e) exons 6 and 7 and the 5' region of exon 18.[70] Exons 6 and 7 encode for the 5'-end portion of the VWFA module of C2 and the mRNAs in which these exons are missing are the only ones, apart from a clone of the human α3(VI) cDNA,[71] in which natural partial deletions of a VWFA module has been described. The variants generated through alternative splicing are likely to represent a substantial fraction of total C2 mRNA[70] since the transcript lacking exons 2 and 3 is abundant and it is the template for a protein of about 70 kD which is found in lysates of all cell types synthesizing and secreting full-length C2.[67] Although lacking part of the leader peptide sequence, this truncated C2 polypeptide can traverse the endoplasmic reticulum membrane, while remaining intracellularly located. Given its relatively high abundance and the fact that the cleavage site activating the C2 serine protease is intact, it seems likely that the truncated C2 polypeptide plays some intracellular function.[67] Alternative splicing giving rise to two C2 transcripts also has been reported in the mouse.[72]

Initial protein sequence and structural analysis of these two proteins was possible only for factor B[6,19,73-77] due to the low plasma levels of C2 which have prevented high yield purifications for protein sequencing. C2 is a 102 kD polypeptide which is cleaved by C1s to yield the N-terminal noncatalytic C2b fragment of 30 kD and the C-terminal catalytic fragment C2a of 70 kD. Factor B is a 90 kD polypeptide which is cleaved by factor D to yield the N-terminal noncatalytic Ba fragment of 30 kD and the C-terminal catalytic fragment Bb of 60 kD. The larger size of C2 when compared to Bb is due to the presence of a higher content of carbohydrates.[78] In fact, although the C2 mRNA is 300 bp longer (2.9 kb) than factor B mRNA (2.6 kb), the unglycosylated forms of the proteins synthesized by peritoneal macrophages in the presence of tunicamycin have similar molecular weights.[79]

Both C2[56,80] and factor B[81] are polymorphic. Although allelic forms have been described on the basis of differences in electrophoretic mobility, this technique is not very useful in the case of C2, as most individuals are homozygous for the common variant. Nevertheless, the use of specific cDNA and genomic probes and Southern blot analysis revealed a number of RFLPs both for C2 and factor B.[80,82-86] Additional polymorphism of C2 is associated with a variable number of tandem repeats of nucleotide sequences,[87] which is part of a SINE-type nonviral retroposon locus[88] termed SINE-R.C2[89] and are located in the third intron. For factor B, the electrophoretic analysis is more informative since the heterogeneity is greater and depends on the presence of two common, two less common, and numerous rare alleles. The two major allelic forms of factor B, that differ only for the residue at position 7,[90] when expressed transiently in a eukaryotic system do not differ significantly in hemolytic activity.[52]

TISSUE EXPRESSION AND FUNCTION

Most complement proteins are synthesized by the liver and their plasma concentration increases following tissue injury and inflammation and belong to the group of acute-phase proteins (APP).[90-92] Factor B, C3 and C4bp, are regulated by IL-1 and belong to the class I APP. C2, which is not an APP since its plasma concentration does not change during the inflammatory acute-phase response, shows greater increases in the extrahepatic sites compared to those detected in the liver. The synthesis of C2 is much higher in monocytes with macrophage maturation, than in freshly isolated monocytes.[93-95] Furthermore, synthesis of C2 is greatly increased in response to γIFN through a PKC-dependent pathway[96] in human monocytes,[97] U937 cells,[98] Hep62 cells,[99] human umbilical vein endothelial cells (HUVEC),[99] fibroblasts,[71,99] alveolar type II cells[100] and the astroglioma cell line U105-MG.[73] In contrast to factor B, C2 is not affected by IL-1 or TNF.[101,102]

In vitro, factor B is synthesized by hepatoma cell lines,[101] monocytes,[103] peritoneal[104] and bronchoalveolar macrophages,[100,105] skin fibroblasts,[71] alveolar type II cells,[100] HUVEC[106] and the astroglioma cell line U105-MG.[73] Several agents stimulate factor B production in numerous cell types. These include IL-1,[01,107-110] γIFN,[96,97,99] IL-6,[110,111] TNF,[106] PDGF,[112] glucocorticoids[113] and LPS.[93] In addition, a marked synergism, affecting both transcriptional and translational activity, is evident when fibroblasts are treated with LPS and γIFN.[71]

The importance of extrahepatic synthesis in local inflammatory processes is exemplified by the widespread cytokine-induced activation of C2 and factor B expression.[71,105-107] An independent contribution to the above observations is derived from the murine model of SLE where upregulation of C2 and factor B genes at sites of inflammation and disease development has been reported.[114,115] Furthermore, both constitutive and IL-1 regulated quantitative tissue-specific and strain-specific differences for C2 and factor B mRNAs are found among inbred mouse strains.[104] The differential strain expression of factor B seems to depend in part upon cis regulatory elements affecting the interaction with a DNA binding protein in a site downstream of the transcription initiation site of the long factor B mRNA.[116] Finally, although C2 and factor B share common biosynthetic and post-translational modifications,[79] factor B is present in plasma at about 10 to 15-fold higher concentrations than C2.

Finally, in addition to its major role in host defense, factor B activation fragments exert several effects on diverse immune cells including stimulation of B cell proliferation and differentiation,[117-120] macrophage spreading[121] and monocyte-dependent cytotoxicity.[122]

STRUCTURE-FUNCTION RELATIONSHIPS

Several proteins interact with C2 and/or compete for binding sites on other complement constituents including C4b, C1s, C4bp, factor I, C3b, CR1, MCP and DAF. Similar proteins interact with factor B and/or compete for its binding sites including C3b, factor D, factor H, factor I, CR1, MCP and DAF.[123] For some of these proteins the binding sites have been identified and in a few cases are located in the VWFA modules of both C2 and factor B.

C2

Following activation of the classical pathway, C4 is cleaved by C1s in C4a and C4b. C2 binds to C4b in a Mg^{2+}-dependent reaction and it also is cleaved in C2a and C2b by C1s resulting in the formation of the C3-convertase $\overline{C4b2a}$. C1s cleaves C2 right at the beginning of the sequence of the VWFA module between R234 and K235. The presence of a C4b binding site on C2b had been suggested by the finding of a C4b-C2b complex in fluid phase[124] and by the noncovalent binding of C2b to Sepharose-coupled C4b after C1s activation.[125] Prevention of C2b binding to C4b is achieved using both intact Ig or the Fab fragment of a monoclonal antibody recognizing an epitope on the C2b fragment.[126] This antibody also inhibits the hemolytic activity of purified C2 and of C2 present in normal serum. Although a precise epitope mapping has not been reported, the antibody is known to recognize an epitope on or near the binding site on C2b for C4b, making a likely location in one of the three SCR/CCP repeats. Since this antibody does not alter the kinetics of decay of the C3-convertase nor the convertase function but only the interaction between C4b and C2, the C4b-binding site on C2b must be important in the initial interaction of C2 with C4b.

The presence of another possible C4b binding site in the N-terminus of C2a was hypothesized by its structural homology with VWFA modules present in Mac-1 (CR3)[24] and p150,95 (CR4)[25] integrins, both of which bind iC3b. Furthermore, and in analogy with similar findings with C2a, they both require Mg^{2+} to bind to their respective Active ligands. Human C2 treated with iodine acquires, after binding to C4b, a 20-fold higher hemolytic activity than native C2.[127] This higher hemolytic activity is the consequence of a decreased rate of decay of the C4b2a complex and the higher affinity binding of C2a to C4b has been attributed to the oxidation, followed by its removal, of the bulky C241 free thiol group.[128] This latter residue is located right after the first Asp (D240) of the recently described MIDAS motif,[129] at the N-terminus of the VWFA module of C2a. Mutagenesis of C241 does not lead to an increase in the C2a hemolytic activity after iodine treatment, providing direct evidence that it is the oxidation of the free thiol group which is responsible for the increase in activity. Furthermore, substitutions of D240 and S244 also result in a 100-fold reduction of specific hemolytic activity suggesting that this region (residues 240-244) might be included in the C4b binding site.[130] It should be stressed that the relevance of the conserved (DxSxS) residues of the MIDAS motif of C2 for the function of this protein was recognized far before[130-132] similar mutagenesis approaches led to the identification that these sites represent a new type of cation-binding motif.[133] Among all the VWFA modules known to date only the human C2 has a cysteine in this position and the guinea pig C2, which instead has an A241, forms a C3 convertase with a 10-fold slower decay rate than the human C2.[134] Based on the findings obtained by more extensive mutagenesis approaches in VWFA modules in other proteins[135-139] it seems that rather than participating in the actual contact sites for C4b,[130] the presence of the C241 and the higher activity that follows oxidation by I_2, might contribute to a higher metal ion affinity of the C2a MIDAS motif.

FACTOR B

Activation of the alternative pathway proceeds through the cleavage of C3 and the formation of the $\overline{C3bB}$ complex. The binding site for factor B on C3b is comprised between residues 730-739[4] and 933-942[140] of the α chain. Binding of factor B to C3b can be inhibited in a dose-dependent manner by function blocking antibodies against the Ba fragment.[18] Since one of these antibodies also inhibits the earlier steps in the hemolytic sequence and it is most efficient when unbound B is removed from the assay, it is likely that it recognizes a site at or very near the C3b binding site of Ba. Therefore, analogous to the findings with C2b, a C3b-binding site may be present in Ba. However, there are some data that do not fit into this scheme and imply the existence of other binding sites for C3b on factor B: (a) after cleavage by factor D between R234 and K235, Bb and not Ba remains bound to C3b; (b) metal ions are required for binding of factor B to C3b and a Ni^{2+} binding site has been localized on Bb;[141] (c) both Ba and Bb are unable to bind by themselves to C3b using nonequilibrium conditions; and (d) finally, unlike the association of C3b with intact factor B, the interaction between Ba and C3b can be demonstrated by the use of chemical cross-linkers even in the presence of 5mM EDTA.[142] Since Mg^{2+} is necessary for a proper assembly of the C3bBb convertase and the C3b-Ba interaction appears to be metal ion independent, it appears that there is a Mg^{2+} dependent binding site for C3b on factor B and it seems very likely that this site is comprised in the MIDAS motif of the VWFA module in Bb (Fig. 5.3).

Function blocking antibodies against Bb have been described which do not inhibit the binding of factor B to C3b, but rather increase the rate of inactivation of $\overline{C3bBb}$.[12] Thus, they play a role similar to that of the regulatory protein H and CR1 and enhance the dissociation of Bb from the $\overline{C3bBb}$ complex destabilizing the C3b binding site of Bb indirectly perhaps through a conformational change. Instead, other antibodies can stabilize a high affinity state of the $\overline{C3bBb}$ complex[143] and appear to function in a way similar to

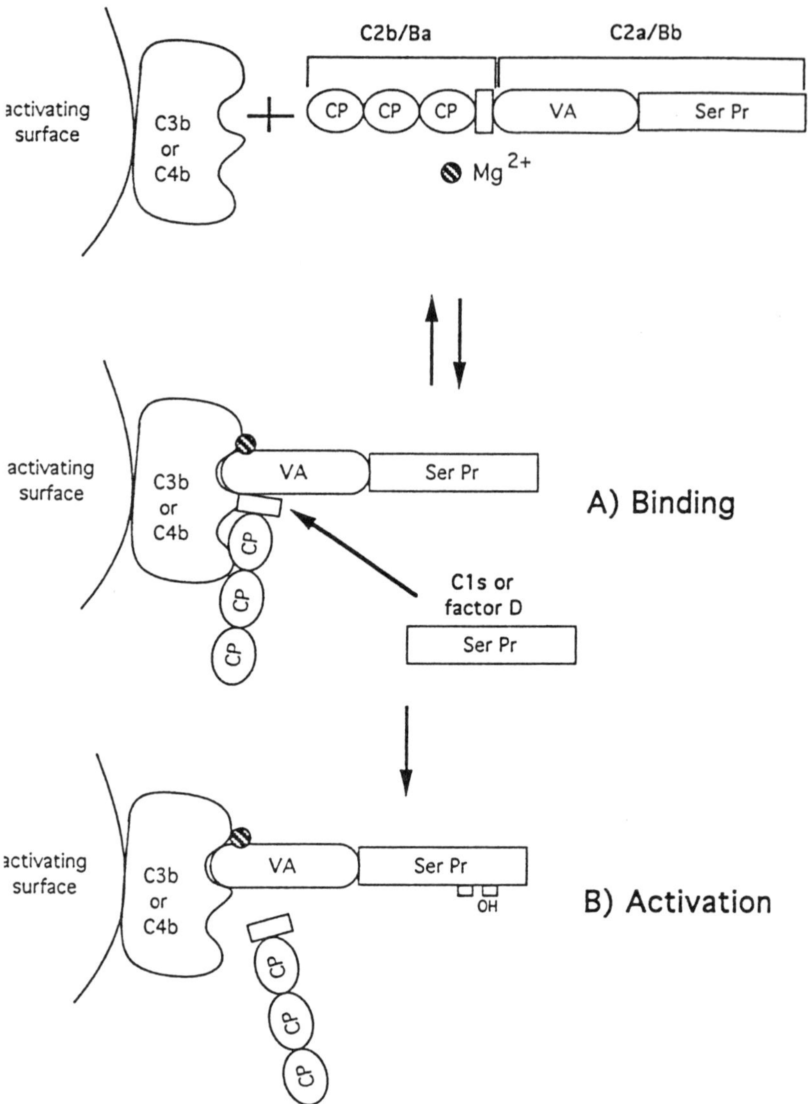

Fig. 5.3. Proposed model for the generation of C3 convertases. Two low affinity binding sites on C3b/C4b are illustrated which interact in a cation-independent (through the CP modules) and in a cation-dependent mechanism (through the MIDAS motifs of the VWFA modules), respectively. After cleavage of C2/factor B by C1s/factor D the C2b/Ba fragments dissociate from C3b/C4b and the catalytic C-terminal domain is activated (shown by a change in the shape of the Ser Pr module).

antibodies against the VWFA module of the β2 integrins.[144-146]

An important observation to consider is that the C3 convertase C3bBb dissociates unidirectionally. Thus, to reconcile the above data and offer an explanation for the dissociation phenomenon it could be hypothesized that the C3b-B interaction is mediated by two discrete cooperative binding sites, one in Ba and one in Bb (Fig. 5.3).[18,142] The two binding sites would be of low affinity, and their low affinity would account for the lack of measurable binding of either Ba and Bb to C3b. However, when cooperating they would provide sufficient avidity to allow the binding of factor B to C3b. The binding site present on Ba is metal ion independent and the other, on Bb, is strongly metal ion dependent[130] and is likely to involve a functional MIDAS motif. Following activation of C3bB by factor D-mediated proteolytic cleavage, most of the Ba fragments dissociate from C3b prior to the dissociation of Bb[141] and the activation of the catalytic C-terminal domain of Bb.[142] The high affinity configuration of the recognition site on Bb is further stabilized by binding of properdin.

Factor D, which is found in plasma only in its activated form, is highly specific for the RK bond present at the N-terminal end of the VWFA module of fragment Bb. This protease is rather unique among the serine protease family since for its full proteolytic activity the C3bB substrate should induce a transient conformational change[147] so that following cleavage of the C3bB complex, factor D reverts to its inactive state. The finding of two molecular conformations in the crystal structure of factor D is in agreement with the above prediction.[148] Furthermore, recent investigations on the structural determinants of the residues participating in the formation of the catalytic pocket and in the formation of the primary and extended substrate binding sites[149] have indicated that one of the three walls that constitute the primary specificity binding pocket of factor D expands upward resulting in a narrowing of the pocket compared to that of other serine proteases such as trypsin. This finding, together with the unique very low reactivity of factor D with small synthetic substrates,[150] suggests that other contact points with C3bB might be important for the active conformation of factor D: residue R218 is likely to provide a contact point for the C3bB complex.[149] Similarly, the contact between factor D and the C3bB complex is through the VWFA domain of the Bb fragment, the spatial organization of the residues of factor D belonging to the primary specificity pocket is reminiscent of the spatial arrangement of the site on type IV collagen which is recognized by the VWFA modules of β1 integrins.[151] There is in fact the possibility that the recognition site on factor D comprises, in addition to R218, G228 and D194 that might form a nonlinear RGD recognition site. The low efficiency of binding of synthetic peptides to factor D along with the known inability of linear collagen peptides to inhibit β1 integrin collagen interactions, is in agreement with suggestion that the recognition of fibrillar collagens and factor D might be using similar recognition sites.

DISEASE ASSOCIATION

The relevance of complement effector functions in maintaining a proper healthy condition is underscored by the frequent association of complement deficiencies with increased susceptibility to infection and/or other immune disregulations.[152] Deficiency of C2 is the most common (1 in 10,000) genetic defect of the complement system[153,154] while factor B deficiency is very rare. Almost 50% of the homozygous C2-deficient individuals present symptoms of SLE or other autoimmune disorders. Heterozygous individuals also have defects in complement functions.

REFERENCES

1. Reid KBM, Day AJ. Structure-function relationship of the complement components. Immunol Today 1989; 10:177-180.
2. Volanakis JE. Transcriptional regulation of complement genes. Annu Rev Immunol 1995; 13:277-305.
3. Dodds AW, Day AJ. The phylogeny and evolution of the complement system. In: Whaley K, Loos M, Weiler JM, eds. Complement in Health and Disease. Kluver Academic Publishers, 1993: 39-88.
4. Fishelson Z. Complement C3: a molecular mosaic of binding sites. Mol Immunol 1991; 28:545-552.
5. Reid KBM. Complete amino-acid sequences of the three collagen-like regions present in subcomponent C1q of the first component of human complement. Biochem J 1979; 179:367-371.
6. Kerr MA. Limited proteolysis of complement components C2 and Factor B. Structural analogy and limited sequence homology. Biochem J 1979; 183:615-622.

7. Kristensen T, D'Eustachio P, Ogata RT et al. The superfamily of C3b/C4b-binding proteins. Fed Proc 1987; 46:2463-2469.

8. Hillarp A, Dahlback B. Novel subunit in C4b-binding protein required for protein S binding. J Biol Chem 1988; 263: 12759-12764.

9. Fearon DT. Identification of the membrane glycoprotein that is the C3b receptor of the human erythrocyte, polymorphonuclear leukocyte, B lymphocyte and monocyte. J Exp Med 1980; 152:20-30.

10. Klickstein LB, Wong WW, Smith JA et al. Human C3b/C4b receptor (CR1): demonstration of long homologous repeating domains. J Exp Med 1987; 165:1095-1112.

11. Lublin DM, Liszewski MK, Post TW et al. Molecular cloning and chromosomal localization of human membrane cofactor protein (MCP): evidence for inclusion in the multi-gene family of complement-regulatory proteins. J Exp Med 1988; 168:181-194.

12. Seya T, Turner J, Atkinson JP. Purification and characterization of a membrane protein (gp45-70) which is a cofactor for cleavage of C3b and C4b. J Exp Med 1986; 163:837-855.

13. Davitz MA, Low MG, Nussenzweig V. Release of decay-accelerating factor (DAF) from the cell membrane by phosphatidylinositol-specific phospholipase C (PIPLC). Selective modification of a complement regulatory protein. J Exp Med 1986; 163:1150-1161.

14. Lublin DM, Atkinson JP. Decay-accelerating factor and membrane cofactor protein. Curr Top Microbiol Immun 1989; 153:123-145.

15. Fujita T, Inoue T, Ogawa K et al. The mechanism of action of decay-accelerating factor (DAF). DAF inhibits the assembly of C3 convertases by dissociating C2a and Bb. J Exp Med 1987; 167:1221-1228.

16. Kinoshita T, Medof ME, Nussenzweig V. Endogenous association of decay-accelerating factor (DAF) with C4b and C3b on cell membranes. J Immunol 1986; 136: 3390-3395.

17. Pangburn MK. Differences between the binding sites of the complement regulatory proteins DAF, CR1 and factor H on C3 convertases. J Immunol 1986; 136: 2216-2221.

18. Ueda A, Kearney JF, Roux KH et al. Probing functional sites on complement protein B with monoclonal antibodies—evidence for C3b-binding sites on Ba. J Immunol 1987; 138:1143-1149.

19. Curman B, Sandberg-Tragardh L, Peterson PA. Chemical characterization of human factor B of the alternate pathway of complement activation. Biochemistry 1977; 16:5368-5378.

20. Yamauchi Y, Stevens JW, Macon KJ et al. Recombinant and native zymogen forms of human complement factor D. J Immunol 1994; 152: 3645-3653.

21. Koistinen V, Wessberg S, Leikola J. Common binding region of complement factors B, H and CR1 on C3b revealed by monoclonal anti-C3d. Complement Inflamm 1989; 6:270-280.

22. Becherer JD, Alsenz J, Esparza I et al. Segment spanning residues 727-768 of the complement C3 sequence contains a neoantigenic site and accomodates the binding of CR1, factor H and factor B. Biochemistry 1992; 31:1787-1794.

23. Alsenz J, Avila D, Huemer HP et al. Phylogeny of the third component of complement, C3: analysis of the conservation of human CR1, CR2, H and B binding sites, concanavalin A binding sites, and thiolester bond in the C3 from different species. Dev Comp Immunol 1992; 16:63-76.

24. Wright SD, Rao PE, Van Voorhis WC et al. Identification of the C3bi receptor of human monocytes and macrophages by using monoclonal antibodies. Proc Natl Acad Sci USA 1983; 80:5699-5703.

25. Micklem KJ, Sim RB. Isolation of complement-fragment-iC3b-binding proteins by affinity chromatography. Biochem J 1985; 231:233-236.

26. Smith CA, Vogel CW, Mueller-Eberhard HJ. MHC Class III products: an electron microscopic study of the C3 convertase of human complement. J Exp Med 1984; 159:324-329.

27. Ishii Y, Zhu ZB, Macon KJ et al. Structure of the human C2 gene. J Immunol 1993; 151:170-174.

28. Morley BJ, Campbell RD. Internal homologies of the Ba fragment from human comple-

ment component Factor B, a class III MHC antigen. EMBO J 1984; 3:153-157.

29. Sackstein R, Colten HR, Woods DE. Phylogenetic conservation of a class III major histocompatibility complex antigen Factor B. J Biol Chem 1983; 258:14693-14697.

30. Carroll MC, Campbell RD, Bentley DR et al. A molecular map of the human major histocompatibility complex Class III region linking complement genes C4, C2, and factor B. Nature 1984; 307:237-241.

31. Campbell RD, Bentley DR. The structure and genetics of the C2 and Factor B genes. Immunol Rev 1985; 87:19-37.

32. Campbell RD, Trowsdale J. Map of the human MHC. Immunol Today 1993; 14:349-352.

33. Chaplin DD, Woods DE, Whitehead AS et al. Molecular map of the murine S region. Proc Natl Acad Sci USA 1983; 80: 6947-6951.

34. Muller U, Stephan D, Philippsen P et al. Orientation and molecolar map position of the complement genes in the mouse MHC. EMBO J 1987; 6:369-373.

35. Kato Y, Salter-Cid L, Flajnik MF et al. Isolation of the *Xenopus* complement factor B complementary DNA and linkage of the gene to the frog MHC. J Immunol 1994; 153:4546-4554.

36. Kato Y, Salter-Cid L, Flajnik MF et al. Duplication of the MHC-linked *Xenopus* complement factor B gene. Immunogenetics 1995; 42:196-203.

37. Wu L-C, Morley BJ, Campbell RD. Cell-specific expression of the human complement protein Factor B gene: evidence for the role of two distinct 5' flanking elements. Cell 1987; 48:331-342.

38. Bentley DR, Campbell RD. C2 and Factor B: structure and genetics. Biochem Soc Symp 1986; 51:7-18.

39. Campbell RD, Porter RR. Molecular cloning and characterization of the gene coding for human complement protein Factor B. Proc Natl Acad Sci USA 1983; 80: 4464-4468.

40. Craik CS, Choo Q-L, Swift GH et al. Structure of two related rat pancreatic trypsin genes. J Biol Chem 1984; 259: 14255-14264.

41. Campbell RD, Bentley DR, Morley BJ. The Factor B and C2 genes. Phil Trans R Soc Lond 1984; B306:367-378.

42. Horiuchi T, Macon KJ, Kidd VJ et al. Translational regulation of complement protein C2 expression by differential utilization of the 5'-untranslated region of mRNA. J Biol Chem 1990; 265:6521-6524.

43. Nonaka M, Ishikawa N, Passwell J et al. Tissue-specific initiation of murine complement Factor B mRNA transcription. J Immunol 1989; 142:1377-1382.

44. Garnier G, Circolo A, Colten HR. Translational regulation of murine complement factor B alternative transcripts by upstream AUG codons. J Immunol 1995; 154: 3275-3282.

45. Nonaka M, Gitlin JD, Colten HR. regulation of human and murine complement: comparison of 5' structural and functional elements regulating human and murine complement factor B gene expression. Mol Cell Biochem 1989; 89:1-14.

46. Ashfield R, Enriquez-Harris P, Proudfoot NJ. transcriptional termination between the closely linked human complement genes C2 and Factor B: common termination factor for C2 and *c-myc*? EMBO J 1991; 10: 4197-4207.

47. Bossone SA, Asselin C, Patel AJ et al. MAZ, a zinc finger protein, binds to *c-myc* and C2 gene sequences regulating transcriptional initiation and termination. Proc Natl Acad Sci USA 1992; 89:7452-7456.

48. Moreira A, Wollerton M, Monks J et al. Upstream sequence elements enhance poly(A) site efficiency of the C2 complement gene and are phylogenetically conserved. EMBO J 1995; 14:3809-3819.

49. Gagnon J. Structure and activation of complement components C2 and factor B. Philos Trans R Soc Lond-B Biol Sci 1984; B306:301-309.

50. Mole JE, Anderson JK, Davison Ea et al. Complete primary structure for the zymogen of human complement factor B. J Biol Chem 1984; 259:3407-3412.

51. Woods DE, Markham AF, Ricker AT et al. Isolation of cDNA clones for the human complement protein factor B, a Class III major histocompatibility complex gene

product. Proc Natl Acad Sci USA 1982; 79:5661-5665.

52. Horiuchi T, Kim S, Matsumoto M et al. Human complement Factor B: cDNA cloning, nucleotide sequencing, phenotypic conversion by site-directed mutagenesis and expression. Mol Immunol 1993; 30: 1587-1592.

53. Sackstein R, Colten HR, Woods DE. Phylogenetic conservation of a class III major histocompatibility complex antigen Factor B. J Biol Chem 1983; 258:14693-14697.

54. Sackstein R, Colten HR. Molecular regulation of MHC Class III (C4 and factor B) gene expression in mouse peritoneal macrophages. J Immunol 1984; 133:1618-1626.

55. Bentley DR, Porter RR. Isolation of cDNA clones for human complement component C2. Proc Natl Acad Sci USA 1984; 81:1212-1215.

56. Woods DE, Edge MD, Colten HR. Isolation of a complementary DNA clone for the human complement protein C2 and its use in the identification of a restriction fragment length polymorphism. J Clin Invest 1984; 74:634-638.

57. Bentley DR. Primary structure of human complement component C2. Homology to two unrelated protein families. Biochem J 1986; 239:339-345.

58. Horiuchi T, Macon KJ, Kidd VJ et al. cDNA cloning and expression of human complement component C2. J Immunol 1989; 142:2105-2111.

59. Ishikawa N, Nonaka M, Wetsel RA et al. Murine complement C2 and factor B genomic and cDNA cloning reveals different mechanisms for multiple transcripts of C2 and B J Biol Chem 1990; 265: 19040-19046.

60. Kjalke M, Welinder KG, Koch C. Structural analysis of chicken Factor B-like protease and comparison with mammalian complement proteins Factor B and C2. J Immunol 1993; 151:4147-4152.

61. Koch C. A genetic polymorphism of the complement component factor B in chickens not linked to the major histocompatibility complex (MHC). Immunogenetics 1986; 23:364-367.

62. Nonaka M, Takahashi M, Sasaki M. Molecular cloning of a lamprey homologue of the mammalian MHC class III gene, complement Factor B. J Immunol 1994; 152:2263-2269.

63. Hashimoto K, Nakanishi T, Kurosawa Y. Isolation of carp genes encoding major histocompatibility complex antigens. Proc Natl Acad Sci USA 1990; 87:6863-6867.

64. Hashimoto K, Nakanishi T, Kurosawa Y. Identification of a shark sequence resembling the major histocompatibility complex class I alpha 3 domain. Proc Natl Acad Sci USA 1992; 89:2209-2212.

65. Perlmutter DH, Cole FS, Goldberger G et al. Distinct primary translation products from human liver mRNA give rise to secreted and cell-associated forms of complement protein C2. J Biol Chem 1984; 259:10380-10385.

66. Katz Y, Cole FS, Strunk RC. Synergism between γ-interferon and lipopolysaccharide for synthesis of Factor B, but not C2, in human fibroblasts. J Exp Med 1988; 167:1-14.

67. Akama H, Johnson CAC, Colten HR. Human complement protein C2. Alternative splicing generates templates for secreted and intracellular C2 proteins. J Biol Chem 1995; 270:2674-2678.

68. Barnum SR, Ishii Y, Agrawal A et al. Production and interferon-γ-mediated regulation of complement component C2 and Factor B and D by the astroglioma cell line U105-MG. Biochem J 1992; 287:595-601.

69. Zhu ZB, Hsieh SL, Bentley DR et al. A variable number of tandem repeats locus within the human complement C2 gene is associated with a retroposon from a human endogenous retrovirus. J Exp Med 1992; 175:1783-1787.

70. Cheng J, Volanakis JE. Alternatively spliced transcripts of the human complement C2 gene. J Immunol 1994; 152:1774-1782.

71. Chu M.-L, Zhang R-Z, Pan T et al. Mosaic structure of globular domains in the human type VI collagen α3 chain: similarity to von Willebrand Factor, fibronectin, actin, salivary proteins and aprotinin type protease inhibitors. EMBO J 1990; 9:385-393.

72. Ishikawa N, Nonaka M, Wetsel RA et al. Murine complement C2 and Factor B ge-

nomic and cDNA cloning reveals different mechanisms for multiple transcripts of C2 and B. J Biol Chem 1990; 265: 19040-19046.

73. Kerr MA, Porter RR. The purification and properties of the second component of human complement. Biochem J 1978; 171:99-107.

74. Christie DL, Gagnon J, Porter RR. Partial sequence of human complement component Factor B: novel type of serine protease. Proc Natl Acad Sci USA 1980; 77:4923-4927.

75. Mole JE, Niemann MA. Structural evidence that complement factor B constitutes a novel class of serine protease. J Biol Chem 1980; 255:8472-8476.

76. Christie DF, Gagnon J. Amino acid sequence of the Bb fragment from complement Factor B. Biochem J 1983; 209:61-70.

77. Caporale LH, Woods D, Gagnon J et al. A computer generated model of the serine proteinase domain of human complement factor B. Immunobiol 1983; 164:213.

78. Tomana M, Niemann M, Garner C et al. Carbohydrate composition of the second, third and fifth components and Factors B and D of human complement. Mol Immunol 1985; 22:107-111.

79. Matthews WJ, Goldberger G, Marino JT et al. Complement proteins C2, C4, and Factor B. Effect of glycosylation on their secretion and catabolism. Biochem J 1982; 204:839-846.

80. Bentley DR, Campbell RD, Cross SJ. DNA polymorphism of the C2 locus. Immunogenetics 1985; 22:377-390.

81. Alper CA, Boenisch T, Watson L. Genetic polymorphism in human glycine rich beta-glycoprotein. J Exp Med 1972; 135:68-80.

82. Cross SJ, Edwards JH, Bentley DR et al. DNA polymorphism of the C2 and factor B genes: detection of a restriction fragment lenght polymorphism which subdivides haplotypes carrying the C2C and factor BF alleles. Immunogenetics 1985; 21:39-48.

83. Sargent CA, Dunham I, Campbell RD. Identification of multiple HTF-island associated genes in the major histocompatibility complex Class III region. EMBO J 1989; 8:2305-2312.

84. Campbell RD. Molecular genetics of C2 and Factor B. Br Med Bull 1987; 43:37-49.

85. Mejia JE, Jahn I, de la Salle H et al. Human factor B. Complete cDNA sequence of the BF*S allele. Hum Immunol 1994; 39:49-53.

86. Campbell RD, Morley BJ, Sargent CA et al. Molecular basis of allelic variations at the Factor B locus. Complement 1985; 2:14-5.

87. Zhu ZB, Volanakis JE. Allelic associations of multiple restriction fragment length polymorphisms of the gene encoding complement protein C2. Am J Hum Genet 1990; 46:956-962.

88. Zhu ZB, Hsieh SL, Bentley DR et al. A variable number of tandem repeats (VNTR) locus within the human complement C2 gene is associated with a retroposon derived from a human endogenous retrovirus. J Exp Med 1992; 175:1783-1787.

89. Zhu ZB, Jian B, Volanakis JE. Ancestry of SINE-R.C2, a human specific retroposon. Human Genet 1994; 93:545-551.

90. Campbell RD. The molecular genetics and polymorphism of C2 and factor B. Br Med Bull 1987; 43:37-49.

91. Colten HR, Strunk RC. Synthesis of complement components in liver and at extrahepatic sites. In: Whaley K, Loos M, Weiler JM, eds. Complement in Health and Disease. 2nd ed. Kluwer Academic Publishers, 1993:127.

92. Baumann H, Gauldie J The acute phase response. Immunol Today 1994; 15:74-80.

93. Cole FS, Schneeberger EE, Lichtenberg NA et al. Complement biosynthesis in human breast milk macrophages and blood monocytes. Immunology 1982; 46:429-441.

94. Einstein LP, Schneeberger EE, Colten HR. Synthesis of the second component of complement by long-term primary cultures of human monocytes. J Exp Med 1976; 143:114-126.

95. Cole FS, Auerbach HS, Goldberger G et al. Tissue-specific pretranslational regulation of complement production in human mononuclear phagocytes. J Immunol 1985; 134:2610-2616.

96. Watanabe I, Horiuchi T, Fujita S. Role of protein kinase C activation in synthesis of complement components C2 and factor B

in interferon-γ-stimulated human fibroblasts, glioblastoma cell line A172 and monocytes. Biochem J 1995; 305:425-431.

97. Strunk R, Cole S, Perlmutter D et al. γ-Interferon increases expression of class III complement genes C2 and Factor B in human monocytes and in murine fibroblasts transfeceted with human C2 and Factor B genes. J Biol Chem 1985; 260: 15280-15285.

98. Littman BH, Hall RE, Muchmore AV. Lymphokine and phorbol (PMA) regulation of complement (C2) synthesis using U937. Cell Immunol 1983; 76:189-195.

99. Lappin DF, Guc D, Hill A et al. Effect of interferon-γ on complement gene expression in different cell types. Biochem J 1992; 281:437-442.

100. Strunk RC, Eidlen DM, Mason RJ. pulmonary alveolar type II epithelial cells synthesize and secrete proteins of the classical and alternative complement pathways. J Clin Invest 1988; 81:1419-1426.

101. Perlmutter DH, Goldberger G, Dinarello CA et al. Regulation of class III major histocompatibility complex gene products by interleukin-1. Science 1986; 232: 850-852.

102. Perlmutter DH, Dinarello CA, Punsal PI et al. Cachectin/tumor necrosis factor regulates hepatic acute-phase gene expression. J Clin Invest 1986; 78:1349-1354.

103. Whaley K. Biosynthesis of the human complement components and the regulatory proteins of the alternative proteins of the alternative complemnt pathway by human peripheral blood monocytes. J Exp Med 1980; 151: 501-516.

104. Falus A, Beuscher HU, Auerbach HS et al. Constitutive and Il-1-regulated murine complement gene expression is strain and tissue specific. J Immunol 1987; 138:856-60.

105. Cole FS, Matthews WJ, Rossing TH et al. Complement biosynthesis by human bronchoalveolar macrophages. Clin Immunol Immunopathol 1983; 27:153-159.

106. Ripoche J, Mitchell JA, Erdei A et al. Interferon-γ induces synthesis of complement alternative pathway proteins by human endothelial cells in culture. J Exp Med 1988; 168:1917-1922.

107. Katz Y, Strunk RC. IL-1 and tumor necrosis factor: similarities and differences in stimulation of expression of alternative pathway of complement and IFN-β2/IL-6 genes in human fibroblasts. J Immunol 1989; 142: 3862-3867.

108. Perlmutter DH, Goldberger G, Dinarello CA et al. Regulation of Class III major histocompatibility complex gene products by interleukin-1. Science 1986; 232:850-2.

109. Nonaka M, Huang ZM. Interleukin-1-mediated enhancement of mouse factor B gene expression via NF$_K$B-like hepatoma nuclear factor. Mol Cell Biol 1990; 10:6283-6289.

110. Falus A, Rokita H, Walcz E et al. Hormonal regulation of complement biosynthesis in human cell lines-II. Upregulation of the biosynthesis of complement components C3, Factor B and C1 inhibitor by interleukin-6 and interleukin-1 in human hepatoma cell line. Mol Immunol 1990; 27:197-201.

111. Perlmutter DH, Colten HR, Adams SP et al. A cytokine-selective defect in interleukin-1β-mediated acute-phase gene expression in a subclone of the human hepatoma cell line (HEPG2). J Biol Chem 1989; 264: 7669-7674.

112. Circolo A, Pierce GF, Katz Y et al. Antiinflammatory effects of polypeptide growth factors. Plateled-derived growth factor, epidermal growth factor, and fibroblast growth factor inhibit the cytokine-induceed expression of the alternative complement pathway activator Factor B in human fibroblasts. J Biol Chem 1990; 265:5066-5071.

113. Lappin DF, Whaley K. Modulation of complement gene expression by glucocorticoids. Biochem J 1991; 280:117-123.

114. Passwell J, Schreiner GF, Nonaka M et al. Local extrahepatic expression of complement genes C3 factor B, C2, and C4 is increased in murine lupus nephritis. J Clin Invest 1988; 82:1676-1684.

115. Passwell JH, Schreiner GF, Wetsel RA et al. Complement gene expression in hepatic and extrahepatic tissues of NZB and NZBxW (F1) mouse strains. Immunology 1990; 71:290-294.

116. Garnier G, Ault B, Kramer M et al. *cis* and *trans* elements differ among mouse strains with high and low extrahepatic complement

Factor B gene expression. J Exp Med 1992; 175:471-479.

117. Peters MG, Ambrus JL Jr, Fauci AS et al. The Bb fragment of complement Factor B acts as a B cell growth factor. J Exp Med 1988; 168:1225-1235.

118. Praz F, Ruuth E. Growth-supporting activity of fragment Ba of the human alternative complement pathway for activated murine B lymphocytes. J Exp Med 1986; 163: 1349-1354.

119. Ambrus JL Jr, Chesky L, Chused T et al. Intracellular signaling events associated with the induction of proliferation of normal human B lymphocytes by two different antigenically related human B cell growth factors (high molecular weight B cell growth factor (HMW-BCGF) and the complement factor B. J Biol Chem 1991; 266: 3702-3708.

120. Praz F, Ruuth E. Growth-supporting activity of fragment Ba of the human alternative complement pathway for activated murine B lymphocytes. J Exp Med 1986; 163: 1349-1354.

121. Gotze O, Bianco C, Cohn ZA. The induction of macrophage spreading by Factor B of the properdin system. J Exp Med 1979; 149:372-386.

122. Hirani S, Fair DS, Papin RA et al. Leukocyte complement: interleukin-like properties of factor Bb. Cell Immunol 1985; 92: 235-246.

123. Farries TC, Seya T, Harrison RA et al. Competition for binding sites on C3b by CR1, CR2, MCP, factor B and factor H. Complem Inflamm 1990; 7:30-41.

124. Kerr MA. The human complement system: assembly of the classical pathway C3 convertase. Biochem J 1980; 189:173-181.

125. Nagasawa S, Stroud RM. Cleavage of C2 by C1 into the antigenically distinct fragments C2a and C2b : demonstration of binding of C2b to C4. Proc Natl Acad Sci USA 1977; 74:2998-3001.

126. Oglesby TJ, Accavitti MA, Volanakis JE. Evidence for a C4b binding site on the C2b domain of C2. J Immunol 1988; 141:926-931.

127. Polley MJ, Mueller-Eberhard HJ. Enhancement of the hemolytic activity of the second component of human complement by oxidation. J Exp Med 1967; 126:1013-1025.

128. Parkes C, Gagnon J, Kerr MA. The reaction of iodine and thiol-blocking reagents with human complement components C2 and factor B. Biochem J 1983; 213:201-209.

129. Lee J-O, Rieu P, Arnaout MA et al. Crystal structure of the A domain from the α subunit of integrin CR3 (CD11b/CD18). Cell 1995; 80:631-638.

130. Horiuchi T, Macon KJ, Engler JA et al. Site-directed mutagenesis of the region around Cys-241 of complement component C2: evidence for a C4b binding site. J Immunol 1991; 147:584-589.

131. Volanakis JE. C3 convertases of complement. Molecular genetics, structure and function of the catalytic domains, C2 and factor B. In: Cruse JM and Lewis RE, eds. The Year in Immunology 1988. Basel, Karger 1989; 4:218-230.

132. Sànchez-Corral P, Antòn LC, Alcolea JM et al. Proteolytic activity of the different fragments of factor B on the third component of complement (C3): involvement of the N-terminal domain of Bb in magnesium binding. Mol Immunol 1990; 27:891-900.

133. Michishita M, Videm V, Arnaout MA. A novel divalent cation-binding site in the α domain of the β2 integrin CR3 (CD11b/CD18) is essential for ligand binding. Cell 1993; 72:857-867.

134. Kerr MA, Gagnon J. The purification and properties of the second component of guinea-pig complement. Biochem J 1982; 205:59-67.

135. Matsushita T, Sadler JE. Identification of amino acid residues essential for von Willebrand factor binding to platelet glycoprotein Ib. J Biol Chem 1995; 270: 13406-13414.

136. Huang C, Springer TA. A binding interface on the I domain of Lymphocyte function-associated antigen-1 (LFA-1) required for specific interaction with intercellular adhesion molecule 1 (ICAM-1). J Biol Chem 1995; 270:19008-19016.

137. Edwards CP, Champe M, Gonzalzs T et al. Identification of amino acids in the CD11a I-domain important for binding of the leukocyte function-associated antigen-1

(LFA-1) to intercellular adhesion molecule-1 (ICAM-1). J Biol Chem 1995; 270: 12635-12640.

138. Kamata T, Wright R, Takada Y. Critical threonine and aspartic acid residues within the I domains of β2 integrins for interactions with intercellular adhesion molecule 1 (ICAM-1) and C3bi. J Biol Chem 1995; 270:12531-12535.

139. Cooney KA, Ginsburg D. Comparative analysis of type 2b von Willebrand disease mutations: implications for the mechanism of von Willebrand factor binding to platelets. Blood 1996; 87: 2322-2328.

140. O'Keefe MC, Caporale LH, Vogel CW. A novel cleavage product of human complement component C3 with structural and functional properties of cobra venom Factor. J Biol Chem 1988; 263:12690-12697.

141. Fishelson Z, Pangburn MK, Mueller-Eberhard HJ. C3 convertase of the alternative complement pathway: demonstration of an active, stable C3b, Bb (Ni) complex. J Biol Chem 1983; 258:7411-7415.

142. Pryzdial ELG, Isenman DE. Alternative complement pathway activation fragment Ba binds to C3b. Evidence that the formation of the factor B-C3b complex involves two discrete points of contacts. J Biol Chem 1987; 262:1519-1525.

143. Daha MR, Deelder AM, Van Es LA. Stabilization of the amplification convertase of complement by monoclonal antibodies directed against human factor B. J Immunol 1984; 132:2538-2542.

144. Diamond MS, Springer TA. A subpopulation of Mac-1 (CD11b/CD18) molecules mediated neurophil adhesion to ICAM-1 and fibrinogen. J Cell Biol 1993; 120:545-556.

145. Landis RC, Bennett RI, Hogg N. A novel LFA-1 activation epitope maps to the I domain. J Cell Biol 1993; 120:1519-1527.

146. van Kooyk Y, Weder P, Hogervorst F et al. Activation of LFA-1 through Ca²⁺-dependent epitope stimulates leukocyte adhesion. J Cell Biol 1991; 112:345-354.

147. Lesavre PH, Muller-Eberhard HJ. Mechanism of action of factor D of the alternative complement pathway. J Exp Med 1978; 148:1498-1509.

148. Narayana SVL, Carson M, El-Kabbani O et al. Structure of human factor D. A complement system protein at 2.0 A resolution. J Mol Biol 1994; 235:695-708.

149. Kim S, Narayana VL, Volankis JE. Catalytic role of a surface loop of the complement serine protese fator D. J Immunol 1995; 154:6073-6079.

150. Kam CM, McRae BJ, Harper JW et al. Human complement protein D, C2, and B: active site mapping with peptide thioester substrates. J Biol Chem 1987; 262: 3444-3451.

151. Vanderberg P, Kern A, Ries A et al. Characterization of a type IV collagen major cell binding site with affinity to the α1β1 and the α2β1 integrins. J Cell Biol 1991; 113:1475-1483.

152. Agnello V. Complement deficiency states. Medicine 1978; 57:1-23.

153. Glass D, Raum D, Gibson D et al. Inherited deficiency of the second component of complement. J Clin Invest 1976; 58: 853-861.

154. Mortensen JP, Buskjaer L, Lamm LU. Studies on the C2-deficiency gene in man. Immunol 1980; 39:541-549.

155. Bork P, Bairoch A. Extracellular protein modules. Trends Biochem Sci 1995; 3.

CHAPTER 6

Extracellular Matrix Proteins

INTRODUCTION ON COLLAGENS

This chapter deals mainly with collagens that incorporate VWFA modules and hence are included in the von Willebrand factor (vWF) superfamily. However, in order to better understand the structural and functional role of these molecules a short overview of the major steps in the process leading to a triple helical collagenous structure is provided.

Although even bacteria may synthesize low amounts of collagen-like proteins,[1] collagens, which are a large family of proteins, collectively represent the major part of extracellular proteins of all multicellular organisms. Collagens constitute major members of organized structures of extracellular matrix (ECM) such as fibers, basement membranes, microfilaments and anchoring fibrils. Collagens participate in the assembly of ECM, playing not only a structural role in tissue architecture and tensile strength, but also in the organization and maintenance of a wide variety of functions. Cells can interact directly with collagens via specific cell surface receptors and these interactions may play major roles in diverse processes such as cell migration during early development and organogenesis, wound healing, tumor cell local invasion and hemostasis to name a few.[2,3]

Numerous molecules fitting into the general definition of collagen, i.e., a protein composed of three helical polypeptide chains (designated α-chains) coiled into an unique type of semirigid right-handed triple helical structure, have been described in recent years. Thus, although several proteins such as acetylcholinesterase,[4] type I and type II macrophage scavenger receptors,[5] C1q component of the complement cascade,[6] and lung surfactant proteins[7] (referred to as collectins[8]) contain triple helical domains, they are not involved in ECM assembly and ECM-cell interactions and do not belong to the collagen superfamily. Conversely, some of the most recently discovered collagens, which are clearly structurally and functionally distinct from the well known fibril-forming collagens, and in which the triple helical domain may amount to only 10% of the mass of the whole molecule, are comprised within the collagen superfamily due to the presence of a triple helix and to the fact that they interact with other ECM members.[9]

Collagens are classified into subfamilies according to the structure of their genes and the domain organization of the protein.[10,11] Presently there are about 20 collagen types and more than 30 genes.[3] Roman numerals indicate a collagen type, i.e., type I, and Arabic numerals are used for the individual α chain constituents, i.e., α1(III) indicates the α1 chain of type III collagen, while the gene for any particular collagen chain is indicated in the following way : COL6A3 is the gene for the α3 chain of type VI collagen. The characteristic feature of all collagens is a rod-like triple helix domain and all collagens differ from each other by the length of their triple helical domain, by the number of short imperfections and interruptions within the triple helix sequence, and by the size and extension of processing of globular domains at the two ends of the triple helix.

The helical structure of collagen arises as a result of the occurrence of a glycine every third residue (Gly-Xaa-Yaa), while the Xaa and Yaa positions are frequently occupied by proline or hydroxyproline (Fig. 6.1). Steric constraints impose that only glycyl residues can occupy the center of the helix since any other amino acid residue would perturb the formation of the triple helix.[12] The presence of a high content of proline and hydroxyproline residues confers rigidity to the triple helical conformation and stability to the collagen structure. The amino acids in the Xaa and Yaa positions have their side chains pointing outward of the triple helix allowing a high potential for lateral interactions with other triple helices. In addition to the triple helical rod (also defined COL domain), there are N- and C-terminal extensions, which in some collagens can form large globules that serve several functions including initiation of triple helix formation and secretion of the procollagen molecule in the extracellular space. These globular domains are indicated with NC (for noncollagenous) followed by a number where 1 indicates the C-terminal globule where the process of nucleation of the triple helix takes place. Collagens, especially the nonfibrillar ones, are multidomain proteins and the triple helices should be considered as rods that can physically separate globular domains.

FIBRILLAR COLLAGENS

Fibrillar collagens (types I, II, III, V, XI) are characterized by an uninterrupted triple helical domain approximately 300 nm in length and are so defined because they assemble into fibrils that aggregate into larger fiber bundles. The fibrillar structures have a characteristic pattern of periodic cross-striation close to 67 nm. This periodicity is conferred by the parallel and staggered (by one quarter of their length) alignment of fibrillar monomers. The fibrillar collagens are synthesized as a precursor polypeptide, procollagen, including relatively large NC extensions (propeptides) that, once the procollagen monomers are secreted, are cleaved to allow proper fibril formation. The biosynthesis of a collagen molecule is a complex, multistage process whereby at least ten different enzymes are implicated to modify the chains. Necessary modifications are the hydroxylation of prolyl and lysyl residues and the glycosylation of hydroxylysyl residues that must be completed before triple helix formation. These enzymatic modifications allow chain selection and this step is very important particularly in collagens made of different polypeptide chains. Chain selection is followed by the association of the C-terminal propeptides that are then stabilized by disulfide bonds. Alignment of the three chains, nucleation (i.e., initiation of the triple helical folding) and finally the propagation of the triple helix toward the N-terminus completes the formation of the trimer. Procollagen monomers are then secreted, the N- and C-terminal propeptides are cleaved by specific metalloproteinases, and finally the self-assembly process leading to fibril formation can initiate via the lysyl oxidase catalyzed intra- and intermolecular covalent cross-links between lysyl and hydroxylysyl residues.[13] In vitro fibrillar collagens can form homotypic fibrils but in vivo they appear to participate in the formation of heterotypic fibrils, i.e., made by more than one collagen type.[14,15]

While the self-assembly leading to the formation of a fibril is a fundamental process in collagen biochemistry, the process described above is characteristic of the fibrillar collagens and is not a prerequisite for the supramolecular assembly of all collagen types. In fact, the large majority of collagens identified and characterized in the most recent years do not form fibrils but other morphologically distinct structures such as sheets (type IV collagen), microfilaments (type VI collagen), anchoring fibrils (type VII collagen), hexagonal lattice structures (types VIII and X collagens), or associate with fibrillar collagens (FACIT collagens types IX, XII, and XIV).

In spite of the heterogeneous structure of the different collagen types, collagens evolve from a common ancestor. The comparison of DNA sequences among fibrillar collagen genes led to the striking observation that exon arrangements are almost identical in the regions coding for the uninterrupted COL domains. The Gly-Xaa-Yaa coding exons are in general 54 bp long or multiples thereof and all the exons start with an intact codon for Gly.[16-18] The 54 bp exon was initially proposed to represent the primordial coding element of the Gly-Xaa-Yaa triplets, successive amplification processes giving rise to the different collagen genes. It turned out later that the genes for non-fibrillar collagens such as type IV do not conform to the 54 bp rule and that for several genes the exons start with a split codon for Gly.[19]

COLLAGENS FORMING SHEETS

Basement membranes contain a unique collagen, type IV,[20] with a supramolecular organization rather distinct from that of

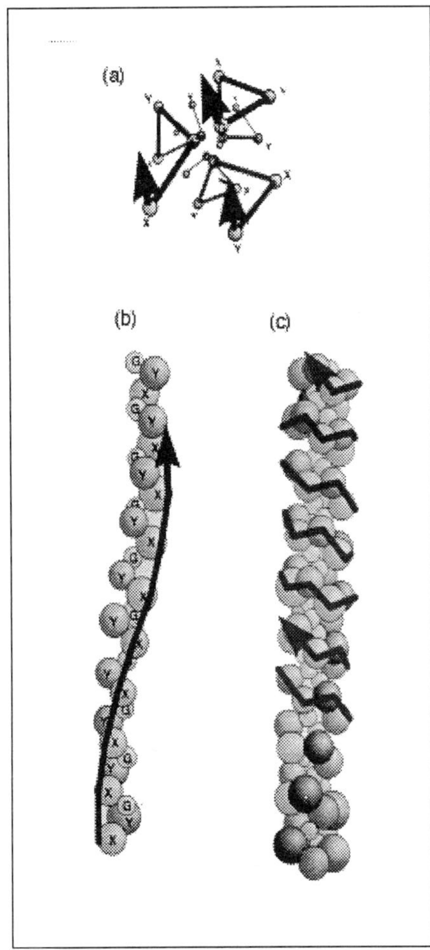

Fig. 6.1. Schematic representation of a collagen triple helix. (a) Cross-section of the triple helix showing that the glycine residues of the Gly-Xaa-Yaa (indicated as G, X and Y) tripeptide unit of collagens are in the center of the helix and the Xaa and Yaa residues project outside of the helix. (b) and (c) show the two different screw-like structures present on the surface of the helix: in (b) the steep right-handed screw formed by each individual ω chain and in (c) the flat left-handed screw formed by the ridge of the side chains of the Xaa and Yaa residues. (With permission from Kuhn K, Eble J: The structural basis of integrin-ligand interactions. Trends Cell Biol 4: 256-261, 1994. Copyright 1994 Elsevier Science Ltd.)

the fibrillar collagens. Limited proteolysis of type IV collagen and analysis of the fragments obtained led to the network model[21] in which two molecules overlap by 25 nm in antiparallel fashion. The dimers then aggregate to tetramers stabilized by disulfide bonds[22] and produce a spider-like structure. Electron microscopic (EM) investigations revealed that after tetramers formation, additional lateral interactions between triple-helical domains take place and strands of two or three triple-helical segments of different type IV molecules are twisted around each other into super-helices.[23] Finally, the formation of reducible and nonreducible intramolecular cross-links creates a continuous network of sheets.

The triple helix of type IV collagen has some short interruptions in the Gly-Xaa-Yaa repeats and these noncollagenous sequences, visible on rotary shadowing EM images as a series of kinks within the triple helical domain, confer a high degree of mechanical flexibility to the individual monomers and hence to the whole assembled aggregated network. Although the triple helix is frequently interrupted, the denaturation temperature of type IV collagen (38°C) is similar to that of type I collagen; apparently the destabilizing effect of the non-triple helical interruptions is compensated by an increased content of hydroxyproline, which is of primary importance for stabilizing the triple helix. Basement membranes, in addition to the open network structure of type IV collagen molecules, include several other constituents such as laminins, nidogen, perlecan and fibulins. These components play an important role and contribute to the formation of a functional basement membrane.[24]

FIBRIL ASSOCIATED COLLAGENS WITH INTERRUPTED TRIPLE HELICES (FACIT)

The FACIT group of collagens includes molecules with two or more short COL domains interrupted by short NC sequences.[9,25] They do not form fibrillar polymers but instead might function as bridges

and couplers organizing and connecting the interstitial collagens in a multi-component three-dimensional pattern. The different members of this group (collagens IX, XII, XIV, XVI and XIX) are characterized by a highly conserved COL1 domain with two cysteine residues at the carboxyl end coded for by a unique exon. The members of the FACIT subgroup of collagens display a broad variation in structure, domain size and organization: in type IX collagen, the three COL domains constitute a large part of the molecule, while in types XII and XIV collagens, the two short COL domains contribute only about 10% of the whole sequence. Only the properties of types XII and XIV that are included in the vWF superfamily of proteins will be described in more detail.

MOLECULAR STRUCTURE

When examined by TEM following rotary shadowing, human type XII collagen displays a cross-shaped structure formed by a kinked 75 nm-long triple helical rod composed of two COL domains interrupted by a small NC2 globule. The rod is attached through a central globule to three 60 nm-long structures ending with a small globule. Each of these long "fingers" corresponds to a single NC3 domain;[27] type XII collagen isolated from chick embryo[28] also display a cross-shaped structure with three thick rods corresponding to the large NC3 domains that are connected to a 70 nm-long collagenase-sensitive segment. At variance with what has been found in type IX and type II collagens, which are covalently attached,[29] no cross links between types XII/XIV and type I collagen have been found although they appear ultrastructurally associated.

Type XII collagen was first discovered at the cDNA level in embryonic chick tendon using the Sau 96I cDNA library screening method.[30] The sequence of the COL1 domain shows a remarkable similarity (50%) to the COL1 domain of α1(IX) collagen chain.[31] In addition, there is a partial homology between the C-terminal NC3 domain of type XII and the NC4 domain of the α1(IX).[30] The contemporary isolation of pepsin-derived fragments from embryonic chick tendon and the fact that their sequence corresponded to the sequence of type XII cDNA, confirmed that the cDNA clones identified and named α1 (XII) belong to a new collagen.[32] Immunological, biochemical and sequence data from human WISH cells,[33] chicken skin fibroblasts,[34] murine cells,[35] newt limb[36] and fetal bovine cartilage[37,38] indicate that there are smaller and larger forms of type XII. These forms result from alternative mRNA splicing by exon skipping[37,38] and the consensus sequence site of splicing has been located at the N-terminus of the third VWFA module[38] so that the two size variants share a common 5' untranslated sequence, the signal peptide, and the initial residues of the mature protein (Fig. 6.2).[39] The shorter variant XIIB/XIIS, which is the major tissue form,[40] consists of the region homologous to the NC4 domain of type IX collagen and of two VWFA modules separated by 10 fibronectin type III modules. The longer variant XIIA/XIIL, which is the major form synthesized by cells in vitro,[33,34,37] consists of two additional VWFA modules separated by eight fibronectin type III modules.[30,38,39] Its ultrastructure is in part distinct from that of the XIIB/XIIS variant since in the distal part of the NC3 "fingers" a double globule likely representing the two VWFA modules is evident.[34]

The existence of type XIV was initially suspected when fragments generated by pepsin digestion of fetal bovine skin yielded collagenous peptides whose sequence was similar to the sequence of the COL 1 domain of α1(IX) and α1(XII) chains.[41] The sequence comparison of type XIV[42-44] indicates that the NC3 arms are slightly shorter than the arms of type XIIB/XIIS, but their overall structure is very similar. At least two variants, which differ in their C-terminal sequences of the NC1 domain, are described in the chick[44,45] and it is possible that N-terminal variants of type XIV also may exist since differences in the nucleotide sequences of the

5'-end of the gene have been reported.[43,45] It became soon evident that undulin,[46] a non-collagenous protein whose sequence had previously been established,[47] represents a proteolytic degradation product of type XIV collagen.[45] Given the high degree of sequence similarity, it is very likely that type XII and type XIV evolved from a common ancestor by gene duplication and multiple module insertions and deletions. The simpler structure of type XIV and its broader distribution[48] suggest that type XIV might resemble the common ancestor more closely. Thus, it is speculated that type XII appeared later in evolution following insertion of several exons into a type XIV-like gene, but no evolutionary data are available to support this hypothesis. If the former gene evolved by insertion of several exons, it maintained an alternatively spliced variant (XIIB/XIIS) that is very much alike type XIV. The human COL12A1 gene has been mapped to chromosome 6q12-q14 syntenic with COL9A1.[35]

The present evidence suggests that both type XII[26] and type XIV[41] collagen exist as disulfide-bonded homotrimers since upon reduction they yield a single polypeptide. Depending upon the tissue, distinct molecular forms of type XII can be isolated: XIIB/XIIS (220kD) is purified from fetal tendon or skin and XIIA/XIIL (320 kD) from cell culture media. From some cell cultures even forms with larger mass (350 kD) that appear to contain glycosaminoglycan (GAG) chains are obtained.[34] The GAG chain is very likely attached to the N-terminus of the NC3 domain which is the domain missing in the XIIB/XIIS variant. Type XIV collagen migrates on reduced gels as a 210 kD polypeptide although occasionally forms with larger mass (340 kD) are observed. In addition, following chondroitinase digestion, type XIV isolated from bovine cartilage is slightly reduced in mass suggesting that it also may be present in some tissues as a proteoglycan.[37] The heterogeneity at least of the type XII molecular forms is even greater since heterotrimers,

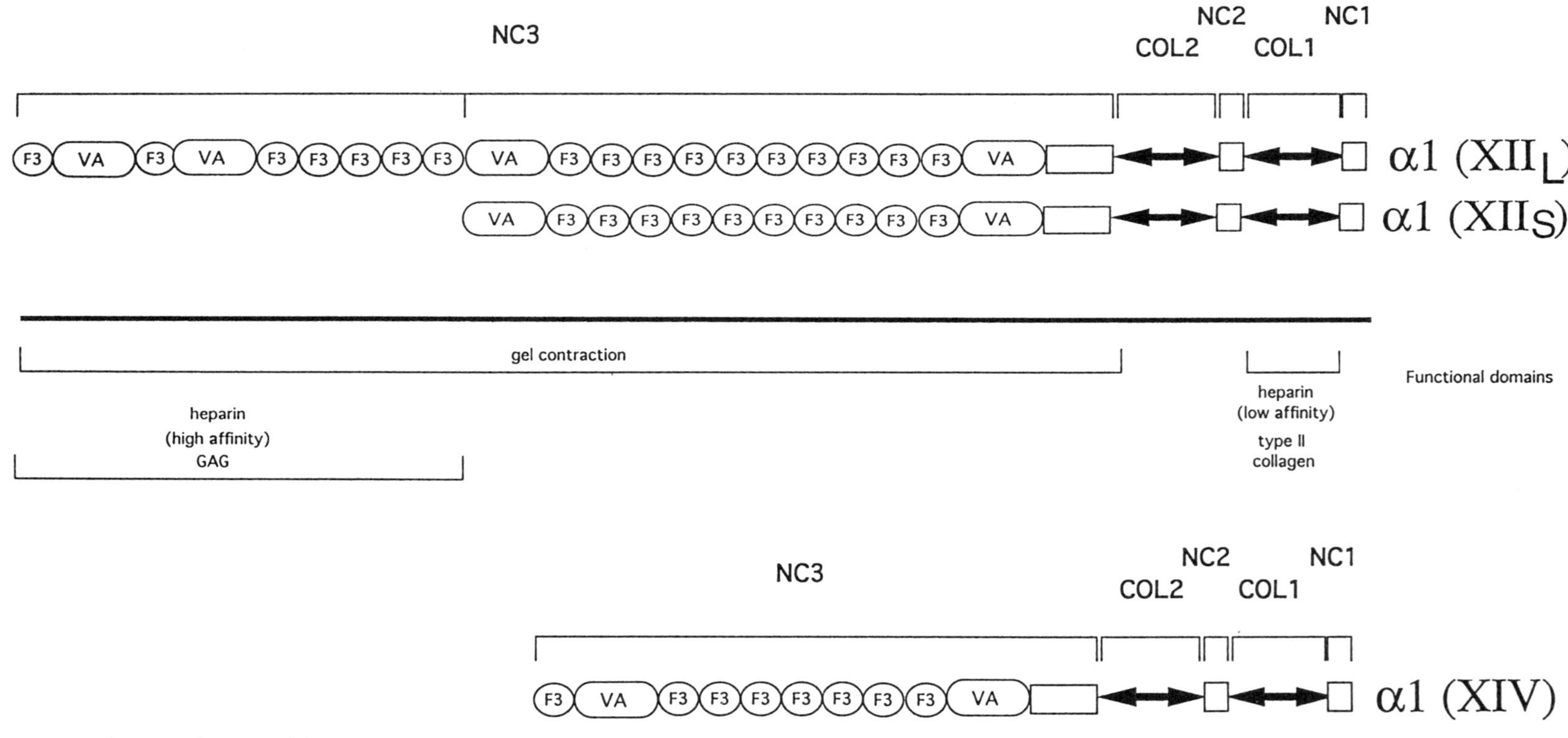

Fig. 6.2. Schematic diagram of the FACIT collagens. The different modules are designated according to the proposed nomenclature of Bork and Bairoch.[238] The location of the major functional sites is indicated. NC, noncollagenous domain; COL, collagenous domain.

i.e., individual collagen molecules consisting of both XIIA/XIIL and XIIB/XIIS chain variants, can be isolated (Fig. 6.3).[49] Type XII (as the other FACIT collagens) is devoid of a C-propeptide like those involved in the initial steps of the assembly of fibrillar collagens and the NC1 domain could play a similar role in chain selection, registration, and trimer assembly. However, trimer and S-S bond formation is not prevented by a deletion of most of the NC1 domain[50] suggesting that very likely only the NC1 residues at the junction between NC1 and COL1 domains are involved in the initial steps of type XII assembly.

TISSUE EXPRESSION

Type XII and type XIV are found in many tissues[33,51-53] but with a differential expression depending upon the developmental stage: thus, type XII is widespread in E6 chick embryos and shows a more restricted distribution (bone, tendon and gizzard) at later stages. In contrast, type XIV is rarely expressed at E6 while it is present virtually in every tissue at later stages. These collagens occur together in some sites, but often they show distinctive regional distributions: for instance, in the skin, type XII is found predominantly in the papillary dermis, while type XIV predominates within the reticular dermis; in blood vessels, type XII is found in the intima and type XIV in the adventitia.[33] Preembedding[54] and postembedding[49] immunogold EM localization studies with antibodies specific for types XII and XIV show gold particles periodic deposition along banded type I fibrils suggesting a possible interaction with type I collagen. However, whether types XII and XIV are really bound to the surface of collagen fibrils is still debated. Particles also are found between fibrils, but this distribution does not appear to constitute an independent network as has been shown for type VI collagen.[55] In addition, while immunolocalization at the ultrastructural level shows that types XIV and VI colocalize in the vicinity of cross-striated collagen fibrils,

type XII displays only limited colocalization with type VI.[54]

FUNCTION

The mechanical stability of different ECMs of tissues is provided by the strength of the various heterotypic fibrils composed of fibrillar collagens and certain properties of these fibers are controlled by the relative proportion of the individual fibrillar collagen types within the fiber.[56] However, both the spatial arrangement that changes among different tissues as well as the fiber diameter might be controlled by the FACIT collagens.[9,25] Insight into the function of type IX was provided initially by its peculiar distribution on the surface of collagen fibers and is supported by recent observations indicating that type IX collagen knock-out homozygous mice appear normal at birth but with increasing age develop a degenerative disease resembling osteoarthritis in man.[57] By functioning as a bridge between collagen fibrils and cartilage proteoglycans, rather than being critical for development type IX collagen might be important for articular cartilage maintenance. Due to their modular structure, both type XII and type XIV collagens could bring new functions to fibrils with which they presumably interact.

STRUCTURE-FUNCTION RELATIONSHIPS

FACIT collagens seem to associate with interstitial collagen fibers by the lateral alignment of their conserved COL1 domain.[49,51,54] The closely located NC1 domain could play a role in the recognition of the appropriate collagen type and/or of the interaction sites. Given that the highest sequence differences among the FACIT collagens are within the NC1 domain, it seems plausible that the specificity of fibrillar collagen recognition or the recognition of a proper fibril arrangement rests more on the variable NC1 domain rather than on the conserved COL1 domain.

Both type XIIB/XIIS and type XIV collagens can promote fibroblast-mediated

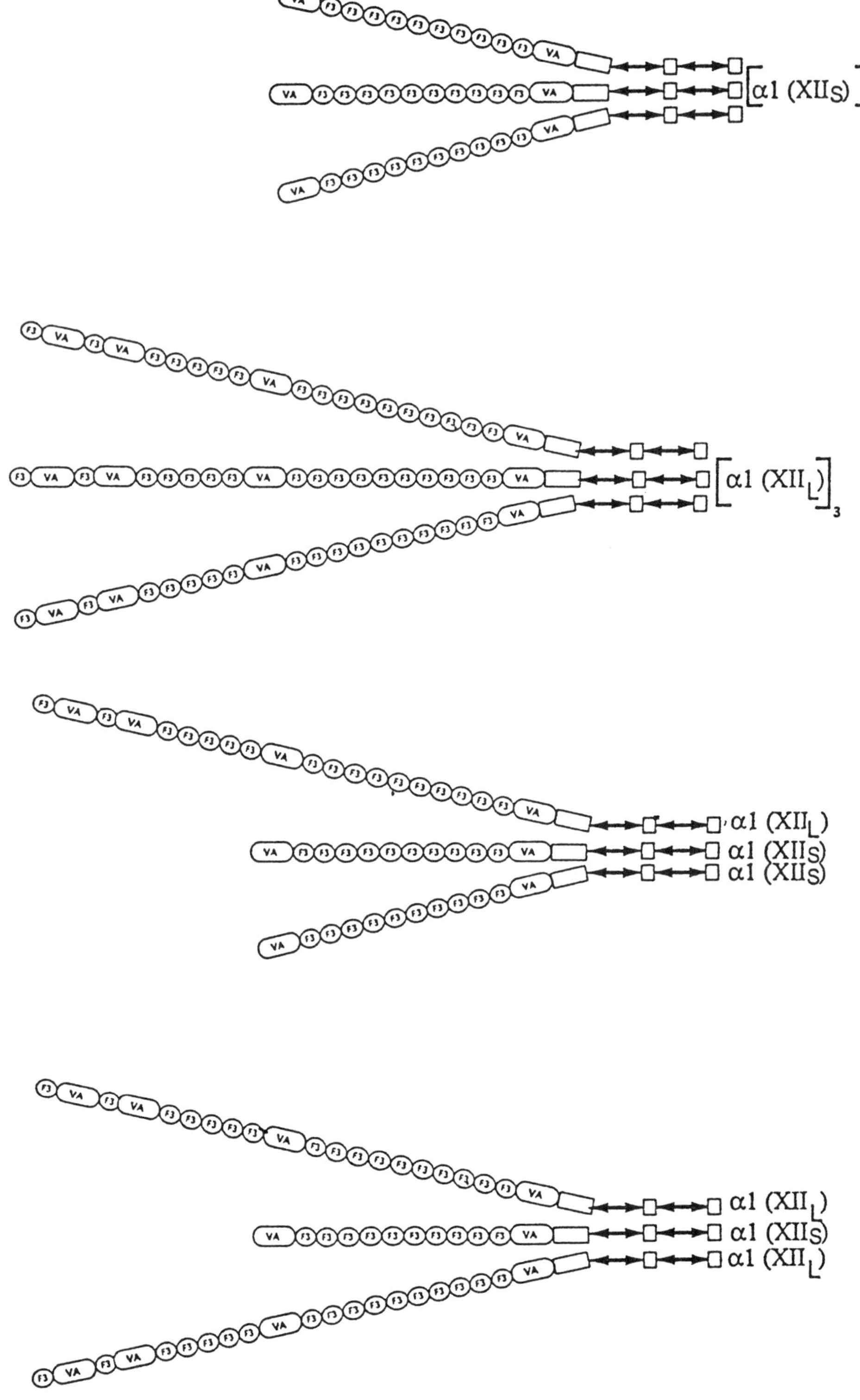

Fig. 6.3. Schematic representation of the heterogeneity of type XII collagen.

collagen gel contraction in dermal equivalents, i.e., fibroblasts cultured within a gel made of type I collagen.[58] This gel contraction model is a suitable dynamic system for studying the interaction of cells with a fibrous collagen substrate in a setting that is similar to the in vivo condition.[59] While no direct interaction between the NC3 domains and neither fibroblasts nor monomeric and fibrillar collagens is measurable, the gel contraction activity of both collagens is provided through their NC3 domains (Fig. 6.2) and requires native type XIIB/XIIL and type XIV collagens as the gel contraction effect is inhibited by their denaturation.[58] The promoting function of type XIIB/XIIL and type XIV collagens might be the result of an increased mobility of the fibrils within the gel secondary to a NC3-mediated competition of the interactions between collagen fibrils. An alternative possibility is that the FACIT collagen-mediated changes in the fibril diameters result in a decreased fibril surface area.

The NC3 arms of both type XII and XIV collagens project outwards from the collagen fibril surfaces[51] where they might interact with other ECM constituents. Furthermore, while both XIIA/XIIL and XIIB/XIIS variants appear to associate with interstitial collagen fibers, the different length of their NC3 domains suggests that they recognize different ligands. Thus, while one low affinity heparin-binding site common to both forms is located in the NC1 and/or COL1 domain, a higher affinity heparin-binding site is present only in the XIIA/XIIL form.[49] The location of this high affinity site is not yet known but VWFA modules are good candidates: in other proteins of the superfamily such as vWF[60] and type VI collagen,[61] VWFA modules are known to interact with heparin. Several other ligands have been recently identified that interact with FACIT collagens; thus, type XIV interacts with the proteoglycan decorin[62] and this binding is saturable, is inhibited by chondroitinase ABC treatment and by an excess of soluble dermatan sulfate that is the major GAG chain of decorin. The precise location of the binding site on type XIV is not known but a direct binding to the NC3 domain is excluded.[62] Therefore, since decorin also interacts with collagen I fibrils[63] this proteoglycan might play the role of a bridging molecule between the FACIT and the fibrillar collagens.

The inability to measure any interaction in vitro between type XIV and pepsin-solubilized monomeric forms of fibrillar types I, III, and V collagens[27] was quite unexpected given the close apposition of type XIV to collagen fibers.[51,54] However, while there is no evidence at present for a direct interaction between type XIV and fibrillar collagens, additional studies are needed. Type XIV interacts with the pepsin-solubilized form of type VI and perlecan while it fails to bind to type I-V collagens and also several other ECM proteins including laminin, nidogen, BM40, fibronectin, vitronectin and vWF are unable to support any interaction.[27] Recent data indicate that rather than interacting with preformed interstitial collagen fibers, type XII coassembles with fibrillar collagen monomers; this interaction is prevented if the collagenous part of type XII is removed by collagenase treatment.[49] It should be pointed out that the VWFA modules of both types XII and XIV collagens are very much like the collagen-binding A1 and A3 modules of vWF as they all possess a single disulfide loop;[64] this loop might play a role in conferring a proper folding to the modules. If the binding to the triple helix of type VI collagen is via the VWFA modules of type collagens XIV, the lack of any interaction between type XIV collagen and triple helices of the fibrillar collagens may indicate a certain degree of specificity in the recognition of different triple helices.

COLLAGEN FORMING MICROFILAMENTS

Type VI collagen is a major component of the ECM of most tissues in several species[65] and molecules with characteristics similar to type VI have been identified in *Xenopus* embryos.[66] Initially, low-yield purification of the peptic fragments of type VI collagen was relatively easy because the high molecular weight complexes that it forms are soluble in physiological buffers.[67] Subsequently Trüeb and collaborators devised a purification protocol allowing at least ten-fold higher yields than previously reported.[68] Since intact nonpepsinized type VI also was initially isolated only in very low quantities,[69] it was assumed that type VI collagen represents a minor ECM constituent. On the contrary, improved extraction procedures and careful control of proteolysis during extraction maneuvers has confirmed that this collagen is a significant ECM component of several tissues,[70,71] notably cornea.[72,73] It forms beaded microfilaments which are organized in tissues into a characteristic highly branched network.[74-77] The microfilaments can be purified under native conditions[78,79] and from some tissues up to about one-third of type VI content is extracted as microfilaments.[80] The molecule has a multidomain structure with a number of potentially functional sites including several cell-binding RGD motifs within the triple-helix. The large N- and C-terminal globular domains flanking the triple helix are unique among collagens and are primarily contributed by the presence of 15-18 VWFA modules. Indeed, type VI collagen is the major representative of the vWF superfamily.

MOLECULAR STRUCTURE

A structural model based upon rotary shadowing EM images has been proposed for type VI collagen microfilaments formation.[75,81] The monomer (three polypeptide chains)[82] appears as a dumb-bell-shaped structure about 110-120 nm long, with a diameter of 3-10 nm: it consists of a short rod-like central triple helical domain linking two large globular domains accounting for more than three-fourths of the mass.[65] Dimers of type VI collagen (six polypeptide chains) are then formed as a result of an antiparallel opposition of monomers whose helices overlap by about 75 nm and are slightly intertwisted in the overlapping region (Fig. 6.4). This organi-

zation allows distinction between the two globular domains of the monomer one of which is located in an inner and the other in an outer position.[83] The inner globular domain represents the C-terminus of the three polypeptide chains since a purified preparation of inner globular domains contains the corresponding sequences, while the outer globular domain contains sequences from the N-terminus of the polypeptide chains.[83] The tetramers (twelve polypeptide chains), the building blocks of microfilaments extracted from tissues, are then formed by the lateral association of two dimers with their ends in register. The assembly of monomers into dimers and tetramers is likely guided by adhesive interactions between globular domains and the adjacent triple helices. Tetramers associate by specific interactions between their outer N-globular domains or between the globular domains and the triple helix, such that they are connected by an overlap of the outer segments that brings all the globular domains close together. The tetramers are for the largest part noncovalently linked to each other,[75,78,81] although the exact nature of their association is not yet clear. Some microfilaments might contain tetramers cross-linked by disulfide bonds as suggested by the persistence of some microfilamentous structures even after extensive pepsin digestion under strong acid conditions.[81,84] In general the microfilaments are beaded[74,77] since they are thicker in the region of the globular domains, but evidence for alternative type VI aggregates occurring as broad-banded fibrils has been provided in both normal and pathological tissues.[74,85,86]

Recently, the genes encoding the three type VI collagen chains were isolated from human,[87-91] chick[92-95] and mouse species[96,97] and most of their gene organization determined. One to three-four exons encode each VWFA module while the COL domains of the genes for the $\alpha1(VI)$ and $\alpha2(VI)$ chains that are fully characterized are encoded by short exon multiples of 9 bp. Since no correlation with the 54 bp building block of the triple helix typical of the fibrillar

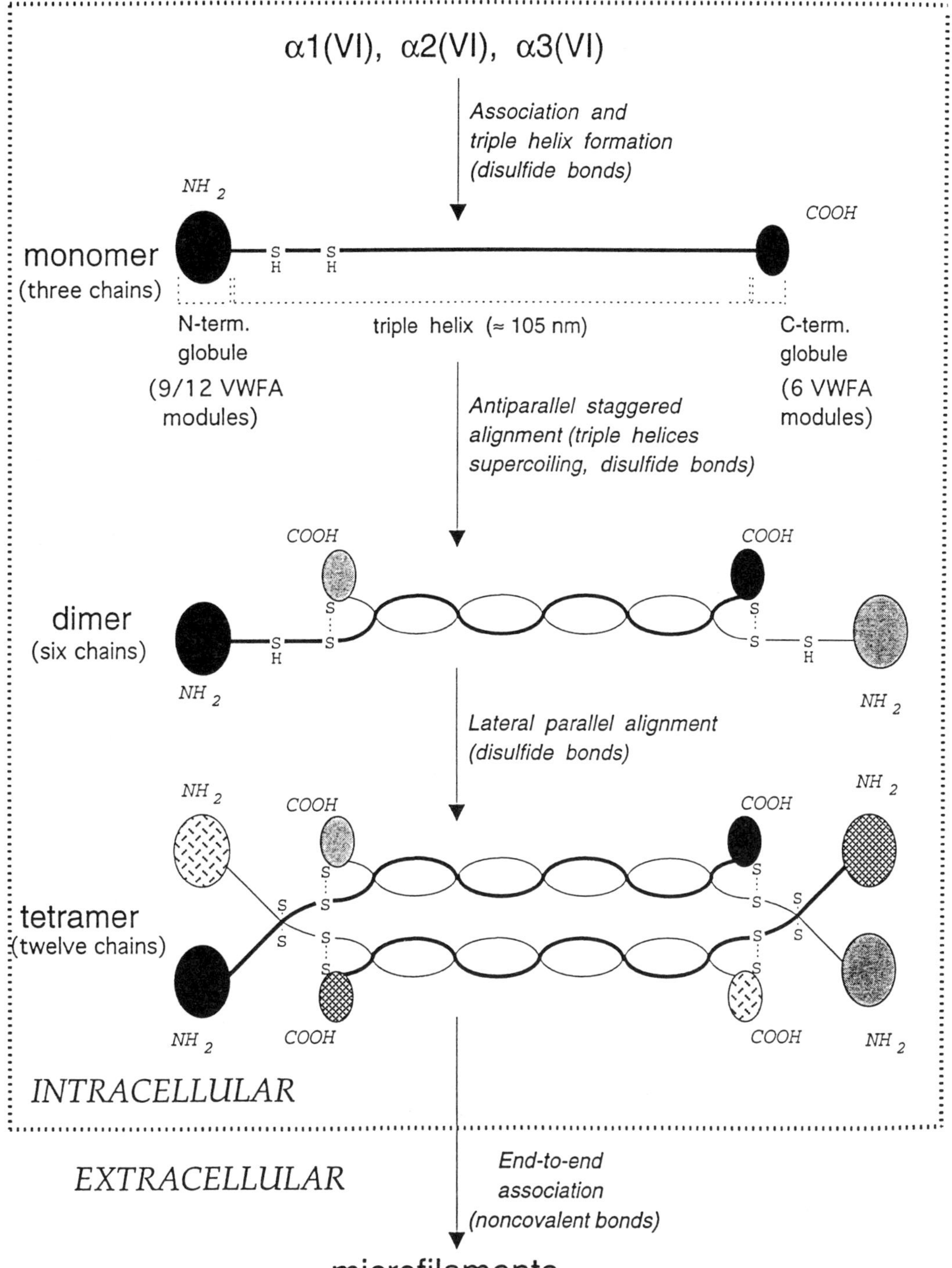

Fig. 6.4. Schematic representation of the assembly of type VI collagen microfilaments. The proposed pathway is based upon in vitro pulse-chase biosynthetic evidences and rotary shadowing EM images. The size of the N- and C-terminal globules and of the triple helix are not drawn to scale.

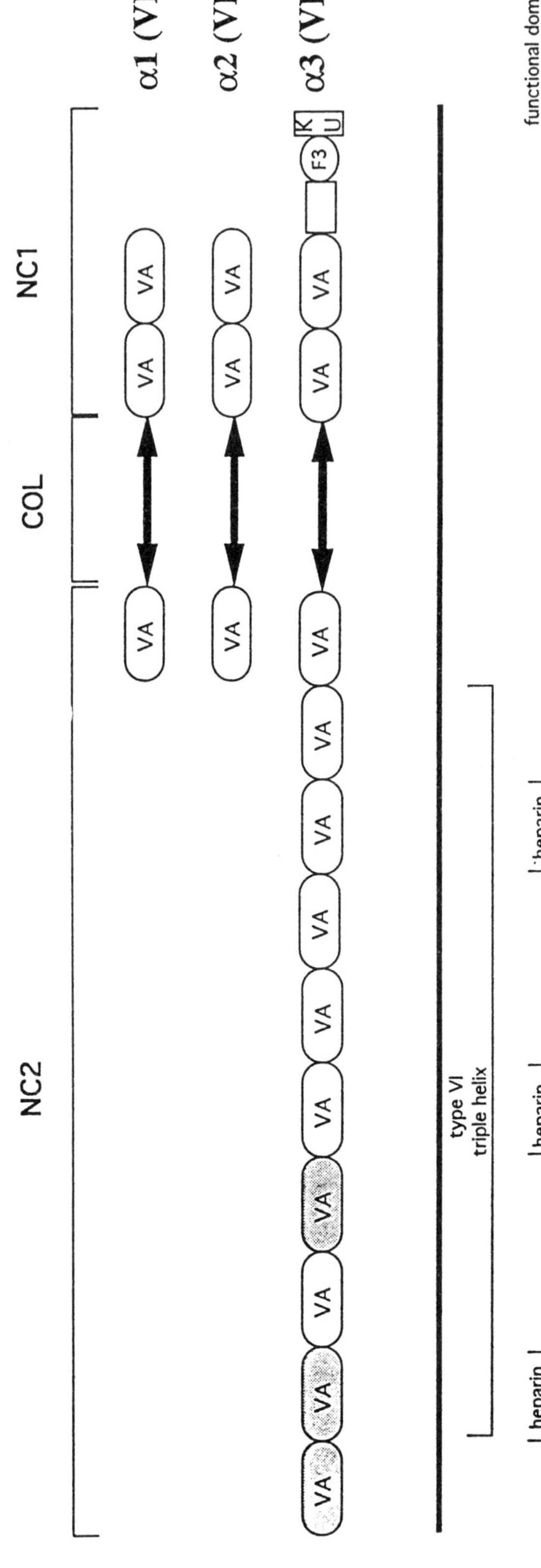

Fig. 6.5. Schematic diagram of type VI collagen. The different modules are designated according to the proposed nomenclature of Bork and Bairoch.[238] Shaded modules undergo alternative splicing. The location of the major functional sites is indicated. NC, noncollagenous domain; COL, collagenous domain.

collagens is detected[18], it could mean that this region of the type VI genes arose by intron recombination of a primordial 9 bp unit. Notwithstanding a high sequence homology of the coding sequences between the different species, significant variation is found between the 5'-end of the genes coding for the human and chicken α2 (VI) chains and the murine α2 (VI) chain, that were studied in more detail. In both human and chicken genes, transcription initiates at multiple sites. However, transcription of the human α2 (VI) starts from two alternative promoters endowed with TATA and CAAT boxes and Sp1 binding elements,[90] while the chicken α2 (VI) gene is transcribed from a single TATA- and CAAT-less promoter.[98] The murine α1 (VI) promoter also lacks canonical TATA and CAAT boxes and Sp1 binding sites but includes sequences for several other transcription factors.[96,97]

The elucidation of the complete sequence of the three constituents chains of type VI based on cDNA cloning has confirmed the results of the structural and biochemical studies suggesting that the chains have quite different molecular masses: about 1000 residues for the α1 (VI) and α2 (VI)[99-102] chains and about 3000 for the α3 (VI) chain,[103-106] which is among the largest collagen chain sequenced to date (Fig. 6.5). Despite this peculiar difference in mass among the three chains the triple helical sequences have nearly identical length (335-336 residues). They are located in the middle portion of the α1 (VI) and α2 (VI) chains and in the C-terminal part of the α3 (VI) chain. The amino acid sequences deduced from the cDNAs indicate that the chains are strongly conserved in human, mouse and chicken and show about 70% identity. Conserved features include the number and position of cysteine residues and the clusters of cysteines at both ends of the COL domain, the triple helix imperfections, the numerous potential cell-binding RGD sites and the putative N-glycosylation sites. The cysteines at the ends of the COL domain might stabilize the triple helix and explain

the resistance to degradation by several metalloproteinases of the non-reduced type VI,[80] while those within the COL domain participate in the dimer and tetramer assembly. The oligosaccharides acceptor sites within the COL domain are fully occupied by oligosaccharides[107] and the role of the sugars may be essential in preventing lateral associations of the individual tetramers or microfilaments. The NC domains of each chain contain VWFA modules (two at the C-terminus and one at the N-terminus), while the extended N-terminal domain of the α3 (VI) chain is contributed by the presence of six[104,105] to nine[91,92] VWFA modules. Furthermore, the α3 (VI) chain differs from the other two chains by the presence of unique additional sequences in the most distal C-terminus. These sequences are not totally homologous between human[104] and chick,[103] but both contain a fibronectin type III module and a serine protease inhibitor of the Kunitz type. Although the overall modular structure of human and chicken α3 (VI) chains is similar, the N-terminal end of the human α3 (VI) chain has several potential glycosylation sites that are absent (except for one) in the chicken molecule and that potentially could generate additional molecular heterogeneity by attachment of branched oligosaccharides. In addition, the human most N-terminal portion has two cysteine residues which are both located in different modules (A9/N10 and A6/N7)[91] compared to the single cysteine of the chicken molecule in module A7.[105] In the N-terminus of the chicken α3 (VI) chain the single cysteine is in a constitutive exon and in the human chain both cysteine residues are present in alternatively spliced exons. This localization further augments the possibilities for structural/functional variations of human type VI collagen. In fact, while disulfide bonding is not one of the major mechanisms that participates in the stabilization of microfilaments formed by the end-to-end association of type VI tetramers,[75,78,81] in the human molecule there is a higher potential for covalent S-S bonding between two tetramers or between a tetramer and another ECM molecule.

Using chaotropic agents several laboratories have succeeded in purifying type VI collagen molecules whose main component is a polypeptide migrating on SDS-PAGE under reducing conditions with a mass of about 140 kD.[69,108-110] In addition to the main band a ladder of four or five fainter bands corresponding to polypeptides in the range of 180-280 kD is present in extracts from tissues of several species.[71,78] All these high mass components are collagenous based on their amino acid composition and react with both polyclonal and monoclonal antibodies to the α3(VI) chain. Therefore, unique among the collagens discovered to date, type VI collagen has a significantly different size of one of its three constituent chains, the α1 (VI) and α2 (VI) chains being about 140 kD and the α3 (VI) chain ranging from 180 to 280 kD.

Finally, native microfilaments in intact form also are purified if collagenase treatment under nonreducing conditions[80,111,112] or, in the case of vertebral discs, jaluronidase treatment[78] are used.

Tissue Expression

Still limited data are available on the first expression and late occurrence of type VI collagen during embryogenesis. The collagen is expressed at high levels in early skin development,[113] liver,[114] heart[115] and secondary stroma of cornea.[116] Furthermore, in the chick embryo (E13) strong positivity for type VI is restricted to the articular cartilage, an area of poor proliferation and initiation of chondrogenesis, and little or no type VI collagen is detectable in the remaining areas of the embryo cartilage.[117] This restricted cartilage localization suggests that rather than being involved in maintenance of the cartilage phenotype like type IX,[57] type VI collagen might be involved in promoting chondrogenesis. This last observation is in agreement with the finding that, in an in vitro system of avian chondrocyte differentiation, type VI collagen expression shows a dramatic rise well before the appearance of "cartilage specific" type II and IX collagens.[117] Finally, there is evidence that variant protein forms of the α3 (VI) chain have distinct tissue distribution in the embryo (see below). Except for the calcified matrix of the bone, type VI has been localized to nearly all sites investigated[54,108,118,119] including cartilage.[86,120,121] The tissue distribution of type VI is predominantly interstitial, but positive localization also appears at the surface of some cell types, in particular smooth muscle cells. Light microscopic data suggests that, at least in some developing tissues, type VI might be localized in close association with basement membranes;[122] while ultrastructural studies of nerves, blood vessels, fat and glomerulus[54,123,124] confirm these observations. Basement membrane localization is still controversial. It has been suggested that in some tissues type VI collagen might play an anchoring function similar to that of type VII.[54] In adult articular cartilage, type VI collagen is associated mainly with the mid and deep chondrocytes while in the superficial zones it is localized both around the cells and throughout the matrix.[54,125]

Biosynthesis

The process of type VI collagen assembly is quite unique and distinct from that of any of the other known collagens. Intracellular association of the three chains in a type VI collagen monomer is initiated and stabilized by S-S bonds and is then followed by the formation of S-S bonded dimers (six chains) and tetramers (twelve chains) before secretion (Fig. 6.4).[126,127] The dimers are very likely stabilized by S-S bonds formed between the single cysteine residues within the COL domain of the α1 (VI) and α2 (VI) chains (position 89 of the triple helix), while a cysteine in the α3 (VI) COL domain (position 50 of the triple helix) may participate in tetramer formation.[99-101,104-106,128] The S-S bonds formed between clusters of cysteines at the junctions between the N- and C-termini of the triple helix and the globular domains contribute to the collagenase resistance and the high thermal stability of the type VI collagen triple helix.[68] In fact, although the triple helix of type VI collagen is only about half as long as that of the interstitial collagens, its termal stability is comparable to that of type I collagen.

SDS-PAGE analysis of tissue extracted[68,71,129] and of biosynthetically labeled type VI collagen[126,130] have suggested that the three chains occur stoichiometrically and associate in a 1:1:1 ratio to form stable heterotrimers. Structural considerations,[75,81] sequence data[99-101,104-106] and molecules produced by transfected cells[131] predict that the [α1(VI)-α2(VI)-α3(VI)] heterotrimer is the form with the highest disulfide bonding and triple-helix stability and that aggregates comprising different chain compositions would be more susceptible to degradation. Alternative chain composites might be produced as suggested by the noncoordinated mRNA and protein levels under certain biological conditions[132-134] or in several tumor cell lines:[135] while skin fibroblasts show comparable steady-state levels of all three mRNAs,[132,136] corneal fibroblasts[135] and fetal cells[137] produce reduced amounts of α3(VI) chain mRNA that appears as the rate-limiting component in the deposition of microfilaments. The three mRNAs can be regulated independently as shown by the analysis of α1 (VI), α2 (VI) and α3 (VI) mRNA levels in human skin fibroblasts grown on collagen gels[132] or treated with γ-IFN:[133] γ-IFN selectively down-regulates α3 (VI) mRNA and reduces the synthesis and deposition of type VI. In contrast, TGF-β causes a selective increase in α3(VI) mRNA and an increased secretion of type VI collagen.[138] The independent regulation of α3(VI) and the apparent coregulation of α1 (VI) and α2 (VI) mRNAs could depend on their different chromosomal localization: COL6A3 is on the distal long arm of chromosome 2 band q37[139] while COL6A1 and COL6A2 are on the distal long arm of chromosome 21 band q22.3.[139,140] Further

analysis has indicated that the two latter genes are less than 185 kb apart.[140]

Type VI collagen is not processed in tissue culture as shown by pulse-chase[130] and immunoblotts of cell layers probed with monoclonal antibodies. While no apparent major processing of the α1 (VI) and α2 (VI) chains is detected,[130] size heterogeneity at the protein level had been reported for the α3 (VI) chain both in vivo[71,83,129,141] and in biosynthetic studies in vitro.[126,127,130,134] In addition, using highly specific polyclonal antibodies against epitopes present on the Kunitz-like domain of the most C-terminal end of the human α3 (VI) chain, it was shown that the reactivity is neither detected by immunofluorescence on tissues nor on guanidine-extracted placental type VI collagen.[142] Multiple alternative splicings of α3 (VI) mRNA have been described[87,89,90] giving rise to primary transcripts that, by a mechanism of exon-skipping, lack all or some N-terminal modules, namely A9, A8 and A6 in chick and A9/N10, A8/N9 and A6/N7 in human. At the moment there is no direct evidence that relates individual mRNAs to the heterogeneous α3 (VI) polypeptides isolated from cells grown in vitro and from tissues, but it is tempting to speculate that the multiple polypeptides detected after SDS-PAGE derive from mRNAs that have skipped one or more exons coding for individual VWFA modules. By using exon-specific RNA probes and module-specific monoclonal and polyclonal antibodies, there is evidence that α3 (VI) variant chains have a differential tissue distribution within several late embryonal chicken tissues (Colombatti et al, submitted; Doliana et al, submitted). For instance, all α3 (VI) variants (i.e., A9+, A8+ and A6+) are present in 17-19 day old embryo skin—the only tissue where A9+ variants can be detected at the protein level; in glandular stomach A8+ and A6+ variants are present in the outer muscular layer and in the intraglandular but not in the periglandular connective tissue; only A6+ variants are localized in the stromal tissue of villi; A8+ variants show a signal only in the endomysium while A6+ variants also are present in the perimysium in striated muscle. It could be envisaged that alterations in chain composition as well as alternative splicing of the α3 (VI) mRNA in response to developmental or local conditions might represent a mechanism to increase the plasticity and change the pattern of type VI molecular interactions.

In vivo, individual variants cannot be purified to heterogeneity from any source and to obtain specific spliced α3(VI) variants that include or are deprived of any of the alternatively spliced VWFA modules a model system, making use of murine NIH/3T3 cells stably transfected with cDNAs encoding chicken type VI chains, was developed.[143] Transfected cells that stably synthesize, secrete and deposit into the ECM an apparently normal type VI were obtained,[131] indicating that this approach is potentially suitable to isolate variant molecules for further functional studies. Finally, three α2 (VI) variants involving mutually exclusive utilization of two exons and with potential distinct C-termini have been described in human mRNAs but the evidence for a distinct protein product is still lacking.[87]

FUNCTION

The widespread distribution of type VI microfilaments between collagen fibers and in close apposition to the surface of several cell types, along with the collagen-, heparin-, hyaluronan- and proteoglycan-binding capacities demonstrated in vitro (see below), has led to the proposal that type VI collagen microfilaments perform a bridging function between cells and ECM, the variant forms representing subtly different functional entities.[105] The finding that type VI microfilaments also are detected underlying basement membranes that are not stabilized by anchoring fibrils[54] further suggests that type VI microfilaments might substitute for type VII fibrils and anchor these basement membranes to the stroma.

Indirect observations such as ultrastructural studies showing a close association of type VI microfilaments with cell surfaces[54,76,120] and sequence data indicating the presence of 13 potential cell-binding RGD motifs in the COL domains suggested that type VI might perform cell-adhesive functions. In fact, various molecular forms of type VI, i.e., microfilaments,[79,111] the "intact" tissue form,[144] the pepsin-solubilized central triple helix domain,[103,145-148] but also the isolated terminal globules[111] or individual chains[149] have been shown to promote cell attachment of fibroblasts,[149] smooth muscle cells,[103,148] corneal fibroblasts,[145] hemopoietic cells[148] and several tumor cell lines.[147] While cell attachment to denatured and unfolded type VI is mediated by α5β1, αIIbβ3, and αvβ3 integrins and is inhibited by RGDS containing peptides,[105,145-147] attachment to native forms is RGD-independent and is mediated primarily by α1β1 and α2β1 (see chapter 3).[146] Whether the RGD-dependent adhesion to the unfolded molecule is of any biological significance during various cellular processes where tissue remodeling is taking place is not yet known. Finally, while there are no indications that both intact and native type VI molecules are better substrates than the pepsin-solubilized form for adhesion of several tumor cell lines, in some experimental model systems the intact and native forms of the molecule are the most efficacious in supporting cell attachment:[111] neural crest cells adhere to and migrate with better efficiency on type VI tetramers and on native microfilaments than on the pepsin-digested form lacking the VWFA modules that constitute most of the globular ends. This behavior suggests the presence of multiple and cooperative cell-binding sites distributed along both the triple-helical and the globular domains. Especially neural crest cell migration seems strictly dependent upon the supramolecular organization of the molecule and the presence of intact globules.[111]

In addition to CD44, a chondroitin sulfate integral membrane receptor that mediates cell attachment to type VI collagen,[150] another cell membrane associated chondroitin sulfate proteoglycan (NG2) with a core protein of about 300 kD can complex type VI collagen.[151] Upon transfection of NG2 in negative cell lines that secrete but do not anchor type VI at the cell surface, the transfected cells acquire the ability to maintain cell surface-bound type VI collagen.[152] Therefore, although the functional consequences of the binding of type VI to the core protein of NG2 at the cell membrane remain unclear, NG2 might be a determining factor in regulating the extent of deposition and organization of type VI collagen in the ECM.

Platelet adhesion to the exposed vascular subendothelial matrix proteins at the injury site is a crucial step in initiating the hemostatic and thrombotic processes. The vWF glycoprotein in the subendothelium or immediately deposited at the initiation of hemostasis mediates platelet adhesion to the subendothelium matrix.[153] Type VI collagen colocalizes with vWF in the vascular subendothelium[154] and can be extracted from this tissue.[155] Pepsin-solubilized type VI collagen mediates $\alpha2\beta1$ integrin-dependent platelet adhesion in both static continuous flow systems.[156] Furthermore, Rand and colleagues have shown that under low shear rates (4 dynes/cm²), type VI collagen supports vWF-mediated platelet adhesion with a higher binding affinity than type I,[157] while at high (40 dynes/cm²) rates the adhesive function of type I collagen is prevailing. These findings indicate a likely role for type VI collagen in the process of hemostasis and thrombosis in regions of the vasculature with low shear flow.

STRUCTURE-FUNCTION RELATIONSHIPS

The finding of serine protease inhibitor Kunitz-like sequences in the C-terminus of the $\alpha3$(VI) chain of both chicken[103] and human[104] molecules prompted an analysis of the functional activity of the isolated Kunitz modules. Quite disappointing was the finding that both human[141] and chicken[158] Kunitz modules fail to demonstrate any inhibitory activity against sev-

eral proteases despite the presence of most of the appropriate residues in the potential functional sites[103,104] and the fact that the tertiary structure is very close to that of all other members of the Kunitz family members.[159,160] However, an explanation for the lack of anti-protease function of this particular Kunitz domain emerges from the X-ray diffraction analysis of the crystal structure[159] and the structure in solution as determined by NMR[160] of the human module: these analyses indicate that one of the three disulfide bonds ($C14$-$C38$) conferring the domain its compact structure has a left-handed instead of a right-handed chirality[159] as found in other functional members of the Kunitz family such as BPTI[161] and API[162] and that the module is highly dynamic in solution.[160] The lack of trypsin inhibition very likely arises from the type of side chains of the adjoining residues at the interface between this Kunitz module and trypsin.

Using affinity chromatography with recombinant fragments of the human $\alpha3$(VI) chain containing nearly all the N-terminal part of the polypeptide (i.e., eight VWFA modules) or proteolytically cleaved single and twin VWFA modules, a strong salt-sensitive binding for heparin involving modules A8/N9, A5/N6 and A2/N3 was detected.[61] The same recombinant $\alpha3$(VI) N-terminal domain recognizes the triple helix domain of type VI suggesting that these VWFA modules might be involved in microfilament self-assembly. Similarly, the isolated globular domains have a strong affinity for each other and for the COL domain of type VI collagen.[80]

A hyaluronidase treatment in vitro can lead to the disassembly of fetal bovine skin type VI microfilaments into tetramers, and a subsequent incubation of the disrupted microfilaments in the presence of hyaluronan facilitates a partial repolymerization of the microfilaments.[79] Others using type VI collagen from different sources, bovine cornea, human amnion and pig cartilage instead of fetal bovine skin, were unable to reproduce the stabilization nor the repolymerization process.[80,112] Therefore, although the suggestion that hyaluronan might play some role in the process of microfilament assembly was supported by affinity chromatography data,[60] at present it appears that there is no direct interaction between type VI molecules and hyaluronan. Intact type VI collagen has been shown to interact with hyaluronan in a solid phase assay[163] and the binding of the human α3 (VI) recombinant fragment to an affinity column of hyaluronan appears to be much stronger than the binding to heparin and to the triple helix as it can only be reversed by denaturating urea concentrations.[61] However, if this fragment is incubated with hyaluronan in solution and then visualized after rotary shadowing no binding of the two molecular species to each other is demonstrable.[112] At variance with the finding when hyaluronan is incubated with aggrecans,[164] no complexes are detected at the EM also when intact type VI instead of the α3(VI) recombinant fragment is used.[80,112] It seems likely that the solid phase and affinity binding data might represent an artifact of the experimental procedures.

A recombinant fragment of the chicken α3(VI) chain (containing five of the most N-terminal VWFA modules) binds type I collagen.[105] However, using a similar human recombinant fragment,[61] binding to any of several fibrillar collagens assayed could not be confirmed. Type XIV collagen localizes in close vicinity to the major cross-striated collagen fibrils,[54] in areas where type VI collagen also is distributed.[55,76] While intact type XIV collagen displays a significant binding for pepsin-solubilized type VI collagen,[27] the NC3 domain of type XIV, where all its VWFA modules are located, is not active suggesting that the interaction between type VI and type XIV collagens does not involve VWFA modules on either site of this bimolecular complex. However, in other studies undulin, a splicing variant and/or a degradation product of type XIV collagen, that contains one N-terminal VWFA module but no collagenous sequences, bound very efficiently to fibrillar type I and

III collagens and to pepsin-solubilized type VI collagen.[46]

Since cell attachment to both pepsin-solubilized and intact type VI collagen is similarly efficient with several tumor cell lines[147] it has been suggested that the non-triple helical globular domains do not contribute to the adhesive function of type VI collagen. Accordingly, these cell lines do not display any cell adhesion to the recombinant fragment including most of the N-terminus of the human α3 (VI) chain.[60] However, recent data from our laboratory show that even individual recombinant VWFA modules of the chicken and human α3 (VI) chain can support cell adhesion in a dose-dependent manner (Segat et al, unpublished). In conclusion, despite the experimental evidence that type VI collagen interacts with numerous binding partners including fibrillar types I[105] and II,[165] FACIT type XIV collagen,[27] proteoglycans such as decorin[165] and NG2,[151] hyaluronan,[60,79,112,162] heparin[60] and vWF,[155,157] very little is known of the molecular sites mediating these interactions, although there is increasing evidence that VWFA modules are involved in at least some of the above interactions.

Finally, a close genetic linkage between COL6A1 and COL6A2 in chromosome 21 and COL6A3 in chromosome 2 in patients affected by Bethlem myopathy has recently been found.[166]

COLLAGEN FORMING ANCHORING FIBRILS

The basement membrane region underlying epithelia consists of several structural elements representing a series of interconnected macromolecular networks. These include the hemidesmosomes, which are thickenings of plasma membrane at the basolateral surface that connect the cellular cytoskeleton with the ECM; the anchoring filaments, which are fine filaments projecting perpendicularly from the hemidesmosomes, that traverse the lamina lucida and terminate in the lamina densa; the anchoring fibrils, which are banded fibrils of about 800 nm in length, that originate at the lamina densa and project into the stroma where they terminate in the so called anchoring plaques, or bend back to reinsert into the lamina densa. By providing resistance against shear forces, all the above structures contribute to epithelial cell attachment to the underlying connective tissue. In the skin the anchoring fibril network extending from the basement membrane into the papillary dermis is one of the major structures mediating epithelial-dermal stroma attachment[167-169] and abnormalities of the anchoring fibrils lead to separation of the epithelium from the dermis and to a blistering phenotype.[170]

There are several types of evidence that implicate type VII collagen as the principal component of anchoring fibrils. For instance, the tissue distribution of type VII is superimposable with the location of anchoring fibrils seen at the EM level;[167] the banding pattern of the COL domain in vitro is identical to that of the anchoring fibrils;[171] gold particles-conjugated antibodies to the N-globular domain of type VII deposit to the terminal ends of anchoring fibrils;[167] finally, dystrophic epidermolysis bullosa (EBD) tissues lack ultrastructurally identifiable anchoring fibrils[171] and no immunofluorescence for type VII is similarly detected.[173,174]

MOLECULAR STRUCTURE

Type VII collagen contains a very long (420nm) discontinuous triple helical region that yields two fragments after pepsin digestion.[175] On rotary shadowing EM images the extended triple helix rod is flanked by a small NC2 globular domain located at the C-terminal end and by three 50 nm long arms each corresponding to a single α-chain and terminating in small globules that represent the NC1 N-terminal domain.[176] Therefore, in the case of type VII collagen and differently from all other collagens, for historical reasons the domain defined as NC1 is at the N-terminus of the molecule. At the junction between the NC1 and the COL domain there is another small globule and few interchain disulfide bonds linking the three extended NC1

structures. The trident structure of the NC-1 domain is well suited to allow maximal interactions with lamina densa since each arm is capable of independent interaction. The complete structural organization of the type VII collagen human gene has been reported recently.[177] The gene has 118 exons but is surprisingly small as it encompasses only 31 kb. More than one third of the exons coding for the COL domain have 36 bp and not 54 bp as found in fibrillar collagens. In analogy with fibrillar collagens and differently from most non-fibrillar collagens containing numerous exons beginning with split codons,[10] none of the codons of type VII collagen are split by introns. Nevertheless, the presence of exons of 36 bp suggests that already at an early stage type VII was evolutionarily distinct from the fibrillar collagen genes. The promoter region lacks a TATA box and contains consensus sequences for binding of several nuclear factors including SP1, AP1, AP2 and NF1.[177] The NF1 and AP1 binding sites are very likely functional since transcriptional activation by TGF-β is mediated by these factors[178] and TGF-β stimulates type VII collagen expression in vitro.[179] The human COL7A1 gene has been mapped to chromosome 3p21.[180-182]

The cloning of human cDNA was accomplished by screening a keratinocyte expression library with IgGs of a patient with an acquired autoimmune form of EB:[180] this resulted in the isolation of a clone homologous to the peptide sequences of genuine human placental type VII collagen. Further cloning resulted in the elucidation of the sequences of the large NC-1 domain and the prediction that, contrary to the original assignment of the NC1 domain to the C-terminus of the α1 (VII) chain[183] and in agreement with similar structures at the N-terminus of type XII and XIV collagens,[45] this domain is at the N-terminus (Fig. 6.6).[184-186] More recently, the entire cDNA sequence of the human α1 (VII) chain was obtained[187] and confirmed previous suggestion that the NC1 domain is N-terminal. The full length cDNA contains an 8,833 nucleotide open

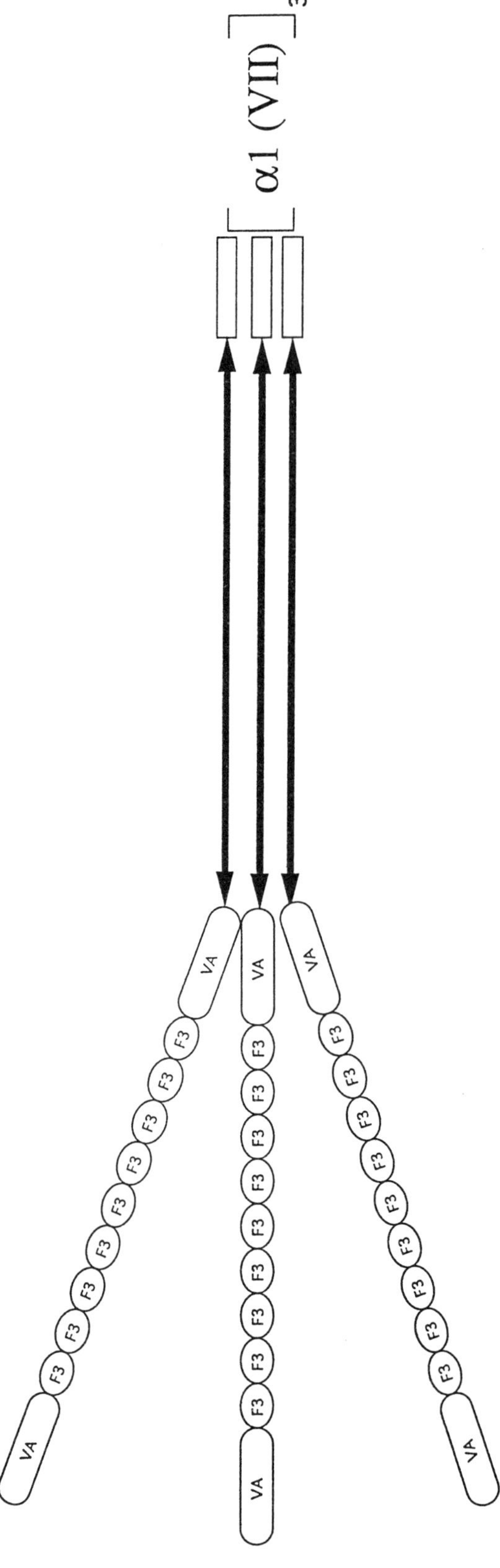

Fig. 6.6. Schematic diagram of type VII collagen. NC, noncollagenous domain; COL, collagenous domain.

reading frame encoding for 2,944 amino acid residues and is transcribed into a 9.2 kb mRNA. The NC1 domain is composed of nine consecutive fibronectin type III (F3) modules flanked at each side by one VWFA module (Fig. 6.6). The VWFA module at the C-terminus of the NC1 domain contains an RGD sequence, the only RGD sequence present in any VWFA module, that is not conserved in the mouse,[188] but it is lacking several residues constituting the MIDAS cation-binding motif.[189] The COL domain has 11 imperfections of 1 or 2 amino acid residues, 7 insertions consisting of 3-10 residues, and a 39 residue-long interruption in the central portion. The presence of this longer interruption had been previously predicted at the protein level by the susceptibility of the COL domain to pepsin digestion under non-denaturing conditions and the resultant two collagenous fragments.[188] At the C-terminus of the COL domain there is one cysteine that might be involved in the formation of the intermolecular S-S bond of the dimer by pairing with the first or the second cysteine in the NC2 domain of an antiparallel type VII molecule. The overlap region of about 60 nm, as determined by rotary shadowing EM images, corresponds to about 200 residues[181] and the actual distance between the two cysteines based on the primary sequence, is 168-170 residues and is in good agreement with the prediction. The NC2 domain consists of 161 residues and its estimated molecular size is considerably smaller than the apparent size (about 30 kD) derived from SDS-PAGE analysis of the purified domain. The most likely explanation for this behavior is the highly acidic nature of this domain. The NC2 domain, in addition to few unrelated sequences, contains a Kunitz type serine protease inhibitor.[184,185] It is not known whether this domain is functionally active or whether it is inactive as the similar domain of the α3 (VI) chain of type VI collagen.[141,158]

Although the conservation at the amino acid level between the human,[185] the hamster[184] and the murine[186] sequences is relatively low, the localization of the imperfections and of the interruptions in the COL domain is highly conserved suggesting that their locations are functionally useful for the proper flexibility of the molecule. In fact, the sometimes tortuous shapes of the anchoring fibrils are likely to result from the discontinuities within the triple-helical domain. Further, the sequence of the NC2 domain is 88% identical between human[185] and hamster[184] and the stretch of 67 residues spanning the junction between the COL and the NC2 domains that is very likely involved in dimer formation is fully conserved.

Type VII is synthesized as a procollagen which is further processed to form the antiparallel dimers. The evidence for this stems from the observation that the molecule extracted from human skin, under strict conditions of inhibition of proteolysis, is smaller than the procollagen synthesized in vitro.[176] This difference does not involve the N-terminal NC1 nor the COL domains but instead it is the C-terminal NC2 domain that is cleaved as seen by the disappearance of the NC2 globule at the EM level from the molecule purified from tissues.[191] The precise sequence of events leading to dimer formation is not fully understood but it seems that the two monomers interact, with an overlap of about 60 nm, via the NC2 domains. In tissues, but not in cell culture, the dimers then become stabilized by S-S bonds and the NC2 domain is finally excised. Since the NC2 domain contains Kunitz-type serine protease inhibitor sequences[180] it might autoregulate its own cleavage. The model predicts that the NC1 domains of the antiparallel dimers are embedded within the type IV containing lamina densa on one side and terminate in the type IV containing anchoring plaques on the other side with the triple helical rod perpendicular to the basement membrane. Finally, the anchoring fibrils are formed by lateral aggregation of individual antiparallel dimers although the details of this process are not yet clarified.

Biochemical analysis indicates a mass of about 340 kD for the intact α1 (VII) chain and of about 150 kD for the NC1 domain. The COL domain is unusually long (424 nm, 170 kD) and is the longest ever found in collagens identified to date. It has been assumed that type VII is a homotrimer mainly because neither the individual chains not their various peptides could be separated by any biochemical approach. Support to this prediction is found in the mapping of EDB mutations to the same genomic region where COL7A1 is located (see below). Nevertheless, there are peptide sequences obtained from purified type VII by Burgeson and coworkers that are not found in the cDNA sequence of α1 (VII) chain and it is possible that there may be additional chains.[192]

TISSUE EXPRESSION

Type VII collagen is present underneath the basement membrane of epithelial cells of several organs,[169] but the tissue most studied both in vivo and in vitro is the skin. Keratinocytes represent the major source of type VII collagen of cutaneous anchoring fibrils in vivo,[193,194] although their biosynthetic function is under control of cellular elements present in the upper dermis.[193,195,196] Fibroblasts also synthesize small quantities of type VII collagen in vitro,[197-199] though they can be stimulated to produce larger amounts under certain conditions, such as in cocultures with keratinocytes.[195] In this latter coculture system a direct cell-cell contact is not required since type VII collagen expression can be enhanced by paracrine mediators even when physical contacts between epithelial cells and fibroblasts are prevented. TGF-β stimulates type VII collagen expression when added to monocultures of fibroblasts, but it is much more efficient if it is added to fibroblast-keratinocyte cocultures suggesting that additional cellular factors (other ECM constituents or other cytokines secreted by keratinocytes released as a consequence of a direct cell-cell contact) may cooperate additively or synergistically to modulate type VII production.[179]

STRUCTURE-FUNCTION RELATIONSHIPS

The formation of the anchoring fibril network requires that the NC1 domain of type VII collagen interacts with constituents present in the lamina densa and the anchoring plaques. Solid-phase binding studies indicate that type VII collagen binds type IV procollagen but not type II collagen.[200] The isolated NC1 domain also can bind type IV collagen and as pepsin digestion of type IV collagen significantly decreases while collagenase digestion does not affect this binding, it is likely that the interaction between these collagens is mediated by their non-triple helical domains. Whether the VWFA or the fibronectin type III modules mediate this interaction or the interaction between the NC1 domain with laminin is still not yet defined.[200] Finally, fibronectin interacts with its N-terminus collagen-binding domain with the triple helix of type VII in a subdomain adjacent to the NC2 domain.[201]

DISEASE ASSOCIATION

Epidermolysis bullosa is a group of heritable diseases characterized by fragility and trauma-induced subepidermal blistering of the skin and mucous membranes resulting in atrophic scars.[170] In the dystrophic (scaring) forms, the tissue separation occurs below the basement membrane at the level of the anchoring fibrils. Both dominant and recessive forms of EDB are described and the most severe forms (recessive) are characterized by mutilating scarring of the extremities, joint contractures and propensity to infections. In recessively inherited EDB, there is a lack of identifiable anchoring fibrils,[172,202] while in dominantly inherited EDB anchoring fibrils have altered morphology and are greatly reduced in number.[172]

As mentioned above, indirect evidence suggested that type VII was the candidate gene in EBD: immunofluorescent studies with anti type VII antibody demonstrated weak, discontinuous or absent staining in the skin of these patients;[173] transmission EM images in affected individuals showing altered morphology, scarcity or absence of anchoring fibrils supported the immunofluorescence studies.[202-204] Finally, the cloning and the chromosomal mapping of the type VII gene has allowed the demonstration of a very close genetic linkage between COL7A1 and both autosomal recessive and dominant forms of EBD.[181,205] Several mutations in the COL7A1 have been described in the highly conserved segment within the NC2 domain,[190,206] in the FN type III modules 1,[207] 2,[208] 5,[209] 7 and 8,[208] and at the N-terminal end[204,208] or in the middle[210] of the COL domain. No mutations have been found so far in the VWFA modules.

Most of the above mutations predict early translation termination and the synthesis of truncated polypeptides. These polypeptides are not incorporated into the type VII trimer and do not result in a clinical phenotype in heterozygous subjects, while full-length mutated polypeptides are incorporated and exert a dominant negative effect.[207] The importance of the stability of the triple-helix notwithstanding the natural 19 imperfections is emphasized by the finding that the substitution of a Gly with a Ser residue in the triple-helical domain results in a dominant form of EBD.[210] This mutation, which is occurring only 62 residues downstream from the large interruption in the middle of the COL domain, suggests that the intact conformation of the triple-helical segment is critical for the proper function of type VII collagen and that alterations of the Gly-Xaa-Yaa triplet, even if they are located close to the long non-helical interruption, greatly affect type VII assembly process.

There is a form of EB called *acquisita* in which autoantibodies against type VII are present in the serum and bound in the region immediately below the lamina densa where type VII is located.[211] These autoantibodies recognize the fibronectin type III modules of the NC1 domain.[211,212] It is likely that in these clinical forms the function of the autoantibodies is to prevent or to relieve the molecular interaction between the NC1 domain of type VII and type IV in the lamina densa.

CARTILAGE MATRIX PROTEIN

MOLECULAR STRUCTURE

Cartilage matrix protein (CMP) is a component expressed specifically during cartilage maturation of still undefined function. The genes of both chicken[213] and human[214] CMP has been isolated and found to be strikingly similar not only in the sequence conservation (79% identity at the amino acid level) but also in the exon and intron sizes and intron phases. The human gene spans approximately 12 kb and is located in chromosome 1p35;[214] the chicken gene is 18 kb long.[213] Both genes have eight exons with exons 2-3 and 5-6 coding for the two VWFA homologous modules (CMP1 and CMP2, respectively) that constitute most of the CMP sequence, and exon four which codes for an EGF-like module. The predicted length of the mature CMP as deduced from cDNA is 471[215] and 474[214] residues for the chicken and human molecule, respectively (Fig. 6.7). Similarly to the organization of the vWF A1 and A3[216,217] modules and of the VWFA modules of the FACIT type XII[30,31] and type XIV[43,44] collagens there is a cysteine residue near each end of both VWFA modules of CMP. In addition, there are two cysteines separated by one residue right after the CMP2 module at the C-terminus of the protein. While the cysteines of the VWFA module make a S-S bridge,[218] it is very unlikely that the two closely spaced cysteines form an intramolecular disulfide bridge. Instead, they might be involved in the oligomerization[219] or in the stabilization[218] of CMP filaments, particularly in view of the fact that these cysteines are preceded by five heptad repeats that are characteristic for coiled-coil proteins and are important for the formation of the CMP trimer.[218]

CMP is an homotrimer constituted by three S-S-linked apparently identical subunits of about 50 kD each.[220,221] CMP cofractionates with cartilage proteoglycans after isolation has been achieved until recently only with the use of denaturing agents such as 4 M guanidine HCl.[220,221]

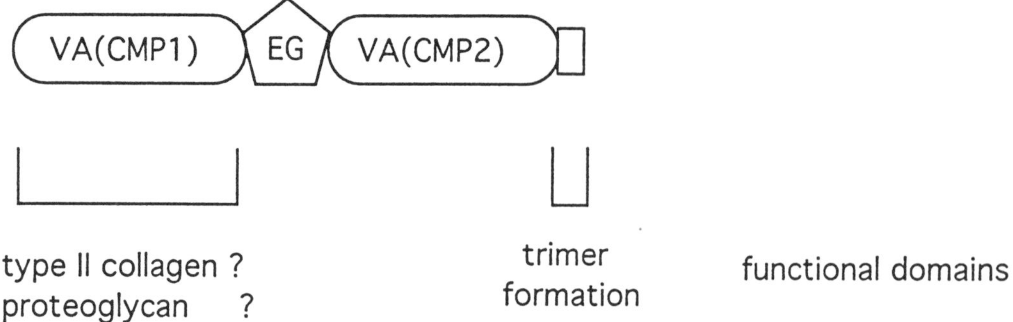

Fig. 6.7. Schematic diagram of CMP. The modules are designated according to the current and the proposed nomenclature of Bork and Bairoch.[238] The proposed location of the binding sites for type II collagen, proteoglycan and the coiled-coil region important for the CMP trimer formation also are indicated. EG, EGF module.

CMP, however, can be selectively extracted from fetal bovine rib cartilage under native conditions in buffers containing EDTA and is then purified by ion exchange and gel filtration chromatography.[219] EM analysis of this native CMP indicates that it is composed of three ellipsoid compact subunits that are connected at one end (presumably the C-terminus).[219] This trimeric assembly is retained even after reduction under native conditions suggesting that the trimeric organization of CMP also results from the noncovalent interactions likely taking place at the C-terminus of the individual chains.

Tissue Expression

The protein is expressed in a limited number of cartilaginous tissues: it is not present in articular cartilage or in the vertebral discs while it is found in tracheal, nasal septal, xiphoid, auricular and epiphysial cartilages.[222] It is distributed in the mature and the hypertrophic zones during endochondral bone formation.[223] CMP is a major component of tracheal cartilage, especially at advanced age;[224] in the bovine trachea, where it has been studied most extensively, CMP represents a marker of aging as it shows a linear concentration increase from 2 up to 10 years representing up to 5% of the wet weight of the tissue.[224] However, while the total amounts of CMP in bovine tracheal cartilage in-

creases with age, the extractable pool decreases,[224] suggesting that there is an increase in covalent cross-links, likely to be dependent upon transglutaminase activity, that proceeds in parallel with the maturation of the cartilage matrix, CMP also has been detected by immunohistochemistry in embryonic chick cornea, sclera, choroid and lens capsule.[225] Since the human cDNA has been isolated from a retina library[214] it is likely that human tissues other than cartilage also express CMP. During limb development CMP is transcribed later than other cartilage specific genes[223] when chondrocytes stop their proliferation,[226] suggesting that the main function of CMP is matrix stabilization.

Structure-Function Relationships

The function of CMP is beginning to be understood and this protein might be involved in the organization and assembly of the cartilage matrix.[215,226,227] CMP distributes along the type II collagen fibrils with a periodicity of 59 nm[228] and certainly the copurification with proteoglycans of the aggrecan family,[220] even under strong denaturing conditions, provides indirect evidence that CMP might be tightly bound to proteoglycans. In addition, the protein exposed to 4 M guanidine HCl binds in a solid phase assay to monomeric collagens,[228] and experimental evidence that the binding of CMP depends upon its VWFA modules has been obtained.[229] This finding is highly probable in light of the similar functional and structural arrangement of the A1 and A3 modules of vWF,[230-232] of type VI collagen[105] and of $\alpha1\beta1$ and $\alpha2\beta1$ integrins,[233-236] all of which have collagen-binding function. Recombinant wild type and mutant (C455S and C457S) CMP molecules expressed in primary chondrocytes and fibroblasts[227] using a retroviral expression system[237] can assemble and form filaments even if interchain disulfide bond formation is prevented. In the same model system it was demonstrated that a truncated form of CMP, consisting of the CMP2 VWFA module and the tail domain, undergoes trimerization but it is not able to assemble into filaments.[227] Thus, it seems likely that either the CMP1 VWFA and/or the EGF modules are necessary for interactions leading to filament formation.

REFERENCES

1. Charalambous BM, Keen JN, McPherson MJ. Collagen-like sequences stabilize homotrimers of a bacterial hydrolase. EMBO J 1988; 7:2903-2909.

2. van der Rest M, Garrone R. Collagen family of proteins. FASEB J 1991; 5:2814-2823.

3. Prockop DJ, Kivirikko KI. Collagens: molecular biology, diseases, and potentials for therapy. Ann Rev Biochem 1995; 64:403-34.

4. Mays C, Rosenberry TL. Characterization of pepsin-resistant collagen-like tail subunit fragments of 18S and 14S acetylcholinesterase from *Electrophorus electricus*. Biochemistry 1981; 20:2810-2817.

5. Kodama T, Freeman M, Rohrer L et al. Type I macrophage scavenger receptor contains α-helical and collagen-like coiled coils. Nature 1990; 343:531-535.

6. Reid KBM. Complete amino-acid sequences of the three collagen-like regions present in subcomponent C1q of the first component of human complement. Biochem J 1979; 179:367-371.

7. White RT, Damm D, Miller J et al. Isolation and characterization of the human pulmonary surfactant apoprotein gene. Nature 1985; 317:361-363.

8. Holmskov U, Malhotra R, Sim RB et al. Collectins: collagenous C-type lectins of the innate immune defense system. Immunol Today 1994; 15:67-73.

9. Fukai N, Apte SS, Olsen BR. Nonfibrillar collagen. Methods Enzymol 1994; 245:3-28.

10. Sandell LJ, Boyd CD. Conserved and divergent sequence and functional elements within collagen genes. In: Sandell LJ, Boyd CD, eds. Extracellular Matrix Genes. San Diego: Academic Press, 1991:1-56.

11. Chu M-L, Prockop DJ. Collagen: gene structure. In: Royce PM, Steinmann B eds. Connective tissue and its heritable disorders: molecular, genetic and medical aspects. New York: Wiley-Liss, 1993:149-165.

12. Rachmadaran GN. Structure of collagen at the molecular level. In: Ramachandran GN, ed. Treatise on Collagen. New York: Academic Press, 1967:103-183.

13. Light ND, Bailey AJ. The chemistry of the collagen cross-links. Purification and characterization of cross-linked polymeric peptide material from mature containing unknown amino acids. Biochem J 1980; 185:379-381.

14. Birk DE, Fitch JM, Babiarz JP et al. Collagen type I and V are present in the same fibril in the avian corneal stroma. J Cell Biol 1988; 106:999-1008.

15. Mendler M, Eich-Bender SG, Vaughan L et al. Cartilage contains mixed fibrils of collagen types II, IX and XI. J Cell Biol 1989; 108:191-197.

16. Yamada Y, Kiau G, Mudryj M et al. Conservation of the size for one but not another class of exons in two chick collagen genes. Nature 1984; 310:333-337.

17. Chu M-L, de Wet W, Cing BM. Nature 1984; Human proalpha 1 collagen gene structure reveals evolutionary consevation of a pattern of introns. Nature 1984; 310: 337-340.

18. Upholt WB, Sandell LJ. Exon/intron organization of the chicken type II procollagen gene: Intron size distribution suggests a minimal intron size. Proc Natl Acad Sci USA 1986; 83:2325-2329.

19. Blumberg B, Kurkinen M. Structure and evolution of collagen IV genes. In: Sandell

LJ, Boyd CD, eds. Extracellular Matrix Genes. San Diego: Academic Press, 1990:115-135.

20. Kefalides NA. Isolation of a collagen from basement membrane containing three identical α chains. Biochem Biophys Res Commun 1971; 45:226-234.

21. Timpl R, Wiedemann H, van Delden V et al. A network model for the organization of type IV collagen molecules in basement membranes. Eur J Biochem 1981; 120: 203-211.

22. Siebold B, Qian R-Q, Glanville RW et al. Construction of a model for the aggregation and cross-linking region (7S domain) of type IV collagen based upon an evaluation of the primary structure of the α1 and α2 chains in this region. Eur J Biochem 1987; 168:569-575.

23. Yurchenco PD, Ruben GC. Basement membrane structure *in situ*: evidence for lateral associations in the type IV collagen network. J Cell Biol 1987; 105:2559-2568.

24. Beck K, Gruber T. Structure and assembly of basement membrane and related extracellular matrix proteins. In: Richardson PD, Steiner M, eds. Principles of Cell Adhesion. Boca Raton: CRC Press, 1995: 219-252.

25. Shaw LM, Olsen BR. FACIT collagens: diverse molecular bridges in extracellular matrices. Trends Biochem Sci 1991; 16:191-4.

26. Dublet B, Oh S, Sugrue SP et al. The structure of avian type XII collagen. α1 (XII) chains contain 190-kDa non-triple helical amino-terminal domains and form homotrimeric molecules. J Biol Chem 1989; 264:13150-13156.

27. Brown JC, Mann K, Wiedemann H et al. Structure and binding properties of collagen type XIV isolated from human placenta. J Cell Biol 1993; 120:557-567.

28. Aubert-Foucher E, Font B, Eichenberger D et al. Purification and characterization of native type XIV collagen. J Biol Chem1992; 267:15759-15764.

29. van der Rest, Mayne R. Type IX collagen proteoglycan from cartilage is covalently cross-linked to type II collagen. J Biol Chem 1988; 263:1615-1618.

30. Gordon MK, Gerecke DR, Olsen BR. Type XII collagen: distinct extracellular matrix component discovered by a cDNA cloning. Proc Natl Acad Sci USA 1987; 84: 6040-6044.

31. Gordon MK, Gerecke DR, Dublet B et al. Type XII collagen. A large multidomain molecule with partial homology to type IX collagen. J Biol Chem 1989; 264: 19772-19778.

32. Dublet B, van der Rest M. Type XII collagen is expressed in embryonic chick tendons. Isolation of pepsin-derived fragments. J Biol Chem 1987; 262:17724-17727.

33. Lunstrum GP, McDonough AM, Marinkovic MP et al. Identification and partial purification of large, variant form of type XII collagen. J Biol Chem 1992; 267:20087-20092.

34. Koch M, Bernasconi C, Chiquet M. A, major oligomeric fibroblast proteoglycan identified as a novel large form of type-XII collagen. Eur J Biochem 1992; 207:847-856.

35. Oh SP, Taylor RW, Gerecke DR et al. The mouse alpha 1(XII) and human alpha 1(XII)-like collagen genes are localized on mouse chromosome 9 and human chromosome 6. Genomics 1992; 14:225-231.

36. Wei Y, Yang EV, Klatt KP et al. Monoclonal antibody MT2 identifies the urodele α1 chain of type XII collagen, a developmentally regulated extracellular matrix protein in regenerating newt limbs. Dev Biol 1995; 168:503-513.

37. Watt SL, Lunstrum GP, McDonough AM et al. Characterization of collagen types XII and XIV from fetal bovine cartilage. J Biol Chem 1992; 267:20093-20099.

38. Yamagata M, Yamada KM, Yamada S et al. The complete primary structure of type XII collagen shows a chimeric molecule with reiterated fibronectin type III motifs, von Willebrand factor A motifs, a domain homologous to a noncollagenous region of type IX collagen, and short collagenous domains with an Arg-Gly-Asp site. J Cell Biol 1991; 115:209-221.

39. Trueb J, Trueb B. The two splice variants of collagen XII share a common 5' ends. Biochim Biophys Acta 1992; 117:97-98.

40. Lunstrum GP, Morris NP, McDonough AM et al. Identification and partial character-

ization of two type XII-like collagen molecules. J Cell Biol 1991; 113:963-969.

41. Dublet B, van der Rest M. Type XIV collagen, a new homotrimeric molecule extracted from fetal bovine skin and tendon, with a triple helical disulfide-bonded domain homologous to type IX and type XII collagens. J Biol Chem 1991; 266:6853-6858.

42. Gordon MK, Castagnola P, Dublet B et al. Cloning of a cDNA for a new member of the class of fibril-associated collagens with interrupted triple helices. Eur J Biochem 1991; 201:333-338.

43. Gerecke DR, Foley JW, Castagnola P et al. Type XIV collagen is encoded by alternative transcripts with distinct 5' regions and is a multidomain protein with homologies to von Willebrand factor, fibronectin, and other matrix protein. J Biol Chem 1993; 268:12177-12184.

44. Waelchli C, Trueb J, Kessler B et al. Complete primary structure of chicken collagen XIV. Eur J Biochem 1993; 212:483-490.

45. Trueb J, Trueb B. Type XIV is a variant of undulin. Eur J Biochem 1992; 207:549-557.

46. Schuppan D, Cantaluppi MC, Becker J et al. Undulin, an extracellular matrix glycoprotein associated with collagens fibrils. J Biol Chem 1990; 265:8823-8832.

47. Just M, Herbst H, Hummel M et al. Undulin is a novel member of the fibronectin-tenascin family of extracellular matrix glycoproteins. J Biol Chem 1991; 266:17326-17332.

48. Castagnola P, Tavella DR, Gerecke B et al. Tissue-specific expression of type XIV collagen—a member of the FACIT class of collagens. Eur J Cell Biol 1992; 59:340-7.

49. Koch M, Bohrmann B, Matthison M et al. Large and small splice variants of collagen XII: differential expression and ligand binding. J Cell Biol 1995; 130:1005-1014.

50. Mazzorana M, Giry-Lozingues C, van der rest M. Trimeric assembly of collagen XII: effect of deletion of the C-terminal part of the molecule. Matrix Biol 1994; 14:583-588.

51. Sugrue SP, Gordon MK, Seyer J et al. Immunoidentification of type XII collagen in embryonic tissues. J Cell Biol 1989; 109:939-945.

52. Oh SP, Griffith CM, Hay ED et al. Tissue-specific expression of type XII collagen during mouse embryonic development. Dev Dyn 1993; 196:37-46.

53. Waelchli C, Koch M, Chiquet M et al. Tissue-specific expression of the fibril-associated collagens XII and XIV. J Cell Sci 1994; 107:669-681.

54. Keene DR, Lunstrum GP, Morris NP et al. Two type XII-like collagens localize to the surface of banded collagens fibrils. J Cell Biol 1991; 113:971-978.

55. Keene DR, Engvall E, Glanville RW. Ultrastructure of type VI collagen in human skin and cartilage suggests an anchoring function for this filamentous network. J Cell Biol 1988; 107:1995-2006.

56. Mendler M, Eich-Bender SG, Vaughan L et al. Cartilage contains mixed fibrils of collagen types II, IX and XI. J Cell Biol 1989; 108:191-197.

57. Faessler R, Schnegelsberg PNJ, Dausman J et al. Mice lacking α11 (IX) collagen develop noninflammatory degenerative joint disease. Proc Natl Acad Sci USA 1994; 91:5070-5074.

58. Nishiyama T, McDonough AM, Bruns RR et al. Type XII and Type XIV collagens mediate interactions between banded collagens fiber in vitro and may modulate extracellular matrix deformability. J Biol Chem 1994; 269:28193-28199.

59. Grinnel F. Fibroblasts, myofibroblasts, and wound contraction. J Cell Biol 1994; 124:401-404.

60. Mohri H, Yoshioka A, Zimmerman TS et al. Isolation of the von Willebrand factor domain interacting with platelet glycoprotein Ib, heparin, and collagen, and characterization of its three distinct functional sites. J Biol Chem 1989; 264:17361-17367.

61. Specks U, Mayer U, Nitsch R et al. Structure of recombinant N-terminal globule of type VI collagen alpha 3 chain and its binding to heparin and hyaluronan. EMBO J 1992; 11:4281-4290.

62. Font B, Aubert-Foucher E, Goldschmidt D et al. Binding of collagen XIV with the dermatan sulfate side chain of decorin. J Biol Chem 1993; 268:25015-25018.

63. Fleischmejer R, Fisher LW, MacDonald DE et al. Decorin interacts with fibrillar collagen of embryonic and adult human skin. J Struct Biol 1991; 106:82-90.

64. Marti T, Roesselet S, Titani K et al. Identification of disulfide-bridge substructure within human von Willebrand factor. Biochemistry 1987; 26:8099-8109.

65. Timpl R, Chu M-L. Microfibrillar collagen type VI. In: Yurchenco PD, Birk DE, Mecham RP. Extracellular Matrix Assembly and Structure. San Diego: Academic Press, 1994: 207-234.

66. Otte AP, Roy D, Siemerink M et al. Characterization of a maternal type VI collagen in *Xenopus* embryos suggests a role for collagen in gastrulation. J Cell Biol 1990; 111:271-278.

67. Chung E, Rhodes RK, Miller EJ et al. Isolation of three collagenous components of probable basement membrane origin from several tissues. Biochem Biophys Res Commun 1976; 71:1167-1174.

68. Trueb B, Schreier T, Bruckner P et al. Type VI collagen represent a major fraction of connective tissue collagens. Eur J Biochem 1987; 166:699-703.

69. Gibson MA, Cleary EG. CL glycoprotein is the tissue form of type VI collagen. J Biol Chem 1985; 260:11149-11159.

70. Trueb B, Winterhalter KH. Type VI collagen is composed of a 200kd subunit and two 140 kd subunits. EMBO J 1986; 5:2815-2819.

71. Colombatti A, Ainger K, Colizzi F. Type VI collagen: High yields of a molecule with multiple forms of α3 chain from avian and human tissues. Matrix 1989; 9:177-184.

72. Zimmermann DR, Trueb B, Winterhalter KH et al. Type VI collagen is a major component of the human cornea. FEBS Lett 1986; 197:55-58.

73. Linsenmayer TF, Mentzer A, Irwin MH et al. Avian type VI collagen: Monoclonal antibody and immunohistochemical identification as a major connective tissue component of cornea and skeletal muscle. Exp Cell Res 1986; 165:518-529.

74. Bruns RR. Beaded filaments and long-spacing fibrils. Relations to type VI collagen. J Ultrastruct Res 1984; 89:136-145.

75. Engel J, Furthmayr H, Odermatt E. Structure and macromolecular organization of type VI collagen. Ann N Y Acad Sci 1985; 460:25-37.

76. Bruns R, Press W, Engvall E et al. Type VI collagen in extracellular, 100-nm periodic filaments and fibrils: identification by immunoelectron microscopy. J Cell Biol 1986; 103:393-404.

77. Kielty CM, Cummings C, Whittaker SP et al. Isolation and ultrastructural analysis of microfibrillar structures from foetal bovine elastic tissues. J Cell Sci 1991; 99:797-807.

78. Wu J-J, Eyre DR, Slayter HS. Type VI collagen of the invertebral disc. Biochemical and electron-microscopic characterization of the native protein. Biochem J 1987; 248:373-381.

79. Kielty CM, Whittaker SP, Grant ME et al. Type VI collagen microfibrils: evidence for a structural association with hyaluronan. J Cell Biol 1992; 118:979-990.

80. Kuo H-J, Keene D, Glanville RW. The macromolecular structure of type-VI collagen. Formation and stability of filaments. Eur J Biochem 1995; 232:364-372.

81. Furthmayr H, Wiedemann H, Timpl R. Electronmicroscopical approach to a structural model of intima collagen. Biochem J 1983; 211,303-311.

82. Odermatt E, Risteli J, van Delden V et al. Structural diversity and domain composition of a unique collagenous fragment (intima collagen) obtained from human placenta. Biochem J 1983; 211:295-302.

83. Kuo H-J, Keene DR, Glanville RW. Orientation of type VI collagen monomers in molecular aggregates. Biochemistry 1989; 28:3757-3762.

84. Fleischmajer R, Perlish JS, Faraggiana T. Rotary shadowing of collagen monomers, oligomers and fibrils during tendon fibrillogenesis. J Histochem Cytochem 1991; 39:51-58.

85. Buckwalter JA, Maynard JA. Banded structure in human nucleous pulposus. Clin Orthop1979; 139:259-266.

86. Ronziére M-C, Ricard-Blum S, Tiollier J et al. Comparative analysis of collagen solubilized from human fetal, and normal, and osteoarthritic adult articular cartilage, with

emphasis on type VI collagen. Biochem Biophys Acta 1990; 1038:222-230.

87. Saitta B, Stokes DG, Vissing H et al. Alternative splicing of the human α2(VI) collagen gene generates multiple mRNA transcripts which predict three protein variants with distinct carboxyl termini. J Biol Chem1990; 265:6473-6480.

88. Saitta B, Wang Y-M, Renkart L. The exon organization of the triple helical coding regions of the human α1 (VI) and α2(VI) collagen gene is highly similar. Genomics 1991; 11:145-153.

89. Stokes DG, Saitta B, Timpl R. Human α3(VI) collagen gene. Characterization of exons coding for the amino-terminal globular domain and alternative splicing in normal and tumor cells. J Biol Chem 1991; 266:8626-8633.

90. Saitta B, Timpl R, Chu M-L. Human α2(VI) collagen gene. Heterogeneity at the 5'-untranslated region generated by an alternative exons. J Biol Chem 1992; 267: 6188-6196.

91. Zanussi S, Doliana R, Segat D et al. The human type VI collagen gene. J Biol Chem 1992; 267:24082-24089.

92. Doliana R, Bonaldo P, Colombatti A. Multiple forms of chicken α3(VI) collagen chain generated by alternative splicing in type A repeat domains. J Cell Biol 1990; 111: 2197-2205.

93. Hayman AR, Koeppel J, Winterhalter KH et al. The triple-helical domain of α2(VI) collagen is encoded by 19 short exons that are multiple of 9 base pairs. J Biol Chem 1990; 265:9864-9868.

94. Hayman AR, Koeppel J, Trueb B. Complete structure of the chicken α2(VI) collagene gene. Eur J Biochem 1991; 197:177-184.

95. Waelchli C, Koller E, Trueb J. Structural comparison of the chicken genes for α1(VI) and α2(VI) collagen. Eur J Biochem 1992; 205:583-589.

96. Bonaldo P, Piccolo S, Marvulli D et al. Murine α1(VI) collagen chain. Complete amino acid sequence and identification of the gene promoter region. Matrix 1993; 13:223-233.

97. Piccolo S, Bonaldo P, Vitale P et al. Tran-

scriptional activation of the α1(VI) collagen gene during myoblast differentiation is mediated by multiple GA boxes. J Biol Chem 1995; 270:19583-19590.

98. Koller E, Hayman AR, Trueb B. The promoter of the chicken α2(VI) collagen gene has features characteristic of house-keeping genes and of proto-oncogenes. Nucleic Acids Res 1991; 19:485-491.

99. Bonaldo P, Russo V, Bucciotti P et al. α1 chain of chick type VI collagen. cDNA sequence reveals a hybrid molecule made of one short collagen and three von Willebrand factor type A like domains. J Biol Chem 1989; 264:5575-5580.

100. Chu M-L, Pan T-C, Conway D et al. Sequence analysis of α1(VI) and α2(VI) chains of human type VI collagen reveals internal triplication of globular domains similar to the A domains of vWF and two α2(VI) chain variants that differ in the carboxyl terminus. EMBO J 1989; 8:1939-1946.

101. Koller E, Winterhalter KH, Trueeb B. The globular domains of type VI collagen are related to the collagen-binding domains of cartilage matrix protein and von Willebrand factor. EMBO J 1989; 8:1073-1077.

102. Ibrahimi A, Bertrand B, Bardon S et al. Cloning of α2 chain of type VI collagen and expression during mouse development. Biochem J 1993; 289:141-147.

103. Bonaldo P, Colombatti A. The c-terminus of the chicken α3 collagen VI is a unique mosaic structure with GPIb-like, fibronectin type III and Kunitz modules. J Biol Chem 1989; 264:20235-20239.

104. Chu M.-L, Zhang R-Z, Pan T et al. Mosaic structure of globular domains in the human type VI collagen α3 chain: similarity to von Willebrand Factor, fibronectin, actin, salivary proteins and aprotonin type protease inhibitors. EMBO J 1990; 9:385-393.

105. Bonaldo P, Russo V, Bucciotti F et al. Structural and functional features of the α3 chain indicate a bridging role for chicken collagen type VI in connective tissues. Biochemistry 1990; 29:1245-1254.

106. Zhang R-Z, Pan T-C, Timpl R et al. Cloning and sequence analysis of cDNAs encoding the α1, α2 and α3 chains of mouse collagen VI. Biochem J 1993; 291:787-792.

107. Fujiwara S, Shinkai H, Timpl R. Structure of N-linked oligosaccharide chains in triple-helical domains of human type VI and mouse type IV collagen. Matrix 1991; 11:307-312.

108. von der Mark H, Aumailley M, Wick G et al. Immunochemistry, genuine size and tissue localization of collagen VI. Eur J Biochem 1984; 142:493-502.

109. Jander R, Troyer D, Rauterberg J. A collagen-like glycoprotein of the extracellular matrix is the undegraded form of type VI collagen. Biochemistry 1984; 23:3675-3681.

110. Heller-Harrison R-A, Carter WG. Pepsin-generated type VI collagen is a degradation of GP140. J Biol Chem 1984; 259:6858-6864.

111. Perris R, Kuo H-J, Glanville R W et al. Neural crest cell interaction with type VI collagen is mediated by multiple cooperative binding sites within triple-helix and globular domains. Exp Cell Res 1993; 209:103-117.

112. Spissinger T, Engel J. Type VI collagen beaded microfibrils from bovine cornea depolymerized at acidic pH, and depolymerization and polymerization are not influenced by hyaluronan. Matrix Biol 1994; 14:499-505.

113. Kielty CM, Berry L, Whittaker SP et al. Microfibrillar assemblies of fetal bovine skin. Developmental expression and relative abundance of type VI collagen and fibrillin. Matrix 1993; 13:103-112.

114. Loreal O, Clement B, Schuppan D et al. Distribution and cellular origin of collagen VI during development and in cirrhosis. Gastroenterology 1992; 102:980-987.

115. Duff K, Williamson R, Richards S-J. Expression of genes encoding two chains of the collagen type VI molecule during human fetal heart development. Int J Cardiol 1990; 27:128-129.

116. Linsenmayer TF, Bruns RR, Mentzer A et al. Type VI collagen: immunohistochemical identification as a filamentous component of the extracellular matrix of the developing avian corneal stroma. Dev Biol 1986; 118:425-431.

117. Quarto R, Dozin B, Bonaldo P et al. Type VI collagen expression is upregulated in the early events of chondrocyte differentiation. Development 1993; 117:245-251.

118. Gibson MA, Cleary EG. Distribution of CL glycoprotein in tissues: an immunohistochemical study. Collagen Relat Res 1983; 3:469-488.

119. Hessle H, Engvall E. Type VI collagen: studies on the localization, structure, and biosynthetic form with monoclonal antibodies. J Biol Chem 1984; 259:3955-3961.

120. Ayad SA, Marriott A, Morgan K et al. Bovine cartilage types VI and IX collagens characterization of their forms in vivo. Biochem J 1989; 262:753-761.

121. Hagiwara H, Schroeter-Kermani C, Merker H-J. Localization of collagen type VI in articular cartilage of young and adult mice. Cell Tissue Res 1993; 272:155-160.

122. Magro G, Grasso S, Colombatti A et al. Distribution of extracellular matrix glycoproteins in the human mesonephros. Acta Histochem 1995; 97:343-351.

123. Carlson EC, Audette JL. Intrinsic fibrillar components of human glomerular basement membranes: A TEM analysis following proteolytic dissection. J Submicrosc Cytol Pathol 1989; 21:83-92.

124. Oomura A, Nakamura T, Arakawa M et al. Alterations in the extracellular matrix components in human glomerular diseases. Virchows Arch (A) Pathol Anat 1989; 415:151-159.

125. Poole CA, Ayad S, Schofield JR. Chondrons from articular cartilage. I. Immunolocalization of type VI collagen in the pericellular capsule of isolated canine tibial chondrons. J Cell Sci 1988; 90:635-643.

126. Engvall E, Hessle H, Klier G. Molecular assembly, secretion and matrix deposition of type VI collagen. J Cell Biol 1986; 102:703-710.

127. Colombatti A, Bonaldo P, Ainger K et al. Biosynthesis of chick type VI collagen. I. Intracellular assembly and molecular structure. J Biol Chem 1987; 262:14454-14460.

128. Chu M-L, Conway D, Pan T-C et al. Amino acid sequence of the triple-helical domain of human collagen type VI. J Biol Chem 1988; 263:18601-18606.

129. Jander R, Rauterberg J, Glanville RW.

Further characterization of the three polypeptide chains of bovine and human short-chain collagen (intima collagen). Eur J Biochem 1983; 133:39-46.

130. Colombatti A, Bonaldo P. Biosynthesis of chick type VI collagen. II. Processing and secretion in fibroblasts and smooth muscle cells. J Biol Chem 1987; 262:14461-14466.

131. Colombatti A, Mucignat MT, Bonaldo P. Secretion and matrix assembly of recombinant type VI collagen. J Biol Chem 1995; 270:13105-13111.

132. Hatamochi A, Aumailley M, Mauch C et al. Regulation of collagen VI expression in fibroblasts. Effects of cell density, cell-matrix interactions, and chemical transformation. J Biol Chem 1989; 264:3494-3499.

133. Hackmann M, Aumailley M, Hatamochi A et al. Down regulation of α3(VI) chain expression by γ-interferon decreased synthesis and deposition of collagen type VI. Eur J Biochem 1989; 182:719-726.

134. Kielty CM, Boot-Handford RP, Ayad S et al. Molecular composition of type VI collagen. Evidence for chain heterogeneity in mammalian tissues and cultured cells. Biochem J 1990; 272:787-795.

135. Chu M-L, Mann K, Deutzmann R et al. Characterization of three constituent chains of collagen type VI by peptide sequences and cDNA clones. Eur J Biochem 1987; 168:309-317.

136. Olsen DR, Peltonen J, Jaakola S et al. Collagen gene expression by cultured human skin fibroblast. Abundant steady-state levels of type VI procollagen messenger RNAs. J Clin Invest 1989; 83:791-795.

137. Kielty CM, Boot-Handford RP, Ayad S et al. Molecular composition of type VI collagen. Evidence for chain heterogeneity in mammalian tissues and cultured cells. Biochem J 1990; 272:787-795.

138. Heckmann M, Aumailley M, Chu M-L et al. Effect of transforming growth factor-β on collagen type VI expression in human dermal fibroblasts. FEBS Lett 1992; 310:79-82.

139. Weil D, Mattei M-G, Passage E et al. Cloning and chromosomal localization of human genes encoding the three chains of type VI collagen. Am J Hum Genet 1988; 42:435-445.

140. Francomano CA, Cutting GR, McCormick MK et al. The COL6A1 and COL6A2 gene exist as a gene cluster and detect highly informative DNA polymorphism in the telomeric region of human chromosome 21q. Hum Genet 1991; 87:162-166.

141. Mayer U, Poeschl E, Nischt R et al. Recombinant expression and properties of the Kunitz-type protease-inhibitor module from human type VI collagen α3 (VI) chain. Eur J Biochem 1994; 225:573-580.

142. Colombatti A, Ainger K, Mucignat MT et al. Monoclonal antibodies for the different chains of chick type VI collagen. Collagen Relat Res 1988; 8:331-337.

143. Colombatti A, Bonaldo P, Bucciotti F. Stable expression of chicken type VI collagen α1, α2 and α3 cDNAs in murine NIH/3T3 cells. Eur J Biochem 1992; 209:785-792.

144. Segat D, Pucillo C, Marotta G et al. Differential attachment of human neoplastic B cells to purified extracellular matrix molecules. Blood 1984; 83:1586-1594.

145. Doane KJ, Yang G, Birk DE. Corneal cell-matrix interactions: type VI collagen promotes adhesion and spreading of corneal fibroblasts. Exp Cell Res 1992; 200:490-499.

146. Pfaff M, Aumailley M, Specks U et al. Integrin and Arg-Gly-Asp dependence of cell adhesion to the native and unfolded triple helix of collagen type VI. Exp Cell Res 1993; 206:167-176.

147. Aumailley M, Mann K, von der Mark H et al. Cell attachment properties of collagen type VI and Arg-Gly-Asp dependent binding to its α2(VI) and α3(VI) chains. Exp Cell Res 1989; 181:463-474.

148. Klein G, Muller CA, Tillet E et al. Collagen type VI in the human bone marrow microenvironment: a strong cytoadhesive component. Blood 1995; 86:1740-1748.

149. Kielty CM, Whittaker SP, Grant ME et al. Attachment of human vascular smooth muscle cells to intact microfibrillar assemblies of collagen VI and fibrillin. J Cell Sci 1992; 103:445-451.

150. Wayner EA, Carter WG. Identification of multiple cell adhesion receptors for type VI

collagen and fibronectin in human fibrosarcoma cells possessing unique α and common β subunits. J Cell Biol 1987; 105:1873-1884.

151. Stallcup WB, Dahlin K, Healy P. Interaction of the NG2 chondroitin sulfate proteoglycan with type VI collagen. J Cell Biol 1990; 111:3177-3188.

152. Nishiyama A, Stallcup WB. Expression of NG2 proteoglycan causes retention of type VI collagen on the cell surface. Mol Biol Cell 1993; 4:1097-1108.

153. Sakariassen KS, Bolhouis PA, Sixma JJ. Human blood platelet adhesion to artery subendothelium is mediated by factor VIII/von Willebrand factor bound to the subendothelium. Nature 1979; 279: 636-638.

154. Rand JH, Wu X-X, Uson RR et al. Co-localization of von Willebrand factor and type VI collagen in human vascular subendothelium. Am J Pathol 1993; 142:843-850.

155. Rand JH, Patel ND, Schwartz E et al. 150-kD von Willebrand factor binding protein extracted from human vascular subendothelium is type VI collagen. J Clin Invest 1991; 88:253-259.

156. Saelman EUM, Nieuwenhuis HK, Hese KM et al. Platelet adhesion to collagen types I through VIII under conditions of stasis and flow is mediated by GPIa/IIa ($\alpha_2\beta_1$-integrin). Blood 1994; 83:1244-1250.

157. Ross JM, McIntire LV, Moake JL et al. Platelet adhesion and aggregation on human type VI collagen surfaces under physiological flow conditions. Blood 1995; 85:1826-1835.

158. Bearz A, Tolazzi G, Leonardi A et al. Expression, purification and functional characterization of a kunitz-type module from chicken type VI collagen. Biochem Biophys Res Commun 1995; 215:1050-1055.

159. Arnoux B, Mérigeau K, Saludjian P et al. The 1.6 A structure of Kunitz-type domain from the α3 chain of human type VI collagen. J Mol Biol 1995; 246:609-617.

160. Zweckstetter M, Czisch M, Mayer U et al. Structure and multiple conformations of the kunitz-type domain from human type VI collagen α3(VI) chain in solution. Curr Biol Struct 1996; 4:195-209.

161. Otting G, Liepinsh E, Wuethrich K. Disulfide bond isomerization in BPTI and BPTI(G36S): an NMR study of correlated mobility in proteins. Biochemistry; 1993; 32:3571-3582.

162. Petersen LC, Biorn SE, Norris F et al. Expression, purification and characterization of a Kunitz-type protease inhibitor domain from human amyloid precursor protein homolog. FEBS Lett 1994; 338:53-57.

163. McDevitt CA, Marcelino J, Tucker L. Interaction of intact type VI collagen with hyluronan. FEBS Lett 1991; 294:167-170.

164. Morgelin M, Engel J, Heinergard D et al. Proteoglycan from the swarm rat chondrosarcoma. Structures of the aggregates extracted with associative and dissociative solvents as revealed by electron microscopy; J Biol Chem 1992; 267:14275-14284.

165. Bidanset DJ, Guidry C, Rosemberg LC et al. Binding of the proteoglycan decorin to collagen type VI. J Biol Chem 1992; 267:5250-5256.

166. Jobsis GJ, Barth PG, Boers JM et al. Bethlem myopathy: clinical and genetic aspects. Neurology 1995; 45 (suppl 4): A407.

167. Regauer S, Seiler GR, Burrandon Y et al. Epithelial origin of cutaneous anchoring fibrils. J Cell Biol 1990; 111:2109-2115.

168. Sakai LY, Keene DR, Morris NP et al. Type VII collagen is a major structural component of anchoring fibrils. J Cell Biol 1986; 103:1577-1586.

169. Keene DR, Sakai LY, Lunstrum GP et al. Type VII collagen forms an extended network of anchoring fibrils. J Cell Biol 1987; 104:611-621.

170. Lin AN, Carter DM. In: Lin AN, Carter DM, eds. Epidermolysis Bullosa: Basic and Clinical Aspects. New York: Springer-Verlag, 1992: 3-165.

171. Burgeson RE, Morris NP, Murray LW et al. The structure of type VII collagen. Ann NY Acad Sci 1986; 460:47-57.

172. Tidman MJ, Eady RAJ. Evaluation of anchoring fibrils and other components of the dermal-epidermal junction in dystrophic epidermolysis bullosa by a quantitative ultrastructural technique. J Invest

Dermatol 1985; 84:374-377.

173. Bruckner-Tuderman L, Ruegger S, Odermatt B et al. Lack of type VII collagen in unaffected skin of patients with severe recessive dystrophic epidermolysis bullosa. Dermatologica (Basel) 1988; 176:57-64.

174. Bruckner-Tuderman L, Mitsuhashi Y, Schnyder UW et al. Anchoring fibrils and type VII collagen are absent from skin in severe recessive dystrophic epidermolysis bullosa. J Invest Dermatol 1989; 93:3-9.

175. Christiano AM, Hoffman GG, Chung-Honet LC et al. Structural organization of the human type VII collagen gene (COL7A1), composed of more exons than any previously characterized gene. Genomics 1994; 21:169-179.

176. Massague J. The transforming growth factor-β family. Annu Rev Cell Biol 1990; 6:597-641.

177. Koenig A, Bruckner-Tuderman L. Transforming growth factor-β stimulates collagen VII expression by cutaneous cells in vitro. J Cell Biol 1992; 117:679-685.

178. Parente MG, Chung LC, Ryynanen J et al. Human type VII collagen: cDNA cloning and chromosomal mapping of the gene. Proc Natl Acad Sci USA 1991; 88:6931-6935.

179. Ryynaenen M, Knowlton RG, Parente MG et al. Human type VII collagen: genetic linkage of the gene (COL7A1) on chromosome 3 to dominant dystrophic epidermolysis bullosa. Am J Hum Genet 1991; 49:797-803.

180. Greenspan DS, Byers MG, Eddy RL et al. Localization of the human collagen gene COL7A1 to 3p21.3 by fluorescence *in situ* hybridization. Cytogenet Cell Genet 1993; 62:35-36.

181. Morris NP, Keene DR, Glanville RW et al. The tissue form of type VII collagen is an antiparallel dimer. J Biol Chem 1986; 261:5638-5644.

182. Christiano AM, Rosenbaum LM, Chung-Honet LC et al. The large non-collagenous domain (NC-1) of type VII collagen is amino terminal and chimeric. Homology to cartilage matrix protein, the type III domain of fibronectin and the A domain of von Willebrand factor. Hum Mol Genet 1992; 7:475-481.

183. Gammon WR, Abernethy ML, Padilla KM et al. Noncollagenous (NC1) domain of collagen VII resembles multidomain adhesion proteins involved in tissue-specific organization of extracellular matrix. J Invest Dermatol 1992; 99:691-696.

184. Greenspan DS. The carboxyl-terminal half of type VII collagen, including the noncollagenous NC-2 domain and intron/exon organization of the corresponding region of the COL7A1 gene. Hum Mol Genet 1993; 2:273-278.

185. Christiano AM, Greenspan DS, Lee S et al. Cloning of human type VII collagen. J Biol Chem 1994; 269:20256-20262.

186. Li K, Christiano AM, Copeland NG et al. cDNA cloning and chromosomal mapping of the mouse type VII collagen gene (Col7a1):evidence for rapid evolutionary divergence of the gene. Genomics 1993; 16:733-739.

187. Lee J-O, Rieu P, Amin Arnaout M et al. Crystal structure of the A domain from the a subunit of integrin CR3 (CD11b/CD18). Cell 1995; 80:631-638.

188. Bentz H, Morris NP, Murray LW et al. Isolation and partial characterization of a new human collagen with an extended triple-helical structural domain. Proc Natl Acad Sci USA 1983; 80:3168-3172.

189. Lunstrum GP, Kuo H-J, Rosenbaum LM et al. Anchoring fibrils contain the carboxyl-terminal globular domain of type VII procollagen, but lack the amino-terminal globular domain. J Biol Chem 1987; 262:13706-13712.

190. Bruckner-Tuderman L, Nilssen O, Zimmermann DR et al. Immunohistochemical and mutation analyses demonstrate that procollagen VII is processed to collagen VII through removal of the NC-2 domain. J Cell Biol 1995; 131:551-559.

191. Baechinger HP, Morris NP, Lunstrum GP et al. The relationship of the biophysical and biochemical characteristics of type VII collagen to the function of anchoring fibrils. J Biol Chem 1990; 365:10095-10101.

192. Burgeson RE. Type VII collagen, anchoring fibrils, and epidermolysis bullosa. J Invest Dermatol 1993; 101:252-255.

193. Regauer S, Seiler GR, Barrandon Y et al.

Epithelial origin of cutaneous anchoring fibrils. J Cell Biol 1990; 111:2109-2115.

194. Smith LT, Sybert VP. Intra-epidermal retention of type VII collagen in a patient with recessive dystrophic epidermolyses bullosa. J Invest Dermatol 1990; 94: 261-264.

195. Konig A, Bruckner-Tuderman L. Epithelial-mesenchymal interactions enhance expression of collagen VII in vitro. J Invest Dermatol 1991; 96:803-808.

196. Ryynanen J, Sollberg S, Parente MG et al. Type VII collagen expression by cultured human cells and in fetal skin. J Clin Invest 1992; 89:163-168.

197. Stanley JR, Rubinstein N, Klaus-Kortun V. Epidermolysis bullosa acquisita antigen is synthesized by both human keratinocytes and human dermal fibroblasts. J Invest Dermatol 1985; 85:542-545.

198. Lunstrum GP, Sakai LY, Keene DR et al. Large complex globular domains of type VII procollagen contribute to the structure of anchoring fibrils. J Biol Chem 1986; 261:9042-9048.

199. Bruckner-Tuderman L, Schnyder UW, Winterhalter KH et al. Tissue form of type VII collagen from human skin and dermal fibroblasts in culture. Eur J Biochem 1987; 165:607-611.

200. Burgeson RE, Lunstrum GP, Rokosova B. The structure and function of type VII collagen. Ann NY Acad Sci 1990; 580:32-43.

201. Lapiere JC, Chen JD, Iwasaki T et al. Type VII collagen specifically binds fibronectin via an unique subdomain within the collagenous triple helix. J Invest Dermatol 1994; 103:637-641.

202. Briggaman RA, Wheeler CE Jr. Epidermolysis bullosa Dystrophica-recessive: a possible role of anchoring fibrils in the pathogenesis. J Invest Dermatol 1975; 65:203-211.

203. Leigh IM, Eady RAJ, Heagerty HM et al. Type VII collagen is a normal component of epidermal basement membrane which shows altered expression in recessive distrophic epidermolysis bullosa. J Invest Dermatol 1988; 90:639-642.

204. McGrath JA, Ishida-Yamamoto A, O'Grady A et al. Structural variations in anchoring fibrils in dystrophic epidermolysis bullosa: correlation with type VII collagen expression. J Invest Dermatol 1993; 100:366-372.

205. Hovnanian A, Duquesnoy O, Blanchet-Bardon C et al. Genetic linkage of recessive dystrophic epidermolysis bullosa to the type VII collagen gene. J Clin Invest 1992; 90:1032-1036.

206. Christiano AM, Greenspan DS, Hoffman GG et al. A missense mutation in type VII collagen in two affected siblings with recessive dystrophic epidermolysis bullosa. Nature Genet 1993; 4:62-66.

207. Hovnanian A, Hilal L, Blanchet-Bardon C et al. Recurrent nonsense mutations within the type VII collagen gene in patients with severe recessive dystrophic epidermolysis bullosa. Am J Human Genet 1994; 55: 289-296.

208. Christiano AM, Anhalt G, Gibbons S et al. Premature termination codons in the type VII collagen gene (COL7A1) underlie severe, mutilating recessive dystrophic epidermolysis bullosa. Genomics 1994; 21:160-168.

209. Hilal L, Rochat A, Duquesnoy P et al. A homozygous frameshift mutation in COL7A1 predicts a shortened protein in the generalized mutilating (Hallopeau-Siemens) form of recessive dystrophic epidermolysis bullosa. Nature Genet 1993; 5:287-293.

210. Christiano AM, Ryynaenen M, Uitto J. Dominant dystrophic epidermolysis bullosa: identification of a Gly—Ser substitution in the triple-helical domain of type VII collagen. Proc Natl Acad Sci USA 1994; 91:3549-3553.

211. Woodlet DT, Burgeson RE, Lunstrum G et al. Epidermolysis bullosa acquisita antigen is the globular carboxyl terminus of type VII procollagen. J Clin Invest 1988; 81:683-687.

212. Gammon WR, Murrell DF, Jenison MW et al. Autoantibodies to type VII collagen recognize epitopes in a fibronectin-like region of the noncollagenous (NC-1) domain. J Invest Dermatol 1993; 100:618-622.

213. Kiss I, Deàk F, Holloway RG Jr et al. Structure of the gene for cartilage matrix protein, a modular protein of the extracellular matrix. Exon/Intron organization, unusual

splice sites, and relations to a chains of β2-integrins, von Willebrand factor, complement factors B and C2, and epidermal growth factor. J Biol Chem 1989; 264: 8126-8134.

214. Jenkins RN, Osborne-Lawrence SL, Sinclair AK et al. Structure and chromosomal location of the human gene encoding cartilage matrix protein. J Biol Chem 1990; 265:19624-19631.

215. Agraves WS, Deàk F, Sparks KJ et al. Structural features of cartilage matrix proteins deduced from cDNA. Proc Natl Acad Sci USA 1987; 84:464-468.

216. Marti T, Roesselet S, Titani K et al. Identification of disulfide-bridge substructure within human von Willebrand factor. Biochemistry 1987; 26:8099-8109.

217. Andrews RK, Gorman JJ, Booth WJ et al. Cross-linking of a monomeric 39/34-kDa dispase fragment of von Willebrand factor (Leu-480/Val-481-Gly-718) to the N-terminal region of the α-chain of membrane glycoprotein Ib on intact platelets with bis (sulfosuccinimidyl) suberate. Biochemistry 1989; 28:8326-8336.

218. Haudenschild DR, Tondravi MM, Hofer U et al. The role of coiled-coil α-helices and disulfide bonds in the assembly and stabilization of cartilage matrix protein. A mutational analysis. J Biol Chem 1995; 270: 32150-23154.

219. Hauser N, Paulsson M. Native cartilage matrix protein (CMP). J Biol Chem 1994; 269: 25747-25753.

220. Paulsson M, Heinegard D. Matrix proteins bound to associatively prepared proteoglycans from bovine cartilage. Biochem J 1979; 183:539-545.

221. Paulsson M, Heinegard D. Purification and structural characterization of a cartilage matrix protein. Biochem J 1981; 197:367-375.

222. Paulsson M, Heinegard D. Radioimmunoassay of the 148-kilodalton cartilage protein. Distribution of the protein among bovine tissues. Biochem J 1982; 207:207-213.

223. Stirpe NS, Goetinck PF. Gene regulation during cartilage differentiation: temporal and spatial expression of link protein and cartilage matrix protein in the developing limb. Development 1989;107:23-33.

224. Paulsson M, Inerot S, Heinegard D. Variation in quantity and extractability of the 148-kilodalton cartilage protein with age. Biochem J 1984; 221: 623-630.

225. Tsonis PA, Goetinck PF. Expression of cartilage-matrix genes and localization of their translation products in the embryonic chickeye. Exp Eye Res 1988; 46:753-764.

226. Chen Q, Johnson DM, Haudenschild DR et al. Progression and recapitulation of the chondrocyte differentiation program: cartilage matrix protein is a marker for cartilage maturation. Dev Biol 1995; 172:293-306.

227. Chen Q, Johnson DM, Haudenschild DR et al. Cartilage matrix protein forms a type II collagen-independent filamentous network: analysis in primary cell cultures with a retrovirus expression system. Mol Biol Cell 1995; 6:1743-1753.

228. Winterbottom N, Tondravi MM, Harrington TL et al. Cartilage matrix protein is a component of the collagen fibril of cartilage. Dev Dyn 1992; 193:266-276.

229. Tondravi MM, Winterbottom N, Haudenschild DR et al. Cartilage matrix protein binds to collagen and plays a role in collagen fibrillogenesis. In: Fallon JF, Goetinck PF, Kelly RO, Stocum DL, eds. Limb Development and Regeneration. New York: Wiley-Liss, 1993: 515-522.

230. Pietu G, Meulien P, Cherel G et al. Production in *Escherichia coli* of a biologically active subfragment of von Willebrand factor corresponding to the platelet glycoprotein Ib, collagen and heparin binding domains. Biochem Biophys Res Commun 1989; 164:1339-1347.

231. Cruz MA, Yuan H, Lee JR et al. Interaction of the von Willebrand Factor (vWF) with collagen. J Biol Chem 1995; 270:10822-10827.

232. Denis C, Baruch D, Kielty CM et al. Localization of von Willebrand factor binding domains to endothelial extracellular matrix and to type VI collagen. Arterioscler Thromb 1993; 13:396-406.

233. Underwood PA, Bennet FA, Kirkpatrick A et al. Evidence for the location of a binding sequence for the α2β1 integrin of endothelial cells, in the β1 subunit of laminin.

Biochem J 1995; 309:765-771.

234. Vanderberg P, Kern A, Ries A et al. Characterization of a type IV collagen major cell binding site with affinity to the α1β1 and the α2β1 integrins. J Cell Biol 1991; 113:1475-1483.

235. Gullberg D, Gehlsen KR, Turner DC et al. Analysis of α1β1, α2β1 and α3β1 integrins in cell-collagen interactions: identification of conformation dependent α1β1 binding sites in collagen type I. EMBO J 1992; 11:3865-3873.

236. Kern A, Eble J, Goblik R et al. Interaction of type IV collagen with the isolated integrins α1β1 and α2β1. Eur J Biochem. 1993; 215:151-159.

237. Hughes SH, Greenhouse JJ, Petropulos CJ et al. Adaptor plasmids simplify the insertion of foreign DNA into helper-independent retroviral vectors. J Virol 1987; 61:3004-3012.

238. Bork P, Bairoch A. Extracellular protein modules. Trends Biochem Sci 1995; 3.

CHAPTER 7

OTHER MEMBERS OF THE SUPERFAMILY

αEβ7 INTEGRIN

The mucosal and skin immune system represents a subset of the immune system consisting of cutaneous lymphocytes and lymphocytes of the gastrointestinal, genitourinary, the upper respiratory tract and the mammary gland. It consists of organized lymphoid tissues such as Peyer's patches of intestine and isolated lymphocytes diffusely distributed in the epithelia. These lymphocytes derive from hematopoietic precursors that either enter the thymus and undergo partial maturation and selection before migrating into the skin or mucosa or home directly into the peripheral organs where they mature in situ.[1] Intraepithelial lymphocytes (IEL) reside in the lamina propria of the basement membrane adjacent to the basolateral surface of epithelial cells. IEL are predominantly CD8[+], either CD8αβ with T cell receptor (TCR) αβ or CD8αα with TCR αβ or TCR γδ, and have a restricted repertoire of variable region exon usage compared to peripheral blood lymphocytes.[2,3] Thus, IEL represent a distinct lymphocyte subpopulation functioning in immunological defense against pathogenic insults from the mucosal microenvironment. The first evidence that IEL express selectively a cell surface marker antigen (αEβ7) was provided in the rat.[4] Later on it was confirmed in humans,[5-8] mouse,[9,10] and more recently in chicken.[11]

MOLECULAR STRUCTURE

The cDNA of the human αE has been isolated and sequenced entirely[12] while only partial sequences of the murine αE are known.[13] The full length human sequence of 3.5 kb comprises 1160 amino acid residues coding for the mature protein. A comparison with other integrin α subunits indicates that αE is more closely related to the α subunits containing a VWFA module: αE contains a VWFA module, it has three cation binding motifs and lacks the membrane proximal cleavage site (Fig. 7.1). However, while resembling other integrin α subunits in overall similarity, αE is unique in two features: it contains an extra domain,

The Superfamily with von Willebrand Factor VA Domains, edited by
Alfonso Colombatti and Roberto Doliana. © 1996 R.G. Landes Company.

X, located just N-terminal to the VWFA module that harbors the unique proteolytic cleavage site (Arg-Arg) followed by a stretch of 18 negatively charged residues. These amino acids are likely well exposed to the solvent and might participate in ligand recognition. The αE subunit has ten potential glycosylation sites two of which are in the VWFA module. The VWFA module presents in its N-terminus two cysteines separated by two residues. Analysis of mRNA transcripts of the αE subunit indicates a high level of expression in cultured IEL and in tissues known to harbor IELs, such as small intestine, colon, lung but also in the thymus.[12] Surprisingly, αE transcripts are detected in pancreas, testis and in few cell lines in the absence of detectable β7 mRNA suggesting either that in these tissues αE is expressed only at the mRNA level or that it associates with a β subunit different from β7.

The αE integrin subunit identified by immunoprecipitation with several monoclonal antibodies and SDS-PAGE migrates at about 175 kD under nonreducing conditions. The αE, like many other integrin α subunits, is composed of two disulfide-bonded polypeptides and it migrates as two fragments at about 150 and 25 kD under reducing conditions.[7,8,11,14,15] The αE pairs predominantly, if not exclusively, with the β7 subunit,[16] although in several occasions other polypeptides of apparent mass of 135-150 kD are detectable:[8,16] one possible explanation for the presence of additional polypeptides in the immunoprecipitates might be that they represent alternatively spliced variant forms or that they are derived from distinct post-translational processing.

Tissue Expression

Various monoclonal antibodies raised against IEL preparations from different species[4-8,10,11,14] or against human neoplastic cells[17,18] recognize the same molecule or the same heterodimeric complex. Among the reagents more widely used to study the expression and function of αEβ7 (also known in humans as CD103 according to the 5th International Workshop on Human Leukocyte Differentiation Antigens) are the antibodies HML-1[5] and Ber-ACT8[6] which recognize the human molecule, and M290[10] which recognizes the murine molecule.

As mentioned above, αEβ7 is expressed almost selectively by IEL (85-90% IEL cells are positive) although few lymphoid cells at other sites also are positive: it is expressed on a small minority of peripheral blood T cells,[5] on activated T and B lymphocytes[21] and on some T lymphomas[19,20] and hairy cell leukemias.[17,18] In addition, in the mouse, few (3-5%) fetal or adult TCR γδ and TCR αβ medullary thymocytes express αEβ7.[22]

This integrin also is expressed at high levels on dendritic interdigitating cells in

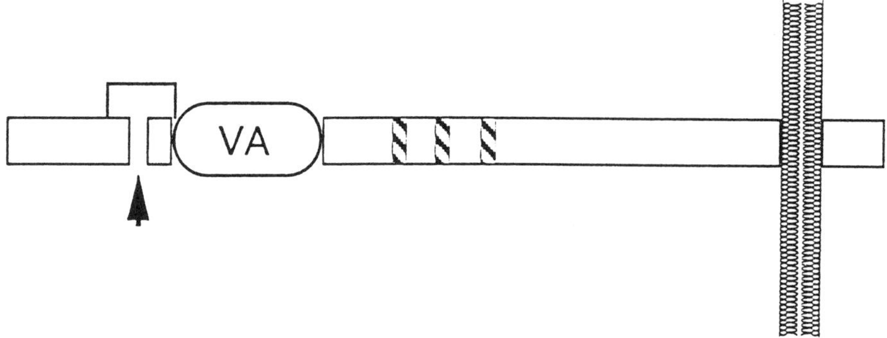

Fig. 7.1. Schematic diagram of the αE chain. The disulfide linked (shown as a connecting line) cleavage site (indicated by an arrow) occurs in the acidic sequence upstream of the VWFA/I (designated VA according to the proposed nomenclature of Bork and Bairoch[202]) module. The striped boxes represent the EF hand-like cation binding sites.

the mesenteric lymph nodes and in the gut mucosa and on 50-60% of dendritic interdigitating cells from lymph nodes draining nonmucosal tissues.[23] While monocytes do not express αEβ7 unless stimulated in vitro with PMA or IFN-γ,[24] macrophages associated with pneumocytes in the lungs, Kuppfer cells in the liver and sinus macrophages in lymph nodes express high levels of this integrin.[24] In addition, the promyelocytic HL-60 and histiocytic THP-1 cell lines express αEβ7 when induced to differentiate into macrophages following treatment with TPA or if stimulated with IFN-γ.[24] Finally, most T lymphocytes in the mouse can be induced to express αEβ7 following in vitro activation with TGF-β[14,25] or with soluble factors released by activated mast cells.[13]

FUNCTION

Naive IELs bear a relatively nonspecific array of homing receptors; but once a lymphocyte has been activated in a given tissue and has been exposed to cytokines within that specific microenvironment, it will express adhesion receptors useful for homing to or functioning in similar tissues. Like all other memory lymphocytes, IEL recirculate through the bloodstream and then return to mucosal tissues through the process of homing. This process is facilitated by the expression of the homing receptor α4β7 which confers unique migratory capacities since it directs lymphocytes to adhere to a counter-receptor expressed on endothelial cells in the gut and associated lymphoid organs.[26-28] To arrive at the gut wall, IEL or their precursors must traverse the basement membrane and then localize within the intraepithelial spaces. It is noteworthy that IELs also express α1β1 integrin,[29] which is a receptor for laminin and type IV collagen, two of the major constituents of basement membranes (see chapter 3).[15] Once there, IELs require a mechanisms for retention in the epithelium since the columnar epithelial cells turn over and are released into the intestinal lumen at a much greater rate than the homing of new IELs to the same site. Therefore, IELs

must adhere to the luminal side of the villus basement membrane and/or to the epithelial cells and perhaps high levels of αEβ7 are required for retention of IEL within the epithelium.

αEβ7 exhibits several characteristics that make it an excellent candidate for an adhesion molecule that could be involved in anchorage or retention of cells within the mucosae:[30] it is not expressed on T and B cells in the peripheral blood; except for a few cells in the thymus, spleen and peripheral blood on which low levels of αEβ7 are present; it is expressed at relatively high levels on T cells primarily after they reach the mucosae; it behaves as a late activation antigen for all T cells provided the right stimuli are delivered and its expression can be activated by IFN-γ[24] and by TGF-β1.[10,14,25] The effect of TGF-β1 is notable since this growth and differentiation-promoting factor may be produced by epithelial cells.[31,32] The presence of αEβ7 on thymic TCR γδ and αβ T cells[22] suggests a common function for this integrin during early T cell differentiation in the thymus especially in light of the finding that expression is skewed in the adult thymus toward the more mature cells present in the medulla.[22]

The high expression of αEβ7 on IELs and dendritic epidermal cells in the mouse[23] and resident mature macrophages in lungs, liver, and lymphnodes[24] compared to other cells suggests that its expression is regulated in a tissue-specific manner and that αEβ7 might play some role in antigen presentation or antigen capture at epithelial surfaces. Since both intestinal and skin epithelial cells produce TGF-β1,[31,32] it is likely that upregulation of αEβ7 takes place in situ: this is supported by the finding that TGF-β1 upregulates αEβ7 on several cell types in vitro.[10,14,15] Therefore, an adhesion/retention system can be envisaged in which dendritic antigen presenting cells are in contact with epithelial cells and this facilitates uptake of viruses or antigenic molecules by dendritic cells. Activated TCR γδ IELs also produce keratinocyte growth factor[33] and this in turn can modulate epithelial cell growth and function. Initiation of immune responses against local pathogens in sites of IEL homing could take place in the following way : dendritic and other antigen presenting cells expressing αEβ7 adhere to epithelial cells and are in close contact with IELs; IELs also are in direct contact with epithelial cells via αEβ7 and counter-receptors on the epithelial cell membrane so that the maximum of stimulation can occur. Furthermore, αEβ7 functions as a costimulatory molecule since some antibodies to αEβ7 can impart a costimulatory signal to IELs.[7,16,34]

STRUCTURE-FUNCTION RELATIONSHIPS

αEβ7 fails to recognize the α4β7 ligands such as fibronectin,[37] VCAM-1[38] and MAdCAM-1,[27,28] whereas it recognizes surface molecules of epithelial cells. It mediates T lymphocyte adhesion on murine[35] and human[29,36] carcinoma cell lines and this adhesion is inhibited by several antibodies. This inhibition can prevent IEL-mediated cytotoxicity against cultured epithelial cells.[35] More recently, the ligand of αEβ7 on epithelial cells has been convincingly identified as E-cadherin both in human[39] and in murine[40] cells. This finding is quite unexpected since cadherins are known to mediate homotypic and homophilic interactions.[41,42] Which are the sites mediating the recognition between αEβ7 and E-cadherin? This binding is cation dependent and the metal ion dependent adhesion site (MIDAS)[43] of the VWFA module as well as other sites on the module might be involved as shown for other VWFA containing integrins.[44-52] In light of the recent finding that cadherins contain an aspartate in the middle of the immunoglobulin-like CD loops,[53] that could represent the sixth coordination site of the MIDAS motif, this interaction is very likely to occur. Alternatively, the highly charged stretch of amino acids could represent the actual binding site with the VWFA module maintained in a proper conformation by the presence of the cation and acting indirectly on the charged site.

DHP-SENSITIVE CA²⁺ CHANNEL

Voltage-gated channels are responsible for the generation of conducted electrical signals in a variety of cells. The high voltage-gated L-, N-, P-, Q- and R-type Ca²⁺ channels, by mediating entry of calcium in response to depolarization without significant flux of any other ion, contribute to the general electric status of excitable cells and translate electrical signals on the membrane surface into intracellular chemical signals affecting cellular functions such as contraction and secretion.[54-56] The increase in permeability deriving from depolarization consists of a rapid (few milliseconds) increase (activation) followed by a decrease (inactivation) to baseline levels. Ca²⁺ ions are conducted across the membrane at rates close to their rates of free diffusion in solution and in fact Ca²⁺ channels are the most selective ion channels known, as they choose Ca²⁺ over Na⁺ by a ratio of about 1000:1. The L-type channels which have a high threshold and a long-lasting response are sensitive to blockers such as dihydropyridine (DHP), phenylalkylamines and benzothiazepines. In particular, DHP modulates the function of the channels critical to cardiac, smooth, striated muscle contraction and excitation-secretion coupling in endocrine cells and some neurons. The striated muscle DHP receptor, which is located in the membrane T-tubules, represents a model that has been most extensively investigated due to the abundance of the DHP-sensitive receptor in this tissue. It is a slow L-type Ca²⁺ channel and it is involved in replenishing Ca²⁺ pools during periods of rapid activity and in serving as a voltage sensor in excitation-contraction coupling.

MOLECULAR STRUCTURE

The major functional subunits of Ca²⁺ channels are members of a large gene family and are expressed in association with auxiliary proteins whose function is to increase the efficiency of the channel. Several channel constituents have been cloned, α1,[57,58] α2,[59,60] β[61,62] and γ,[63] and their function investigated after transfection in different types of cells. The α1 subunit is largely hydrophobic and carries the function of the specific calcium antagonist receptor[64-67] and of the channel forming component.[57] This had been initially suspected by the use of a function blocking antibody which recognized the α1 subunit and inhibited the slow Ca^{2+} current.[68] When the cDNA sequences became available it turned out that the sequence of the α1 subunit is highly similar to that of other ion channels proteins and that the structural organization of the α1 subunit corresponds to the molecular organization common to other ion channels: four homologous transmembrane domains each of which contains six hydrophobic alpha helices and surround a central pore, with the highly charged fourth helix (S4) in each domain serving as the voltage sensor[69,70] (Fig. 7.2).

The α2 subunit consists of 1106 amino acid residues, including 26 residues for the leader peptide, arranged in a N-terminal extracellular domain of 421 residues comprising the VWFA module which is located near the cell membrane. The VWFA module is followed by three hydrophobic, likely transmembrane, sequences separating a large (449 residues) intracellular domain bearing two potential phosphorylation sites and a 5 amino acid long cytoplasmic tail (Fig. 7.3). The second extracellular domain of 135 residues has four potential S-S bonds and is very likely highly compact. The deduced molecular mass of α2 is 125 kD,[59] and this mass is about 20 kD larger than the apparent mass of the fully deglycosylated subunit, suggesting that a portion of the protein, as deduced by the cDNA sequence, is absent from the mature α2 subunit. In fact, the mature α2 is truncated at A934 in the middle of the second extracellular domain and residues A935-L1080 constitute the disulfide-liked δ subunit.[60,71] Therefore, the α2 and δ subunits are coded for by the same gene.[72] The cDNA of the β subunit codes for a protein of 524 residues containing multiple consensus sites for phosphorylation that is lo-

cated intracellularly. There is evidence for only one γ gene coding for a 222 residue component which is expressed primarily in skeletal muscle as a transmembrane protein.[63] Both α2δ and γ subunits are glycosylated. Several homologous genes have been mapped[73] and found to undergo multiple splicings.[74] Multiple β subunits cDNA[55,62,76] have been detected, while only one α2 gene is apparently transcribed but its primary transcripts are alternatively spliced at the 3'-end of the mRNA and give rise to at least five variant subunits.[77-79]

The striated muscle DHP-sensitive receptor[65] is composed of five polypeptides α1, α2, β, γ, and δ with apparent molecular masses of about 170, 140, 50, 32 and 27 kD, respectively.[67,80,81] The specific association of these proteins as a multiprotein complex is supported by the copurification of each subunit with the DHP-binding and the calcium-conductance activities provided by the α1 subunit[82] and by the co-immunoprecipitation of the whole complex with the use of individual subunit specific antibodies.[82,83] Similar complexes, except for the absence of the γ subunit, have been isolated from heart[84] and neurons.[72,85]

EXPRESSION AND FUNCTION

As mentioned above the striated muscle DHP-sensitive channel contains five polypeptides. While during development the α2 subunit appears much earlier and it is followed only later by a rapid postnatal rise in the expression levels of the α1 subunit,[86] in the adult skeletal muscle the two subunits show a superimposable localization.[87] The use of muscle cell cultures from mdg mice, which lack slow DHP-sensitive Ca^{2+} current[88] due to a primary defect in the α1 subunit gene, supported the notion that the α1 subunit is the principal element in the channel since its transfection into homozygous mutant cells can restore a normal voltage function.[89,90] In mdg/mdg cells the α2 subunit is abnormally and diffusely distributed in the perinuclear region and in some parts of the

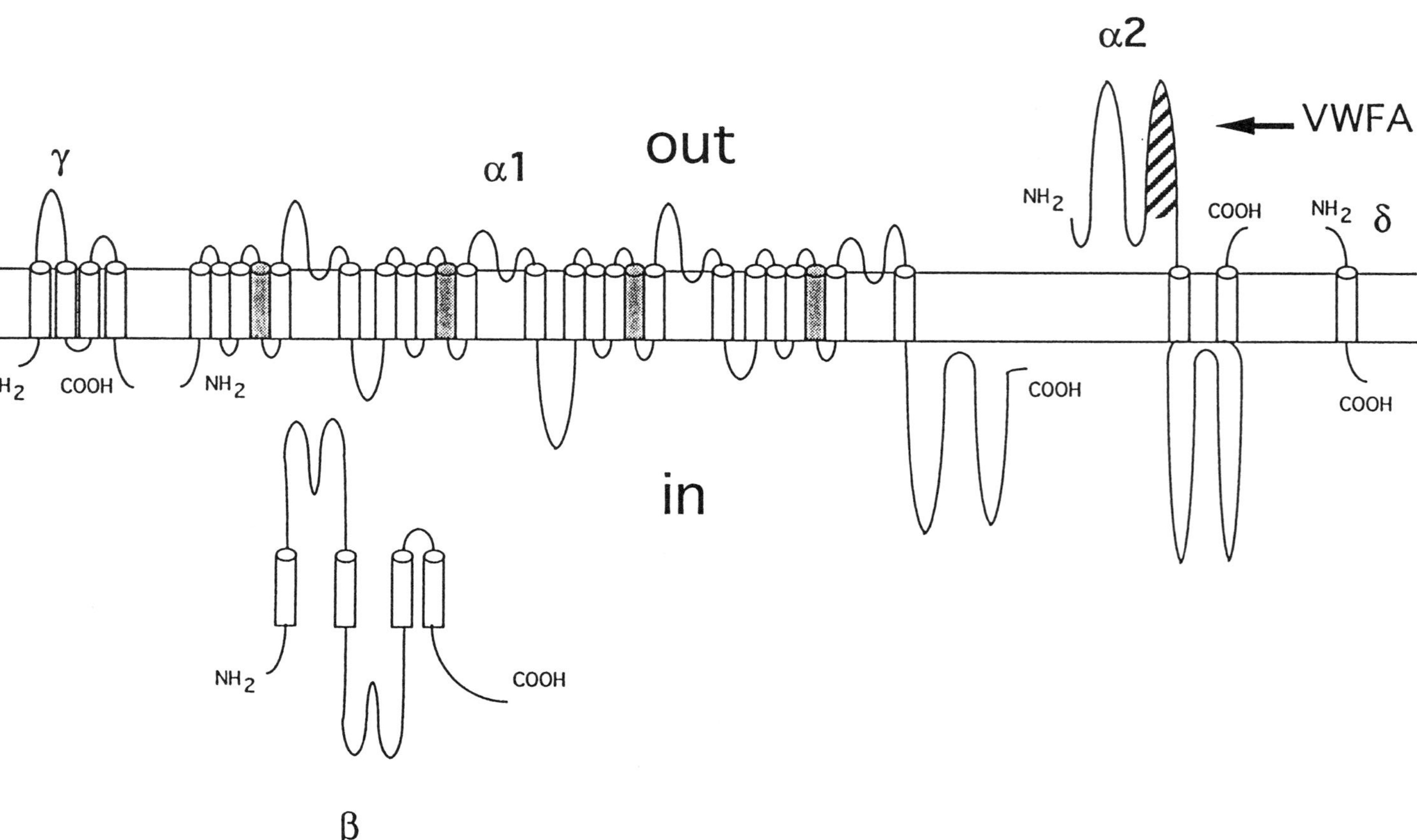

Fig. 7.2. Hypothetical transmembrane organization of the DHP-sensitive Ca^{2+} channel. The subunit arrangement based on the primary structure is illustrated. Cylinders represent α-helical segments within the cell membrane (except for the β chain) with the highly charged fourth helix (S4) serving as the voltage sensor (shaded). Lines represent the polypeptide chains of each subunit.

cell membrane and only after transfection with the α1 subunit the normal clustered codistribution of the two subunits within the T tubules is rescued.[91] This suggests that a direct interaction between α1 and α2 subunits is likely and maybe necessary for the correct organization of the T-tubule membrane. However, the conclusion drawn from the studies with dysgenic myotubes are hampered by the contemporary expression of the other subunits.[92]

More conclusive evidence for the α1 chain being a functional channel came from studies with *Xenopus* oocytes which express functional channel current after injection with the α1 subunit RNA.[58,93] Similarly, transfection of α1 into L cells[94] leads to the appearance of both DHP binding and Ca^{2+} currents, suggesting that this subunit is sufficient for channel activity. In particular, the S3 segment of the linker sequence between segments S3 and S4 of repeat I is critical for activation of the channel.[95] Finally, although the α1 subunit from heart,[93] skeletal muscle[96] and rat brain[97]

possesses the necessary properties of a Ca^{2+} channel and neither α2 nor β subunits are essential both for cell surface expression of the α1 subunit and for its function, coexpression of the α2δ[58,98-100] and of the β[98,100-102] subunits results in a significant increase in DHP binding sites and channel activity. While the current expressed in α1 transfected L cells is at least 10-fold slower than the current detected in skeletal muscle, the kinetics of activation and deactivation is dramatically accelerated if the other subunits are cotransfected.[103-107] These observations suggest that the primary function of the α2 and β subunits is to act synergistically and to confer to the complex a quaternary structural conformation more suitable for a properly functional channel.[108] The DHP-sensitive Ca^{2+} channels, like several other ion channels, associate with the ryanodine-sensitive calcium release channels, which function as effectors during the process of excitation-contraction coupling. The latter channels physically interact with the intracellular

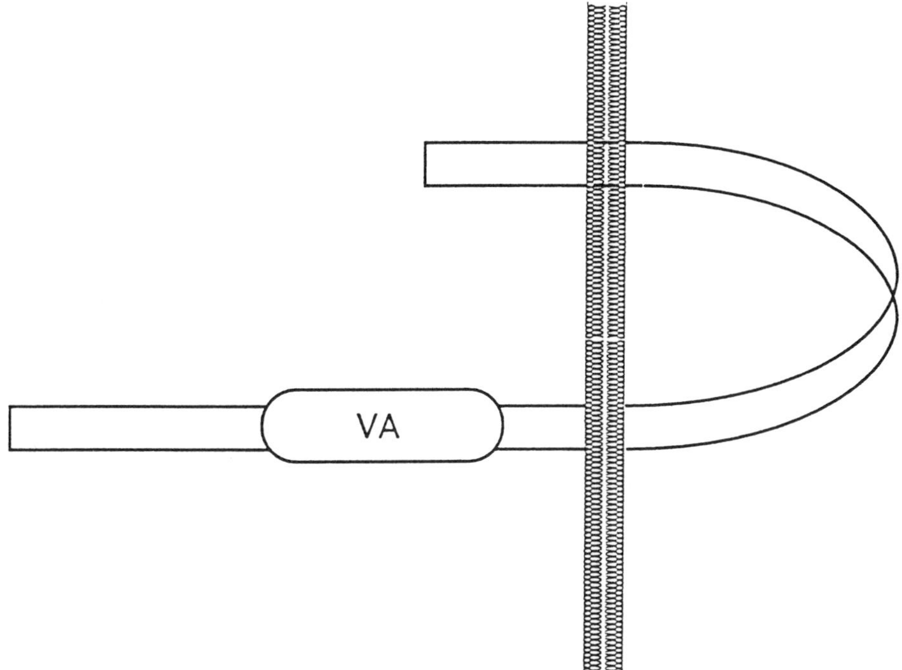

Fig. 7.3. Schematic diagram of the α2 chain of the DHP sensitive Ca^{2+} channel. In and out indicate the cytoplasmic and the extracellular side of the cell membrane.

loop connecting domains II and III of the α1 subunit, as shown by using chimeric DHP receptors,[109] and functions by modulating the kinetics of activation, inactivation, current and drug binding thereby expanding the potential functions of the Ca^{2+} channels.

The β subunit might be involved in phosphorylation/dephosphorylation events and/or in lowering the energy barrier for opening the channel.[110] The binding site on the α1 subunit for a conserved motif on the β subunit[111] has recently been identified.[112] It is a sequence conserved in all the α1 subunits and it is located in the intracellular loop between domains I and II. Recently, skeletal muscle α1 subunit point mutations have been implicated in hypokalemic periodic paralysis.[113] Finally, while several mutagenesis studies have clarified the role of the different segments of the homologous α1 subunits in ion conductance and inactivation,[114] few data are still available that might help define the primary structural elements responsible for the basic function of the other subunits and, particularly of the α2 subunit of the DHP-sensitive Ca^{2+} channel. Finally, another hint in the function of the α2 subunit may come from the observation that the α2δ gene has been mapped in or near the malignant hyperthermia mutation occurring in some families.[115] Maybe the α2 subunit is involved in oligomerization processes which are important for channel function.

INTER-α-INHIBITOR FAMILY

Inter-α-inhibitor (IαI) proteins are a complex group of plasma proteinase inhibitors constituting a family of proteins with serine protease inhibitory activity.[116-118] Collectively IαI concentration in serum is relatively high (0.45 mg/ml), however it accounts for only about 5% of the total serum antiprotease activity. It has been suggested that IαI makes a low affinity complex with proteases, its main function being to shuttle the proteases to other inhibitors.[119-121] While the physiological role of IαI family members remains largely unknown and it is further complicated by the absence of known deficiency syndromes, recent progress has been made to allow some understanding of the function of IαI family members.

MOLECULAR STRUCTURE

The members of IαI family have long been known but until recently the nomenclature referring to the various members has been confusing and sometimes contradictory. We will follow the proposed nomenclature of Salier[118] that has the merit to use a terminology that clearly distinguishes between the precursor polypeptides, the mature polypeptides and the protein complexes formed. IαI family members are synthesized predominantly in the liver from five separate genes coding for the heavy chains H1, H2, H3 and H4[122-127] and for a fifth polypeptide called AMBP (α1-microglobulin/bikunin precursor).[128] AMBP is cleaved into α1-microglobulin[129] and a light chain designated bikunin which consists of a tandemly arranged Kunitz-type protease inhibitor modules.[130-132]

The H1 gene has been recently isolated and preliminarily characterized:[133] it has 22 exons spanning about 14 kb in length, four of which code for the VWFA module and five for the C-terminal peptide which is cleaved in the mature protein. The gene has no typical TATA sequences and the promoter region shows binding sites for IL-6 and hepatocyte nuclear factor that give reason for the restricted tissue-specific transcription and the IL-6 inducibility.[134] The H1 and H3 genes are located in chromosome 3p21.1-p21.2; the H2 gene is on chromosome 10p14-15 and the gene for AMBP is on chromosome 9q32-33.[124] The location of the gene for the fourth heavy chain is not known yet. Furthermore, the genes for the H and bikunin components are in homologous chromosomal locations in humans and mice.[135,136] It is likely that H2 originated from an H ancestor, which more recently duplicated to provide the H1 and H3 genes.[135,136] This suggestion is supported by the tandemly close location of H1 and H3 since they are only 2721 bp apart on the same DNA strand,[137] the higher sequence similarity both at the nucleotide and amino acid level of H1 and H3[127] and the fact that H1 and H2 are the least similar, It is likely that H2 originated from an H ancestor, which more recently duplicated to provide the H1 and H3 genes.[135,136]

The cDNAs for all four human H precursor chains (HxP) have been isolated: H1, H2 and H3 code for precursor molecules that are processed and shed a large C-terminus peptide of about 240-280 residues depending upon the chain (Fig. 7.4).[124,126,127,138] The fourth chain (H4P) is highly homologous to the other H chains only in the N-terminal two-thirds of the sequence; the C-terminus of H4P contains a bradykinin-like domain bracketed by two Arg residues that allow release of a peptide by plasma kallikrein.[122] All four H chains possess a VWFA module located toward the N-terminus of the polypeptides. That H1 also possesses a VWFA module[125,138] had been overlooked by the first authors to report the sequence,[125,127,138] by us[139,140] in our previous reviews on the VWFA superfamily and also by other investigators.[141-143] Although H1 and H3 closely located in chromosome 3[124,137] and the sequence homology among the members of the family is very high in the region including the VWFA module, the inability to identify a VWFA module in a sequence is not too surprising since the overall homology among the different members of the superfamily is rather low. Recently, the murine homologue cDNAs were cloned and found to be about 85% identical for a given H chain.[144]

The HxP chains are processed intracellularly to the mature forms (designated H)[145] by cleavage of a C-terminal sequence at an Asp residue that removes a peptide of about 25 kD. This processing has not been demonstrated for H4P. The processing is comprised of two separate steps which involve first the proteolytic cleavage at the Asp-Pro sequence that releases the large (240-280 residues) C-terminus fragment and by the carbohydrate attach-

ment.[146] In addition, a short (36 residues) peptide is released from the N-terminus of the H2P chain.[126] The AMBP component also is cleaved to release bikunin which can be either free in plasma or become part of IaI family molecules. The members of the family are composed of varying combinations of the different subunits defined as inter-α-inhibitor (IαI), pre-α-inhibitor (PαI), and inter-α-like inhibitor (IαLI).[145,147] The plasma IαI is composed of three chains, H1, H2 and bikunin, joined by a unique protein-glycosaminoglycan-protein (PGP) cross-link; PαI is composed of H3 and bikunin, and IαLI is composed of H2 and bikunin.[145,148-150] Similar components have been isolated from bovine cumulus-oocyte complexes.[151-153] Further, a serum-derived hyaluronan-associated protein (SHAP) that is found covalently linked with hyaluronan corresponds to the H1 and H2 chains in human and to the H2 and H3 chains in bovine.[154] The binding site for hyluronan is located in the H2 chain of both bovine and human IαI. The covalent PGP cross-chain link in IαI molecules can be cleaved by chondroitinase, hyluronidase or mild sodium hydroxide treatment,[145,150,155-158] and a bikunin-free, covalent hyaluronic acid protein complex can be obtained by adding hyaluronic acid to human or bovine serum.[154,159] The PGP link consists of a chondroitin-4-sulfate-glycan bond that cross-links the mature chains terminal aspartic residues (D638 and D648 of H1P and H2P polypeptides, respectively) to S10 of bikunin (Fig. 7.5).[156] IαLI also is found cross-linked by a glycosaminoglycan chain to TSG-6 (TNF-stimulated gene 6),[158] a 30 kD glycoprotein which is a member of a family of hyluronan binding proteins including CD44, cartilage link protein, aggrecan and versican.[160] A unique feature of TSG-6 is the tendency to form reduction-resistant complexes with H2 and bikunin with the release of H1.[158,161] Other peculiar IαI compositions have been detected: in the HepG2 hepatoma cell line two H2 are linked to two bikunin chains by a chondroitin sulfate bridge.[162]

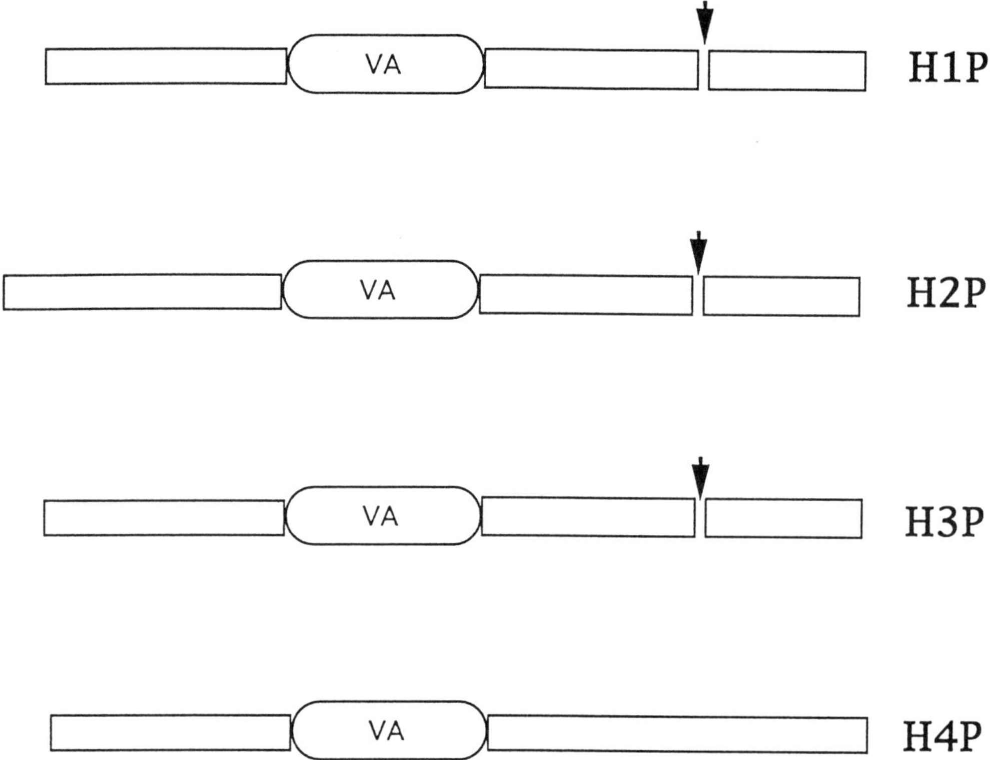

Fig. 7.4. Schematic diagram of the heavy chains of the Iαl family of protease inhibitors. The non-disulfide linked cleavage sites are indicated by the arrow.

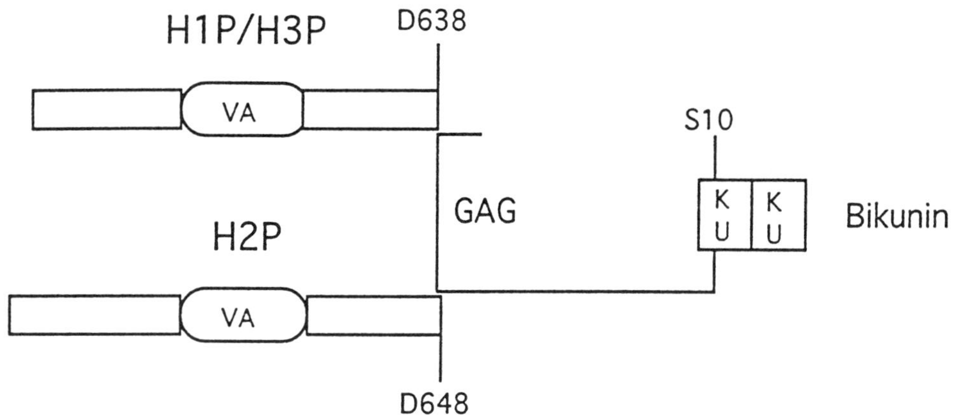

Fig. 7.5. The protein-glycosaminoglycan-protein (PGP) cross link. A glycan bond of a glycosaminoglycan (GAG) chain cross-links the terminal aspartic acid of the mature chains with the serine at position 10 of the first Kunitz module of Bikunin with the formation of the different plasma Iαl family members.

EXPRESSION AND FUNCTION

The IαI genes are primarily transcribed in the liver and their pattern of expression is highly regulated;[14,163] in addition, the H2 and H3 genes are expressed in the brain, whereas H1 is undetectable in this tissue.[163] Changes in serum concentration of the different members of the family during inflammatory processes have been reported.[164] Furthermore, in the synovial fluid of patients with rheumatoid arthritis, IαLI is found associated with hyaluronan whereas no IαLI is detectable in control synovial fluid. In acute inflammatory states the liver responds by down regulating AMBP and H2 genes so that the relevant molecules IαI and IαLI behave as negative acute-phase proteins, while H3 is upregulated and the corresponding PαI member behaves as a positive acute-phase protein.[164] Accordingly, the H2 and H3 genes respond differently to a treatment with IL-6, the major inducer of acute-phase reactions: H2 mRNA is decreased and H3 mRNA is increased in a dose- and time-dependent manner.[134] Still unclear is why the H1 gene is upregulated as is the H3 gene at the mRNA level[134] while no increases in the protein are detected.[164] The similar gene regulation of H1 and H3 is in agreement with their close location on chromosome 3p21.1-21.2.[124,137] The H4 gene also is upregulated in acute inflammation.[165]

It is likely that the antiprotease activity resides exclusively in the polypeptide bikunin. The Kunitz module also is part of several larger molecules endowed with serine protease inhibitory activity such as pancreatic trypsin inhibitor,[166] LACI[167] and β-amyloid precursor protein[168] or devoid of functional activity such as the α3 chain of type VI collagen.[169-171] Trypsin and chymo—trypsin form equimolar complexes with IαTI suggesting that a single inhibitory site is functional in the Kunitz-type bikunin. The noncovalent complexes between hyaluronan and IαI found in cumulus-oocyte complexes (COC)[172] could behave as a proteinase inhibitor for enzymes that might potentially disrupt the cumulus or they could stabilize the ECM of the expanding cumulus by directly binding to the major component hyaluronan. Their function as a structural ECM component would be exerted by complexing with newly secreted hyaluronan which is the major factor in limiting the COC expansion.[173] Recently, IαI members were described that stabilize the hyaluronan pericellular coat also of other cell types such as fibroblasts and mesothelial cells.[164]

H2 lacks sequences homologous to the classical hyaluronan binding proteins such as the link protein[174] and CD44[175] and to the well described RHAMM hyaluronan receptor, unrelated to the link-protein family, that mediates tumor motility.[176] Since H2 has no similarity to either of these families it might represent a novel type of hyaluronan binding protein. There are clusters of positively charged residues that might potentially allow strong ionic interactions with hyaluronan that could then result in a covalent link between H2 and hyaluronan.[154] One of these charged sequences is located in the H2 VWFA module (K376-K385) and similar sequences are present in the same position also in the H1 and H3 chains. However, no structure/function studies which could help clarify how the VWFA module contribute to the function of the IαI members is available yet.

PARASITE PROTEINS: TRAP

The infective function of salivary gland sporozoites is dependent upon the CS protein: this conclusion was derived from the observation that antibodies against the CS protein inhibit infectivity[177] and that recombinant CS protein bound to the hepatocyte basolateral cell membrane in the same area where sporozoites contact the host target cell.[178] However, since non-infective oocyst and hemocoel sporozoites express relevant quantities of the CS protein[179,180] and the expression pattern of CS cannot fully explain the differential infectivity of sporozoites from distinct developmental stages, it is likely that other constituents might participate and play an important role in the complex process of sporozoite infection.

MOLECULAR STRUCTURE

The thrombospondin-related adhesive protein (TRAP) was identified by screening a genomic *Plasmodium falciparum* library with an oligonucleotide probe corresponding to the conserved region II of the CS protein.[181] In addition to TRAP and CS numerous proteins possess the conserved nonamer motif (WSPCSVTCG) such as thrombospondin,[182] F-spondin,[183] properdin,[184] PySSP2[185] and Etp 100 of *Eimeria tenella*.[186] With the above probe several clones were isolated and an open reading frame of 559 amino acid residues was identified, rich in asparagine and proline, and coding for a protein of approximately 63 kD.[181] The TRAP gene is very polymorphic and several nucleotide substitutions have been reported.[187] The sequence includes a VWFA module at the N-terminus, immediately followed by the conserved nonapeptide. Similar structures have been sequenced and isolated from *Plasmodium yoelii* (PySSP2)[188] from *Eimeria tenella* (Etp 100)[189] and from *Eimeria maxima* (Emp 100) (Fig. 7.6).[190] The mature TRAP/PfSSP2 protein has a molecular mass (90 kD) which is much larger than that predicted from the cDNA sequence.[191]

EXPRESSION AND FUNCTION

TRAP is expressed by sporozoites produced by salivary gland[192] and is found on the external parasite membrane and on micronemes.[178] Whether TRAP is expressed in the blood-stage parasites is not yet resolved as contrasting results were reported.[191,192] Salivary gland sporozoite differ from oocyst and hemocoel sporozoites primarily because they can induce a protective immune response.[193] In addition, and differently from the less mature forms that lack or exhibit a low infectivity, the salivary gland sporozoites infect vertebrate host cells very effectively,[194] although they cannot reinfect the salivary gland cells. TRAP/PfSSP2 is a good candidate to fulfill a relevant function in this process. First, it is not expressed in non-infective oocyst and hemocoel sporozoites, while infective salivary gland sporozoites are all TRAP/PfSSP2 positive.[195] Furthermore, the regulated expression might well account for the increasing infectivity of sporozoites depending on their maturation stage. Second, recombinant TRAP/PfSSP2 also binds to the basolateral membrane of hepatocytes where infective sporozoites contact the target cell,[178] as revealed by a careful immuno-electron microscopy study.[195] Third, the possibility that TRAP/PfSSP2 may be one of the "receptor" molecules implicated in hepatocyte infection also is supported by field studies, which indicate that anti TRAP antibodies are found in infected individuals[196] and seem to be involved in the control of the parasite levels.[197] The role of TRAP/PfSSP2 in efficient immunity against plasmodium is further confirmed by results obtained in mice: spleen cells from mice immunized with irradiated sporozoites and restimulated in vitro with different synthetic peptides of the PySSP2 protein, which is the equivalent of TRAP/PfSSP2 in the *Plasmodium yoelii*, induce a strong cytotoxic T cell response.[198]

STRUCTURE-FUNCTION RELATIONSHIPS

Both recombinant CS and TRAP are able to attach to the hepatoma HepG2 cell line and their binding sites map to the region including the conserved WSPCSVTCG motif.[178,199] The current evidence is that proteins containing this motif bind to sulfatides, although different proteins harboring the conserved motif differ in their fine specificity for sulfated glycoconjugates such as heparan sulfate and heparin.[200] Cell surface proteoglycans, such as syndecans, were in fact suggested as potential sporozoites receptors.[201] In the case of TRAP/PfSSP2 the binding to sulfatides is specific and is inhibited competitively by various sulfatides including suramin, an anti-protozoan polysulphonated drug. Also synthetic peptides corresponding to the conserved region bind to sulfatides and to hepatocyte cell membrane[200] but only if present as multimers.[178,201] This interaction is specific, as peptides from other regions of TRAP/

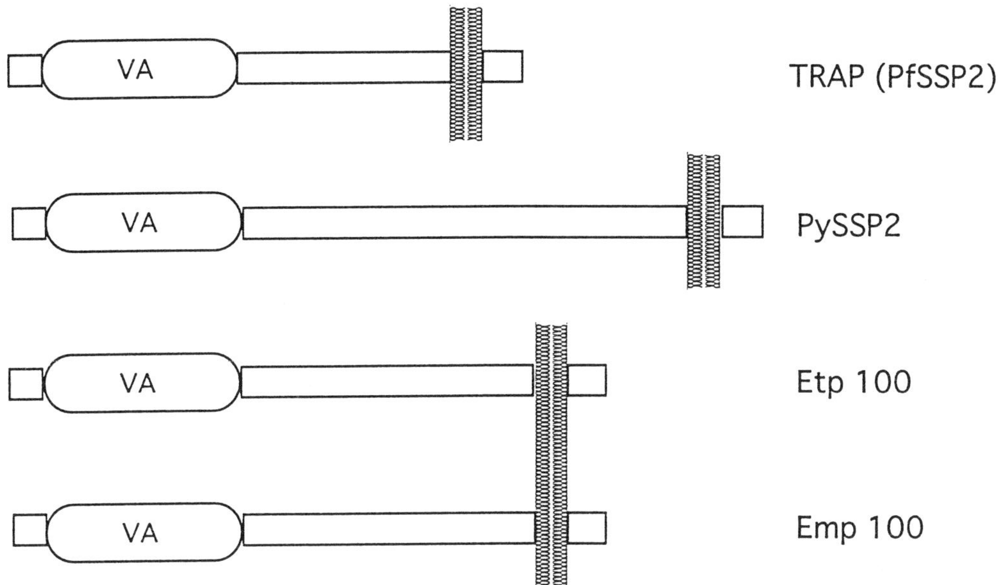

Fig. 7.6. Schematic diagram of the parasite proteins containing a VWFA (VA) module. TRAP (PfSSP2) and PySSP2 are expressed on the membrane of sporozoites of the Plasmodium falciparum *and* Plasmodium yoelii, *respectively. Etp100 and Emp100 are expressed on the membrane of coccidia* Eimeria tenella *and* Eimeria maxima, *respectively.*

PfSSP2 do not bind, and the interaction seems to depend upon the presence of the conserved motif. Using TRAP constructs progressively deleted at their C-terminus has allowed determination the sites necessary for binding to hepatocytes. Thus, only constructs containing the supposed sulfatide-binding motif can bind to hepatocytes.[195] This binding is abolished by pretreatment of hepatocytes with heparitinase and heparinase supporting the notion that glycosaminoglycans may function as ligands for TRAP/PfSSP2. However, although constructs lacking the sulfatide binding motif do not bind to hepatocytes,[195] several polyclonal antisera raised against C-terminus deleted constructs of TRAP inhibit HepG2 cell infection. Quite unexpectedly, a significant level of inhibition is obtained also with an antiserum raised against one of the constructs (R26-C205) which does not contain the WSPCSVTCG motif.[200] This antiserum, which does not recognize the sulfatide binding motif, is directed against a large portion of the VWFA module of TRAP/PfSSP2. Thus, it is likely that while the sulfatide binding motif is contributing to the general recognition of cell surfaces, an important role is exerted by the VWFA module also. This conclusion is relevant especially in view of the observation that synthetic peptides with the WSPCSVTCG motif can bind to hepatocytes cell membranes only if presented as multimers.[178,201] The function of the VWFA module might be to provide additional binding sites and thus contribute to reach a sufficient binding affinity even to the single WSPCSVTCG motif present in the TRAP protein. The contribution of sites close to the VWFA modules to the function of the respective proteins is suggested by findings obtained with LFA-1[203,204] and Mac-1.[205]

References

1. Lefrancois L, Puddington L. Extrathymic intestinal T-cell development: virtual reality? Immunol Today 1995; 16:16-21.
2. Van Kerckhove C, Russel GJ, Deutsch K et al. Oligoclonality of human intestinal intraepithelial T cells. J Exp Med 1991; 175:57-63.

3. Asarnow DM, Goodman T, Lefrancois L et al. Distinct antigen receptor repertoires of two classes of murine epithelium-associated T cells. Nature 1989; 341:60-62.

4. Cerf-Bensussan N, Guy Grand D, Lisowska Grospierre B et al. A monoclonal antibody specific for rat intestinal lymphocytes. J Immunol 1986; 136:76-82.

5. Cerf-Bensussan N, Jarry A, Brousse N et al. A monoclonal antibody (HML-1) defining a novel membrane molecule present on human intestinal lymphocytes. Eur J Immunol 1987; 17:1279-1285.

6. Kruschwitz M, Fritzsche G, Schwarting R et al. Ber-ACT8: a new monoclonal antibody to the mucosal lymphocyte antigen (MLA). J Clin Pathol 1991; 44:636-645.

7. Russel GJ, Parker CM, Cepek KL et al. Distinct structural and functional epitopes of the αEβ7 integrin. Eur J Immunol 1994; 24:2832-2841.

8. Micklem KJ, Dong Y, Willis A et al. HML-1 antigen on mucosa-associated T cells, activated cells, and hairy leukemic cells is a new integrin containing the β7 subunit. Am J Pathol 1991;139:1297-1301.

9. Kilshaw PJ, Baker KC. A unique surface antigen on intraepithelial lymphocytes in the mouse. Immunol Lett 1988; 18:149-154.

10. Kilshaw PJ, Murant SJ. A new surface antigen on intraepithelial lymphocytes in the intestine. Eur J Immunol 1990; 20:2201-2207.

11. Haury M, Kasahara Y, Schaal S et al. Intestinal T lymphocytes in the chicken express an integrin-like antigen. Eur J Immunol 1993; 23:313-319.

12. Shaw SK, Cepek KL, Murphy EA et al. Molecular cloning of the human mucosal lymphocyte integrin αE subunit. J Biol Chem 1994; 269:6016-6025.

13. Smith TJ, Ducharme LA, Shaw SK et al. Murine M290 integrin expression modulated by mast cell activation. Immunity 1994; 1:393-403.

14. Kilshaw PJ, Murant SJ. Expression and regulation of β7(βp) integrins on mouse lymphocytes: relevance to the mucosal immune system. Eur J Immunol 1991; 21:2591-2597.

15. Parker CM, Cepek KL, Russell GJ et al. A family of β7 integrins on human mucosal lymphocytes. Proc Natl Acad Sci USA 1992; 89:1924-1928.

16. Cerf-Bensussan N, Bègue B, Gagnon J et al. The human intraepithelial lymphocyte marker HML-1 is an integrin consisting of a β7 subunit associated with a distinctive α chain. Eur J Immunol 1992; 22:273-277.

17. Visser L, Shaw A, Slupsky J et al. Monoclonal antibodies reactive with hairy cell leukemia. Blood 1989; 74:320-325.

18. Flenghi L, Spinozzi F, Stein H et al. LF61: A new monoclonal antibody directed against a trimeric molecule (150kD, 125kD, 105kD) associated with hairy cell leukaemia. Br J Haematol 1990; 76:451-459.

19. Spencer J, Cerf-Bensussan N, Jarry N et al. Enteropathy-associated T cell lymphoma (Malignant histiocytosis of the intestine) is recognized by a monoclonal antibody (HML-1) that defines a membrane molecule on human mucosal lymphocytes. Am J Pathol 1988, 132:1-5.

20. Moeller P, Mielke B, Moldenhauer G. Monoclonal antibody HML-1, a marker for intraepithelial T cells and lymphomas derived thereof, also recognizes hairy cell leukemia and some B-cell lymphomas. Am J Pathol 1990; 136:509-512.

21. Schieferdecker HL, Ullrich L, Weiss-Breckwoldt AN et al. The HML-1 antigen of intestinal lymphocytes is an activation antigen. J Immunol 1990; 144:2541-2549.

22. Lefrancois L, Barret TA, Havran WL et al. Developmental expression of the αIELβ7 integrin on T cell receptor γδ and T cell receptor αβ T cells. Eur J Immunol 1994; 24:635-640.

23. Kilshaw PJ. Expression of the mucosal T cell integrin αM290β7 by a major subpopulation of dendritic cells in mice. Eur J Immunol 1993; 23:3365-3368.

24. Tiisala S, Paavon T, Renkonen R. αEβ7 and α4β7 integrins associated with intraephitelial and mucosal homing, are expressed on macrophages. Eur J Immunol 1995; 25:411-417.

25. Austrup F, Rebstock S, Kilshaw et al. Transforming growth factor-β1-induced expression of the mucosa-related integrin αE on

lymphocytes is not associated with mucosa-specific homing. Eur J Immunol 1995; 25:1487-1491.

26. Schweigghoffer T, Tanaka Y, Tidswell M et al. Selective expression of integrin α4β7 on a subset of human CD4[+] memory T cells with hallmarks of Gut-Trophism. J Immunol 1993; 151:717-729.

27. Berlin C, Berg L, Briskin MJ et al. α4β7 integrin mediates lymphocyte binding to the mucosal vascular addressin MadCAM-1. Cell 1993; 74:185-195.

28. Strauch UG, Lifka A, Gosslar U et al. Distinct binding specificities of integrins alpha 4 beta 7 (LPAM-1), alpha 4 beta 1 (VLA-4) and alpha IEL beta 7. Int Immunol 1994; 6:263-275.

29. Cepek KL, Parker CM, Madara JL et al. Integrin αEβ7 mediates adhesion of T lymphocytes to epithelial cells. J Immunol 1993; 150:3459-3470.

30. Yuan Q, Jiang W-M, Hollander D et al. Identity between the novel integrin β7 subunit and an antigen found expressed on intraepithelial lymphocyte in the small intestine. Biochem Biophys Res Comm 1991; 176:1443-1449.

31. Koyama SY, Podolsky DK. Differential expression of transforming growth factors α and β in rat intestinal epithelial cells. J Clin Invest 1989; 83:1768-1773.

32. Barnard JA, Beauchamp RD, Coffey RJ et al. Regulation of intestinal epithelial cell growth by transforming factor type β. Proc Natl Acad Sci USA 1989; 86:1578-1582.

33. Boismenu R, Havran WL. Modulation of epithelial cell growth by intraepithelial T cells. Science 1994; 266:1253-1255.

34. Sarnacki S, Bègue B, Buc H et al. Enhancement of CD3-induced activation of human intestinal intraepithelial lymphocytes by stimulation of the β7-containing integrin defined by HML-1 monoclonal antibody. Eur J Immunol 1992; 22:2887-2892.

35. Roberts K, Kilshaw PJ: The mucosal T cell integrin αM290β7 recognizes a ligand on mucosal epithelial cell lines. Eur J Immunol 1993; 23:1630-1635.

36. Roberts AL, O'Connell SM, Ebert EC. Intestinal entraepithelial lymphocytes bind to colon cancer cells by HML-1 and CD11a.

Cancer Res 1993; 53:1608-1611.

37. Postigo AA, Sanchez-Mateos P, Lazarovits AI et al. α4β7 integrin mediates B cell binding to fibronectin and vascular adhesion molecule-1: expression and function of α4 integrins on human B lymphocytes. J Immunol 1993; 151:2471-2483.

38. Chan BMC, Elices MJ, Murphy E et al. Adhesion to vascular cell adhesion molecule 1 and fibronectin: comparison of α4β1 (VLA-4) and α4β7 on the human B cell line JY. J Cell Biol 1992; 267:8366-8370.

39. Cepek KL, Shaw SK, Parker CM et al. Adhesion between epithelial cells and T lymphocytes mediated by E-cadherin and the αEβ7 integrin. Nature 1994; 372:190-193.

40. Karecla PI, Bowden SJ, Green SJ et al. Recognition of E-cadherin on epithelial cells by the mucosal T cell integrin αM290β7(αEβ7). Eur J Immunol 1995; 25:852-856.

41. Takeichi M. Cadherins: a molecular family important in selective cell-cell adhesion. Annu Rev Biochem 1990; 59:237-252.

42. Shirayoshi Y, Nose A, Iwasaki K et al. N-linked oligosaccharides are not involved in the function of a cell-cell binding glycoprotein E-cadherin. Cell Struct Funct 1996; 11:245-252.

43. Michishita M, Videm V, Arnaout MA. A novel divalent cation-binding site in the α domain of the β2 integrin CR3 (CD11b/CD18) is essential for ligand binding. Cell 1993; 72:857-867.

44. Diamond MS, Garcia-Aguilar J, Bickford JK et al. The I domain is a major recognition site on the leukocyte integrin Mac-1 (CD11b/CD18) for four distinct adhesion ligands. J Cell Biol 1993; 120:1031-1043.

45. Randi AM, Hogg N. I domain of β2 integrin lymphocyte function-associated antigen-1 contains a binding site for ligand intercellular adhesion molecule-1. J Biol Chem 1994; 269:12395-12398.

46. Landis RC, McDowall A, Holness CLL et al. Involvement of the "I" domain of LFA-1 in selective binding to ligands ICAM-1 and ICAM-3. J Cell Biol 1994; 126:529-537.

47. Champe M, McIntyre W, Berman PW. Monoclonal antibodies that block the activ-

ity of leukocyte function-associated antigen 1 recognize three discrete epitopes in the inserted domain of CD11a. J Biol Chem 1995; 270:1388-1394.

48. Huang C, Springer TA. A binding interface on the I domain of Lymphocyte function-associated antigen-1 (LFA-1) required for specific interaction with intercellular adhesion molecule 1 (ICAM-1). J Biol Chem 1995; 270:19008-19016.

49. Edwards CP, Champe M, Gonzalzs T et al. Identification of amino acids in the CD11a I-domain important for binding of the leukocyte function-associated antigen-1 (LFA-1) to intercellular adhesion molecule-1 (ICAM-1). J Biol Chem 1995; 270: 12635-12640.

50. Ueda T, Rieu P, Brayer J et al. Identification of the complement iC3b binding site in the β2 integrin CR3 (CD11b/CD18). Proc Natl Acad Sci USA 1994; 91:10680-10684.

51. Kamata T, Wright R, Takada Y. Critical Threonine and aspartic acid residues within the I domains of β2 integrins for interactions with intercellular adhesion molecule 1 (ICAM-1) and C3bi. J Biol Chem 1995; 270:12531-12535.

52. Kamata T, Takada Y. Direct binding of collagen to the I domain of integrin α2β1 (VLA-2, CD49b/CD29) in a divalent cation-independent manner. J Biol Chem 1994; 269:26006-26010.

53. Overduin M, Harvey TS, Bagby S et al. Solution structure of the epithelial cadherin domain responsible for selective cell adhesion. Science 1995; 267:386-389.

54. McCleskey EW. Calcium channels: cellular roles and molecular mechanisms. Curr Op Neurobiol 1994; 4:304-312.

55. Catterall WA. Structure and function of voltage-gated ion channels. Annu Rev Biochem 1995; 64:493-531.

56. Varadi G, Mori Y, Mikala G et al. Molecular determinants of Ca^{2+} channel function and drug action. Trends Pharmacol Sci 1995; 16:43-49.

57. Tanabe B, Takeshima H, Mikami A et al. Primary structure of the receptor for calcium channel blockers from skeletal muscle. Nature 1987; 328:313-318.

58. Mikami A, Imoto K, Tanabe T et al. Primary structure and functional expression of the cardiac dihydropyridine-sensitive calcium channel. Nature 1989; 340:230-233.

59. Ellis SB, Williams ME, Ways N et al. Sequence and expression of mRNAs encoding the α1 and α2 subunits of a DHP-sensitive calcium channel. Science 1988; 241: 1661-1664.

60. de Jongh KS, Warner C, Catterall WA. Subunits of purified calcium channels. J Biol Chem 1990; 265:14738-14741.

61. Ruth P, Rohrkasten A, Biel M et al. Primary structure of the β subunit of the DHP-sensitive calcium channel from skeletal muscle. Science 1989; 245:1115-1118.

62. Castellano A, Wei X, Birnbaumer L et al. Cloning and expression of a neuronal calcium channel β subunit. J Biol Chem 1993; 268:12359-12366.

63. Jay SD, Ellis SB, McCue AF et al. Primary structure of the γ subunit of the DHP-sensitive calcium channel from skeletal muscle. Science 1990; 248:490-492.

64. Borsotto M, Barhanin J, Fosset M et al. The 1,4-dihydropyridine receptor associated with the skeletal muscle voltage-dependent Ca^{2+} channel-purification and subunit composition. J Biol Chem 1985; 260:14255-14263.

65. Flockerzi V, Oeken H-J, Hofmann F et al. Purified dihydropyridine-binding site from skeletal muscle t-tubules is a functional calcium channel. Nature 1986; 323:66-68.

66. Striessnig J, Moosburger K, Goll A et al. Stereosective photoaffinity labeling of the purified 1,4 dihydropyridine receptor of the voltage-dependent calcium channel. Eur J Biochem 1986; 161:603-609.

67. Takahashi M, Seagar MJ, Jones JF et al. Subunit structure of the dihydropyridine-sensitive calcium channels from skeletal muscle. Proc Natl Acad Sci USA 1987; 84:5478-5482.

68. Morton ME, Caffrey JM, Brown AM et al. Monoclonal antibody to the α1-subunit of the dihydropyridine-binding complex inhibits calcium currents in BC3H1 myocytes. J Biol Chem 1988; 263:613-616.

69. Guy HR, Conti F. Pursuing the structure and function of voltage-gated channels. Trends Neurosci 1990; 13:201-206.

70. Stuehmer W, Conti F, Suzuki H et al. Struc-

tural parts involved in activation and inactivation of the sodium channel. Nature 1989; 339:597-603.

71. Jay SD, Sharp AH, Kahl SD et al. Structural characterization of the dihydropyridine-sensitive calcium channel α_2-subunit and the associated δ peptides. J Biol Chem 1991; 266:3287-3293.

72. Takahashi M, Catterall WA. Identification of an α subunit of dihydropyridine-sensitive brain calcium channels. Science 1987; 236:88-91.

73. Hofmann F, Biel M, Flockerzi V et al. Molecular basis for Ca^{2+} channel diversity. Annu Rev Neurosci 1994; 17:399-418.

74. Zhang J-F, Randall AD, Ellinor PT et al. Distinctive pharmacology and kinetics of cloned neuronal Ca^{2+} channels and their possible couterparts in mammalian CNS neurons. Neuropharmacology 1993; 32:1075-1088.

75. Pragnell M, Sakamoto J, Campbell KP. Cloning and tissue-specific expression of the brain calcium channel beta subunit. FEBS Lett 1991; 291:253-258.

76. Hullin R, Singer-Lahat D, Freichel M et al. Calcium channel β subunit heterogeneity: functional expression of cloned cDNA from heart, aorta and brain. EMBO J 1992; 11:885-890.

77. Williams ME, Feldmann DH, McCue AF et al. Structure and functional expression of alpha 1, alpha 2, and beta subunits of a novel human neuronal calcium channel subtype. Neuron 1992; 8:71-84.

78. Kim H-L, Kim H, Lee P et al. Rat brain expresses an alternatively spliced form of the dihydropyridine-sensitive L-type calcium channel α_2 subunit. Proc Natl Acad Sci USA 1992; 89:3251-3255.

79. Brust PF, Simerson S, McCue AF et al. Human neuronal voltage-dependent calcium channels: studies on subunit structure and role in channel assembly. Neuropharmacology 1993; 32:1089-1102.

80. Gutierrez LM, Brawley RM, Hosey MM. Dihydropyridine sensitive calcium channels from skeletal muscle. J Biol Chem 1991; 266:16387-16394.

81. Hamilton SL, Hawkes MJ, Brush K et al. Subunit composition of the purified dihydropyridine binding protein from skeletal muscle. Biochemistry 1989; 28:7820-7828.

82. Takahashi M, Seagar MJ, Jones JF et al. Subunit structure of dihydropyridine-sensitive calcium channels from skeletal muscle. Proc Natl Acac Sci USA 1987; 84:5478-5482.

83. Ahlijanian MK, Westenbroek RE, Catterall WA. Subunit structure and localization of dihydropyridine-sensitive calcium channels in mammalian brain, spinal cord, and retina. Neuron 1990; 4:819-832.

84. Chang FC, Hosey MM. Dihydropyridine and phenylalkylamide receptors associated with cardiac and skeletal muscle calcium channels are structurally different. J Biol Chem 1988; 263:18929-18937.

85. Chin H, Smith MA, Kim HL et al. Expression of dihydropyridine-sensitive brain calcium channels in the rat central nervous system. FEBS Lett 1992; 299:69-74.

86. Morton ME, Froehner SC. The $\alpha1$ and $\alpha2$ polypeptides in the dihydropyridine-sensitive calcium channel differ in developmental expression and tissue distribution. Neuron 1989; 2:1499-1506.

87. Flucher BE, Morton ME, Froehner SC et al. Localization of the $\alpha1$ and $\alpha2$ subunits of the dihydropyridine receptor and ankyrin in skeletal muscle triads. Neuron 1990; 5:339-351.

88. Beam KG, Knudson CM, Powell JA. A lethal mutation in mice eliminates the slow calcium current in skeletal muscle cells. Nature 1986; 320:168-170.

89. Adams BA, Tanabe T, Mikami A et al. Intramembrane charge movement restored in dysgenic skeletal muscle by injection of dihydropyridine receptors cDNAs. Nature 1990; 346:569-572.

90. Tanabe T, Beam KG, Powell JA et al. Restoration of excitation-contraction coupling and slow calcium current in dysgenic muscle by dihydropyridine receptor complementary DNA. Nature 1988; 336:134-139.

91. Flucher BE, Phillips JL, Powell JA. Dihydropirydine receptor a subunits in normal and dysgenic muscle in vitro: expression of $\alpha1$ is required for proper targeting and distribution of $\alpha2$. J Cell Biol 1991;

115:1345-1356.

92. Knudson CM, Chaudhari N, Sharp AH et al. Specific absence of the α1 subunit of the dihydropyridine receptor in mice with muscular dysgenesis. J Biol Chem 1989; 264:1345-1348.

93. Atsushi M, Imoto K, Tanabe T et al. Primary structure and functional expression of the cardiac dihydropyridine-sensitive calcium channel. Nature 1989; 340:230-233.

94. Perez-Reyes E, Kim HS, Lacerda A E et al. Induction of calcium currents by the expression of the α1-subunit of the dihydropyridine receptor from skeletal muscle. Nature 1989; 340:233-236.

95. Nakai J, Adams BA, Imoto K et al. Critical roles of the S3 segment and S3-S4 linker of repeat I in activation of L-type calcium channels. Proc Natl Acad Sci USA 1994; 91:1014-1018.

96. Perez-Reyes E, Kim HS, Lacerda AE et al. Induction of calcium currents by the expression of the α1-subunit of the dihydropyridine receptor from skeletal muscle. Nature 1989; 340:233-236.

97. Stea A, Tomlinson WJ, Soong TW et al. Localization and functional properties of a rat brain α1A calcium channel reflect similarities to neuronal Q-and P-type channels. Proc Natl Acad Sci USA 1994; 91:10576-10580.

98. Itagaki K, Koch WJ, Bodi I et al. Native-type DHP-sensitive calcium channel currents are produced by cloned rat aortic smooth muscle and cardiac α1 subunits expressed in *Xenopus laevis* oocytes and are regulated by α2-and β-subunits. FEBS Lett 1992; 297:221-225.

99. Kim HS, Wei X-Y, Ruth P et al. Studies on the structural requirements for the activity of the skeletal muscle dihydropyridine receptor/slow Ca2+ channel. Allosteric regulation of dihydropyridine binding in the absence of α2 and β components of the purified protein complex. J Biol Chem 1990; 265:11858-11863.

100. Welling A, Bosse E, Cavalié A et al. Stable co-expression of calcium channel alpha 1, beta and alpha 2/delta subunits in a somatic cell line. J Physiol 1993; 471:749-765.

101. Nishimura S, Takeshima H, Hofmann F et al. Requirement of the calcium channel beta subunit for functional conformation. FEBS Lett 1993; 324:283-286.

102. Lory P, Varadi G, Schwartz A. The beta subunit controls the gating and dihydropyridine sensivity of the skeletal muscle Ca2+ channel. Biophys J 1992; 63:1421-1424.

103. Varadi G, Lory P, Schultz D et al. Acceleration of activation and inactivation by the β subunit of the skeletal muscle calcium channel. Nature 1991; 352:159-162.

104. Lacerda AE, Kim HS, Ruth P et al. Normalization of current kinetics by interactions between the α1 and β subunits of the skeletal muscle dihydropyridine-sensitive Ca2+ channel. Nature 1991; 352:527-530.

105. Itagaki K, Koch WJ, Bodi I et al. Native-type DHP-sensitive calcium channel currents are produced by cloned rat aortic smooth muscle and cardiac alpha 1 subunit expressed in *Xenopus laevis* oocytes and are regulated by alpha 2 and beta subunits. FEBS Lett 1992; 297:221-225.

106. Sather WA, Tanabe T, Zhang J-F et al. Distinctive biophysical and pharmacological properties of class A (BI) calcium channel alpha 1 subunits. Neuron 1993; 11:291-303.

107. Ellinor PT, Zhang J-F, Randall AD et al. Functional expression of a rapidly inactivating neuronal calcium channel. Nature 1993; 363:455-458.

108. Singer D, Biel M, Lotan I et al. The roles of the subunits in the function of the calcium channel. Science 1991; 253:1553-1557.

109. Tanabe T, Beam KG, Adams BA et al. Regions of the skeletal muscle dihydropyridine receptor critical for excitation-contraction coupling. Nature 1990; 346:567-569.

110. Neely A, Wei X, Olcese R et al. Potentiation by the β subunit of the ratio of the ionic current to the charge movement in the cardiac calcium channel. Science 1993; 262:575-578.

111. De Waard M, Pragnell M, Campbell KP. Ca2+ channel regulation by a conserved beta subunit domain. Neuron 1994; 13:495-503.

112. Pragnell M, De Waard M, Mori Y et al.

Calcium channel beta-subunit binds to a conserved motif in the I-II cytoplasmic linker of the alpha1-subunit. Nature 1994; 368:67-70.

113. Ptacek LJ, Rabi T, Griggs RC et al. Dihydropyridine receptor mutations cause hypokalaemic periodic paralysis. Cell 1994; 77:863-868.

114. Noda M, Suzuki H, Numa S et al. A single point mutation confers tetrodoxotin and saxitoxin intensivity on the sodium channel II. FEBS Lett 1989; 259:213-216.

115. Iles DE, Segers B, Olde-Weghuis D et al. Refined localization of the alpha-1 subunit of the skeletal muscle L-type voltage-dependent calcium channel (CACNL1A3) to human chromosome 1q32 by in situ hybridization. Hum Mol Genet 1994; 3: 969-975.

116. Salier JP. Inter-alpha-trypsin inhibitor: emergence of a family within the kunitz-type protease inhibitor superfamily. Trends Biochem Sci 1990; 15:435-439.

117. Gebhard W, Hochstrasser K, Fritz H et al. Structure of the inter-alpha-inhibitor (inter-alpha-trypsin inhibitor) and pre-alpha-inhibitor: current state and proposition of a new terminology. Biol Chem Hoppe Seyler 1990; 371:13-22.

118. Salier JP, Rouet P, Raguenez G et al. The Inter-a-Inhibitor family, from structures to regulations. Biochem J 1996; 315:1-9.

119. Nishimura H, Kakizaki I, Muta T et al. cDNA and deduced amino acid sequence of human PK-120, a plasma kallikrein-sensitive glycoprotein. FEBS Lett 1995; 357: 207-211.

120. Saguchi K, Tobe T, Hashimoto K et al. Cloning and characterization of cDNA for inter-alpha-trypsin inhibitor family heavy chain-related protein (IHRP), a novel human plasma glycoprotein. J Biochem (Tokyo) 1995; 117:14-18.

121. Pratt CW, Pizzo SV. In vivo metabolism of inter-alpha-trypsin inhibitor and its proteinase complexes: evidence for proteinase transfer to alpha-2-macroglobulin and alpha 1-proteinase inhibitor. Arch Biochem Biophys 1986; 248:587-596.

122. Pratt CW, Pizzo SV. Mechanism of action of inter-alpha-trypsin inhibitor. Arch Biochem Biophys 1987; 258:591-599.

123. Pratt CW, Roche PA, Pizzo SV. The role of inter-alpha-trypsin inhibitor and other proteinase inhibitors in the plasma clearance of neutrophil elastase and plasmin. Arch Biochem Biophys 1987; 258:591-599.

124. Diarra-Mehrpour M, Bourguignon J, Sesbouée R et al. Human plasma inter-α-trypsin inhibitor is encoded by four genes on three chromosomes. Eur J Biochem 1989; 179:147-154.

125. Diarra-Mehrpour M, Bourguignon J, Bost F et al. Human inter-alpha-trypsin inhibitor: full-length cDNA sequence of the heavy chain H1. Biochem Biophys Acta; 1992; 1132:114-118.

126. Gebhard W, Schreitmueller T, Hochstrasser K et al. Complementary DNA and derived amino acid sequence of the precursor of one of the three protein components of the inter-alpha-trypsin inhibitor complex. FEBS Lett 1988; 229:63-67.

127. Bourguignon J, Diarra-Mehrpour M, Thiberville L et al. Human pre-alpha-trypsin inhibitor-precursor heavy chain cDNA and deduced amino-acid sequence. Eur J Biochem 1993; 212:771-776.

128. Kaumeyer JF, Polazzi JO, Kotick MP. The mRNA for a proteinase inhibitor related to the HI-30 domain of inter-α-trypsin inhibitor also encodes α-1-microglobulin (protein HC). Nucleic Acids Res 1986; 14: 7839-7850.

129. Akerstrom B, Loegdberg L. An intringuing member of the lipocalin protein family: α1-microglobulin. Trends Biochem Sci 1990; 15:240-243.

130. Bourguignon J, Sesboue R, Diarra-Mehrpour M et al. Human inter-alpha-trypsin inhibitor. Synthesis and maturation in hepatoma HepG2 cells. Biochem J 1989; 261:305-308.

131. Odum L. Biosynthesis of inter-alpha-trypsin inhibitor and alpha 1-microglobulin in a human hepatoma cell line. Int J Biochem 1992; 24:215-222.

132. Sjoberg EM, Fries E et al. Biosynthesis of bikunin (urinary trypsin inhibitor) in rat hepatocytes. Arch Biochem Biophys 1992; 295:217-222.

133. Bost F, Bourguignon J, Martin JP et al.

Isolation and characterization of the human inter-alpha-trypsin inhibitor heavy-chain H1 gene. Eur J Biochem 1993; 218:283-291.

134. Sarafan N, Martin JP, Bourguignon J et al. The human inter-alpha-trypsin inhibitor genes respond differently to interleukin-6 in HepG2 cells. Eur J Biochem 1995; 227:808-815.

135. Salier JP, VergaV, Doly J et al. The genes for the inter-alpha-inhibitor family share a homologous organization in human and mouse. Mamm Genome 1992; 2:233-239.

136. Salier JP, Simon D, Rouet P et al. Homologous chromosomal locations of the four genes of inter-alpha-inhibitor and pre-alpha-inhibitor family in human and mouse: assignment of the ancestral gene for the lipocalin superfamily. Genomics 1992; 14:83-88.

137. Diarra-Mehrpour M, Bourguignon J, Sarafan N et al. Tandem orientation of the inter-alpha-trypsin inhibitor heavy chain H1 and H3 genes. Biochem Biophys Acta 1994; 1219:551-554.

138. Gebhard W, Schreitmueller T, Hochstrasser K et al. Two out of the three kinds of subunits of inter-alpha-trypsin inhibitor are structurally related. Eur J Biochem 1989; 181:571-576.

139. Colombatti A, Bonaldo P. The superfamily of proteins with von Willebrand factor type A-like domains: one theme common to components of extracellular matrix, hemostasis, cellular adhesion, and defense mechanisms. Blood 1991; 77:2305-2315.

140. Colombatti A, Bonaldo, P, Doliana R. Type A modules. interacting domains found in several non-fibrillar collagens and in other extracellular matrix proteins. Matrix 1993; 13: 297-306.

141. Bork P, Rohde K. More von Willebrand factor type A domains? Sequence similarities with malaria thrombospondin-related anonymous protein, dihydropyridine-sensitive calcium channel and inter-α-trypsin inhibitor. Biochem J 1991; 279: 908-910.

142. Perkins SJ, Smith KF, Williams SC et al. The secondary structure of the von Willebrand Factor type A domain in factor B of human complement by fourier transform infrared spectroscopy. J Mol Biol 1994;

238:104-119.

143. Lee J-O, Rieu P, Arnaout AM et al. Crystal structure of the A domain from the α subunit of integrin CR3 (CD11b/CD18). Cell 1995; 80:631-638.

144. Chan P, Risler J-L, Raguenez G et al. The three heavy-chain precursor for the inter-alpha-inhibitor family in mouse: new members of the multicopper oxidase protein group with differential transcription in liver and brain. Biochem J 1995; 306:505-512.

145. Enghild JJ, Thoegersen IB, Pizzo SV et al. Analysis of inter-α-trypsin inhibitor and a novel trypsin inhibitor, pre-α-trypsin inhibitor, from human plasma. J Biol Chem 1989; 264:15975-15981.

146. Thoergesen IB, Enghild JJ. Biosynthesis of bikunin proteins in the human carcinoma cell line HepG2 and in primary human hepatocytes. J Biol Chem 1995; 270: 18700-18709.

147. Rouet P, Daveau M, Salier JP. Electrophoretic pattern of the inter-alpha-inhibitor family proteins in human serum, characterized by chain-specific antibodies. Biol Chem Hoppe Seyler 1992; 373:1019-1024.

148. Balduyck M, Laroui S, Mizon C et al. A proteoglycan related to the urinary trypsin inhibitor (UTI) links the two heavy chains of inter-α-trypsin inhibitor. Biol Chem Hoppe Seyler 1989; 370:329-336.

149. Malki N, Balduick M, Maes P et al. The heavy chains of human plasma inter-alpha-trypsin inhibitor: their isolation, their identification by electrophoresis and partial sequencing. Differential reactivity with concanavalin A. Biol Chem Hoppe Seyler 1992; 373:1009-1018.

150. Jessen TE, Faarvang KL, Ploug M. Carbohydrate as covalent crosslink in human inter-alpha-trypsin inhibitor: a novel plasma protein structure. FEBS Lett 1988; 230: 195-200.

151. Chen L, Mao SJ, Larsen WJ. Identification of a factor in fetal bovine serum that stabilizes the cumulus extracellular matrix. A role for a member of the inter-alpha trypsin inhibitor family. J Biol Chem 1992; 267:12380-12386.

152. Chen L, Mao SJ, McLean LR et al. Protein of the inter-alpha-trypsin inhibitor family

stabilize the cumulus extracellular matrix through their direct binding with hyaluronan acid. J Biol Chem 1994; 269:28282-28287.

153. Castillo GM, Templeton DM. Subunit structure of bovine ESF (extracellular-matrix stabilizing factor(s)). A chndroitin sulfate proteoglycan with homology to human IaI (inter-α-trypsin inhibitors). FEBS Lett 1993; 318:292-296.

154. Huang L, Yoneda M, Kimata K. A serum-derived hyaluronan-associated protein (SHAP) is the heavy chain of the inter-α-trypsin inhibitor. J Biol Chem 1993; 268:26725-26730.

155. Morelle W, Capon C, Balduyck M et al. Chondroitin-sulphate covalently cross-links the three polypeptide chains of inter-alpha-trypsin inhibitor. Eur J Biochem 1994; 221:881-888.

156. Enghild JJ, Salvesen G, Hefta SA et al. Chondroitin 4-sulfate covalently cross-links the chains of the human blood protein pre-α-inhibitor. J Biol Chem 1991; 266: 747-751.

157. Enghild JJ, Salvesen G, Thoegersen IB et al. Presence of the protein-glycosaminoglycan-protein covalent cross-link in the inter-α-inhibitor-related proteinase inhibitor heavy chain 2/bikunin. J Biol Chem 1993; 268:8711-8716.

158. Wisniewski H-G, Burgess WH, Oppenheim JD et al. TSG-6, an arthritis-associated hyaluronan binding protein, forms a stable complex with the serum protein inter-alpha-inhibitor. Biochemistry 1994; 33: 7423-7429.

159. Jessen TE, Odum L, Johnsen AH. In vivo binding of human inter-alpha-trypsin inhibitor free heavy chains to hyaluronic acid. Biol Chem Hoppe Seyler 1994; 375: 521-526.

160. Lee TH, Wisniewski H-G, Wilcek J. A novel secretory tumor necrosis factor-inducible protein (TSG-6) is a member of the family of hyaluronate binding proteins, closely related to the adhesion receptor CD44. J Cell Biol 1992; 116:545-557.

161. Blom A, Pertoft H, Fries E. Inter-alpha-inhibitor is required for the formation of the hyaluronan-containing coat on fibro-blasts and mesothelial cells. J Biol Chem 1995; 270:9698-9701.

162. Heron A, Bourguignon J, Calle A et al. Post-translational processing of the inter-alpha-trypsin inhibitor in the human hepatoma HepG2 cell line. Biochem J 1994; 302:573-580.

163. Salier JP, Chan P, Raguenez G et al. Developmentally regulated transcription of the four liver-specific genes for inter-alpha-inhibitor family in mouse. Biochem J 1993; 296:85-91.

164. Daveau M, Rouet P, Scotte M et al. Human inter-α-inhibitor family in inflammation: simultaneous synthesis of positive and negative acute-phase proteins. Biochem J 1993; 292:485-492.

165. Gonzalez-Ramon N, Alava MA, Sarsa JA et al. FEBS Lett 1995; 371:227-230.

166. Fioretti E, Iacopino G, Angeletti A et al. Primary structure and antiproteolytic activity of a Kunitz-type inhibitor from bovine spleen. J Biol Chem 1985; 260: 11451-11455.

167. Lindhout T, Willems G, Blezer R et al. Kinetics of the inhibition of human factor Xa by full-length and truncated recombinant tissue factor pathway inhibitor. Biochem J 1994; 297:131-136.

168. Selkoe DJ. Cell biology of the amyloid β-protein precursor and the mechanism of Alzheimer's disease. Annu Rev Cell Biol 1994; 10:373-403.

169. Mayer U, Poeschl E, Nischt R et al. Recombinant expression and properties of the Kunitz-type protease-inhibitor module from human type VI collagen α3 (VI) chain. Eur J Biochem 1994; 225:573-580.

170. Bearz A, Tolazzi G, Leonardi A et al. Expression, purification and functional characterization of a kunitz-type module from chicken type VI collagen. Biochem Biophys Res Commun 1995; 215:1050-1055.

171. Arnoux B, Mérigeau K, Saludjian P et al. The 1.6 A structure of Kunitz-type domain from the α3 chain of human type VI collagen. J Mol Biol 1995; 246:609-617.

172. Camaioni A, Hascall VC, Yanagishita M et al. Effects of exogenous hyaluronic acid and serum on matrix organization and stability in the mouse cumulus cell-oocyte complex.

J Biol Chem 1993; 268:20473-20481.

173. Powers RW, Chen L, Russell PT et al. Gonadotropin-stimulated regulation of blood-follicle barrier is mediated by nitric oxide. Am J Physiol 1995; 269:E290-E298.

174. Goetinck PF, Stirpe NS, Tsonis PA et al. The tandemly repeated sequences of cartilage link protein contain the sites for interaction with hyaluronic-acid. J Cell Biol 1987; 105:2403-2408.

175. Peach RJ, Hollenbaugh D, Stamenkovic I et al. Identification of hyaluronic acid binding sites in the extracellular domain of CD44. J Cell Biol 1993; 122:257-264.

176. Hardwick C, Hoare K, Owens R et al. Molecular cloning of a novel hyaluronan receptor that mediates tumor cell motility. J Cell Biol 1992; 117:1343-1350.

177. Potocnjak P, Yoshida N, Nussenzweig RS et al. Monovalent fragments (Fab) of monoclonal antibodies to a sporozoite surface antigen (Pb44) protect mice against malarial infection. J Exp Med 1980; 151:1504-1513.

178. Cerami C, Frevert U, Sinnis P et al. The basolateral domain of the hepatocyte plasma membrane bears receptors for the circumsporozoite protein of *Plasmodium falciparum* sporozoites. Cell 1992; 70:1021-1033.

179. Golenda CF, Starkweather WH, Wirtz RA. The distribution of circumsporozoite protein (CS) in *Anopheles stephensi* mosquitoes infected with *Plasmodium falciparum* malaria. J Histochem Cytochem 1990; 38:475-481.

180. Nagasawa H, Aikawa M, Procell P et al. *Plasmodium malarie*: distribution of circumsporozoite protein in midgut oocysts and salivary gland sporozoites. Exp Parasitol 1988; 66:27-34.

181. Robson KJH, Hall JRS, Jennings MW et al. A highly conserved amino acid sequence in thrombospondin, properdin and in proteins from sporozoites and blood stage of human malaria parasite. Nature 1988; 335:79-82.

182. Lawler J, Hynes RO. The structure of human thrombospondin, an adhesive glycoprotein with multiple calcium-binding sites and homologies with several different proteins. J Cell Biol 1986; 103:1635-1648.

183. Klar A, Baldassare M, Jessel TM. F-spondin: a gene expressed at high levels in the floor plate encodes a secreted protein that promotes neural cell adhesion and neurite extension. Cell 1992; 69:95-110.

184. Goundis D, Reid KB. Properdin, the terminal complement components, thrombospondin and the circumsporozoite protein of malaria parasites contain similar sequence motifs. Nature 1988; 335:82-85.

185. Hedstrom RC, Campbell JR, Leef ML et al. A malaria sporozoite surface protein distinct from the circumsporozoite protein. Bull WHO 1990; 68 suppl:152-157.

186. Clarke LE, Tomley FM, Wisher MH et al. Regions of an *Eimeria tenella* antigen contain sequences which are conserved in circumsporozoite proteins from *Plasmodium* spp. and which are related to the thrombospondin gene family. Mol Biochem Parasitol 1990; 41:269-279.

187. Robson KJ, Hall JR, Davies LC et al. Polymorphism of the TRAP gene of *Plasmodium falciparum*. Proc R Soc Lond Biol 1990; 242:205-216.

188. Rogers WO, Rogers MD, Hedstrom RC et al. Characterization of the gene encoding sporozoite surface protein 2, a protective *Plasmodium yoelii* sporozoite antigen. Mol Biochem Parasitol 1992; 53:45-51.

189. Tomley FM, Clarke LE, Kawazoe U et al. Sequence of the gene encoding an immunodominant microneme protein of *Eimeria tenella*. Mol Biochem Parasitol 1991; 49:277-288.

190. Pasamontes L, Hug D, Humbelin M et al. Sequence of a major *Eimeria maxima* antigen homologous to the *Eimeria tenella* microneme protein Etp 100. Mol Biochem Parasitol 1993; 57:171-174.

191. Rogers WO, Malik A, Mellouk S et al. Characterization of *Plasmodium falciparum* sporozoite surface protein 2. Proc Natl Acad Sci USA 1992; 89:9176-9180.

192. Cowan G, Krishna S, Cristanti A et al. Expression of thrombospondin-related anonymous proteins in *Plasmodium falciparum* sporozoites. Lancet 1992; 339:1412-1413.

193. Vanderberg JP, Nussenzweig R, Most H. Protective immunity produced by the injection of X-irradiated sporozoites of *Plasmodium berghei*. V. In vitro effects of im-

mune serum on sporozoites. Mil Med 1969; 134 suppl:1183.

194. Touray MG, Warburg A, Laughinghouse A et al. Developmentally regulated infectivity of malaria sporozoites for mosquito salivary gland and the vertebrate host. J Exp Med 1992; 175:1607-1612.

195. Robson KJH, Frevert U, Reckmann I et al. Thrombospondin-related adhesive protein (TRAP) of *Plasmodium falciparum*: expression during sporozoite ontogeny and binding to human hepatocytes. EMBO J 1995; 14:3883-3894.

196. Scarselli E, Tolle R, Koita O et al. Analysis of the human antibody response to thrombospondin-related anonymous protein of *Plasmodium falciparum*. Infect Immun 1993; 61:3490-3495.

197. Muller HM, Scarselli E, Cristanti A. Thrombospondin related anonymous protein (TRAP) of *Plasmodium falciparum* in parasite-host cell interactions. Parasitologia 1993; 35 sppl:69-72.

198. Wizel B, Rogers WO, Houghten RA et al. Induction of murine cytotoxic T lymphocytes against *Plasmodium falciparum* sporozoite surface protein 2. Eur J Immunol 1994; 24:1487-1495.

199. Frevert U, Sinnis P, Cerami C et al. Malaria circumsporozoite protein binds to heparin sulfate proteoglycans associated with the surface membrane of hepatocytes. J Exp Med 1993; 177:1287-1298.

200. Mueller HM, Reckmann I, Hollingdale MR et al. Thrombospondin related anonymous protein of *Plasmodium falciparum* binds specifically to sulfated glycoconjugates and to HepG2 hepatoma cell suggesting a role for this molecule in sporozoite invasion of hepatocytes. EMBO J 1993; 12:2881-2889.

201. Sinnis P, Clavijo P, Fenyo D et al. Structural and functional properties of region II-plus of the malaria circumsporozoite protein. J Exp Med 1994; 180:297-306.

202. Bork P, Bairoch A. Extracellular protein modules. Trends Biochem Sci 1995; 3.

203. Stanley P, Bates PA, Harvey J et al. Integrin LFA-1 α subunit contains an ICAM-1 binding site in domains V and VI. EMBO J 1994; 13:1790-1798.

204. Huang C, Springer TA. A binding interface on the I domain of Lymphocyte function-associated antigen-1 (LFA-1) required for specific interaction with intercellular adhesion molecule 1 (ICAM-1). J Biol Chem 1995; 270:19008-19016.

205. Diamond MS, Garcia-Aguilar J, Bickford JK et al. The I domain is a major recognition site on the leukocyte integrin Mac-1 (CD11b/CD18) for four distinct adhesion ligands. J Cell Biol 1993; 120:1031-1043.

CHAPTER 8

OVERALL CONCLUSIONS

Approximately 50 distinct VWFA modules included in 27 polypeptides expressed on the cell membrane or in the extracellular space are known to date. The members of the superfamily belong to several classes of proteins playing rather diversified functions and contributing to numerous biological processes, but a large body of experimental evidence indicates that cell-cell and cell-ECM interactions represent their prevailing function (Fig. 8.1).

Several approaches, including the use of function blocking and stimulatory antibodies, synthetic peptides, ligand binding studies with recombinant modules and site-directed mutagenesis have indicated that the VWFA modules contain the sites involved in ligand binding of proteins in which they occur. However, VWFA modules are not the exclusive ligand binding regions of the proteins containing them: experimental evidence accumulated with LFA-1 and Mac-1 suggests that both upstream and downstream sequences[1-3] may participate in ligand binding. A sequential or a cooperative type of binding mechanism can be postulated. For instance, initial binding to the VWFA module may alter the integrin subunit structure and this initial interaction is followed by exposure of other sites and adhesion strengthening. Alternatively, the interaction is mediated by contemporary binding of multiple low affinity sites. That downstream and upstream sequences are important in ligand recognition has been evidenced also in binding studies with recombinant constructs of the malaria sporozoite protein TRAP to hepatocytes[4,5] and in the binding of SSC/CCP and VWFA modules of the complement C2 component to C3b.[6]

Most of the interactions mediated by VWFA modules are heterophilic, meaning here that they occur between VWFA modules and unrelated sequences (Fig. 8.1). Integrin mediated cell-cell and cell-ECM adhesion, as well as migration phenomena, phagocytosis, complement activation, Echovirus infection and parasite infestations, hemostasis and blood coagulation, and finally, the interactions between different ECM components are all heterophilic. However, the interactions between the globular domains of type VI collagen tetramers,[7] which are composed exclusively of VWFA modules, and the vWF dependent platelet adhesion to type VI collagen during the hemostatic process at low shear stress rates[8] are likely to be mediated through homophilic recognition of VWFA modules.

The Superfamily with von Willebrand Factor VA Domains, edited by
Alfonso Colombatti and Roberto Doliana. © 1996 R.G. Landes Company.

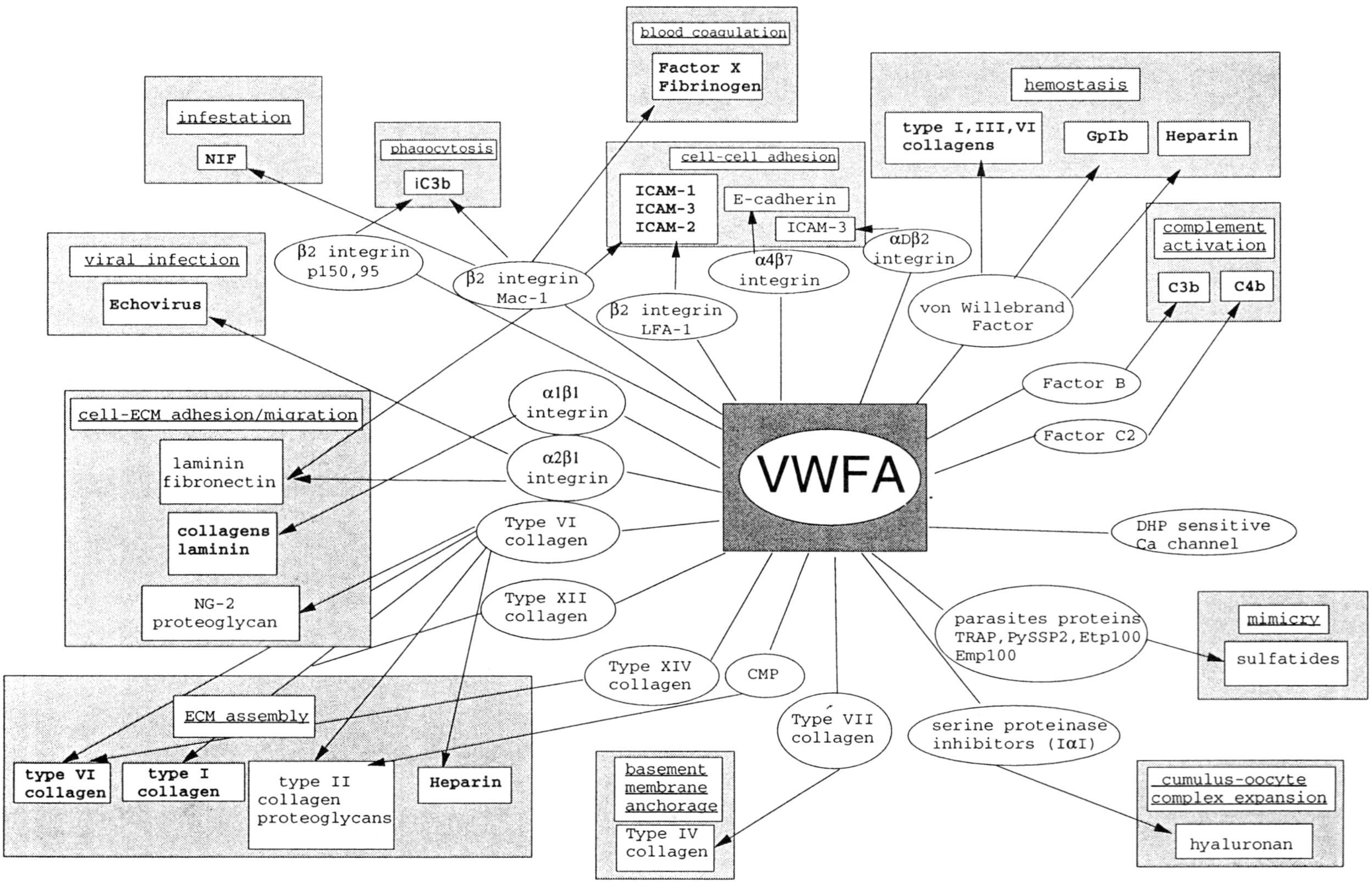

blood coagulation
Factor X
Fibrinogen
infestation
NIF
phagocytosis
iC3b
cell-cell adhesion
ICAM-1
ICAM-3
ICAM-2
E-cadherin
ICAM-3
αDβ2 integrin
hemostasis
type I,III,VI collagens
GpIb
Heparin
complement activation
C3b
C4b
β2 integrin p150,95
β2 integrin Mac-1
β2 integrin LFA-1
α4β7 integrin
von Willebrand Factor
viral infection
Echovirus
Factor B
Factor C2
cell-ECM adhesion/migration
α1β1 integrin
α2β1 integrin
laminin fibronectin
collagens laminin
NG-2 proteoglycan
VWFA
DHP sensitive Ca channel
Type VI collagen
Type XII collagen
Type XIV collagen
CMP
parasites proteins TRAP,PySSP2,Etp100 Emp100
mimicry
sulfatides
ECM assembly
type VI collagen
type I collagen
type II collagen proteoglycans
Heparin
basement membrane anchorage
Type IV collagen
Type VII collagen
serine proteinase inhibitors (IαI)
cumulus-oocyte complex expansion
hyaluronan

The determination of the crystal structure of the VWFA module of Mac-1[9,10] has provided a ground to begin identifying the spatial location of the primary ligand binding sites important for regulating VWFA module-ligand interactions. Due to the well conserved secondary structures among all the VWFA modules,[11,12] it is evident that the tertiary structure of Mac-1 VWFA may serve as a paradigm for the localization of the ligand binding sites within several of the other members of the superfamily. Much information and many questions have emerged from the reported crystal structures: a highly conserved short sequence (DxSxS) and two noncontiguous conserved residues have been precisely located in the three connecting loops at the crevice lined by β strands and α helices that constitute the three-dimensional structure of the module. A cation is present in the crevice and of the six coordination sites involved in ion stabilization, one (in the case of Mg^{2+}) is available for ligand binding (Fig. 8.2). Point mutations in these residues result in abrogation of cation binding to the Mac-1 VWFA module[13] and of the function of Mac-1, LFA-1 integrins and the C2 complement component,[13-15] even when the isolated Mac-1 module is used.[15] The structure of the similar crystal of the Mac-1 VWFA module generated in the presence of Mn^{2+} shows that this cation does not bind ligand associated acidic residues, suggesting that this might represent the inactive form of the module (Fig. 8.3). Crystals of the LFA-1 VWFA modules generated in the presence of Mn^{2+} or Mg^{2+} adopt the inactive conformation.[10] These last two findings are in apparent contradiction with the well known Mn^{2+} stimulation of ligand binding by Mac-1[16] and LFA-1.[17] These two conformations of Mac-1 VWFA modules represent extremes of a dynamic equilibrium. Furthermore, constraints from the ligand(s) and/or other portions of the α and $\beta2$ subunits may affect the transient nature of the activation state. Finally, other cation binding sites are available on the α and β integrin subunits that might bind Mn^{2+} and shift the integrin quaternary structure equilibrium toward the active state.

Although the residues constituting the MIDAS motif are well conserved among the VWFA modules (see Fig. 8.2, chapter 1), not all the ligand interactions are cation dependent. The interaction of vWF A1 module with GPIb and heparin;[18] that of vWF A1 and A3 modules with type I and III[19] and type VI[20] collagens and the homophilic interaction of the globular domains of type VI collagen[6] occurring in the absence of cations, could be explained on the basis of the variant MIDAS motifs of several of these modules. What are then the molecular mechanisms by which these and other VWFA modules bind to their ligands? Moreover, what is the function of the cation in the system? The proposed role of the cation present in the crevice of the MIDAS motif of the Mac-1 integrin is to interact directly with the ligand.[9] Conversely, the three different ligand binding mechanisms of the $\alpha2\beta1$ integrin highlight the multiplicity of the mechanisms of the VWFA-ligand interactions and help delineate their complexity (Fig. 8.4). While binding of the whole heterodimer to collagen is strictly cation dependent,[21] and point mutations in the MIDAS residues of the $\alpha2$ chain abrogate collagen binding,[21] binding of Echovirus is not inhibited by EDTA.[22] Furthermore, the isolated module binds to collagen in a cation independent manner[23] and mutations in the MIDAS residues are ineffective in altering the binding of the mutated module to collagen.

Fig. 8.1. (on opposite page) Overview of the members of the VWFA superfamily and the multiplicity of their interactions. The proteins harboring VWFA modules are circled. The ligands recognized by the various proteins are squared and those for which the interaction is proven to be dependent upon the VWFA module are in bold. Also shown are the functions provided through these interactions.

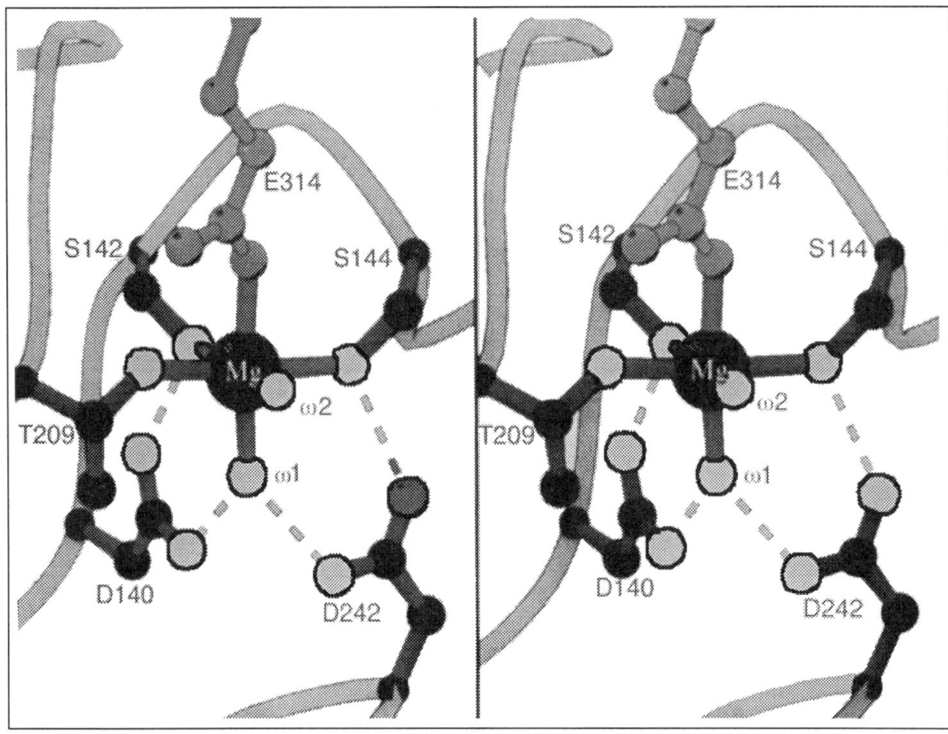

Fig. 8.2. Stereo diagram of the MIDAS motif of the Mac-1 VWFA module. The color code is gray, protein backbone; outlined in black, coordinating oxygen atom; medium gray in center of figure, residue from the ligand/neighboring molecule. Hydrogen bonds are shown by dashed lines. (With permission from Lee J-O, Rieu P, Arnaout MA, Liddington RC : Crystal structure of the A domain from the α subunit of integrin CR3 (CD11b/CD18). Cell 80: 631-638, 1995. Copyright 1995 Cell Press).

Fig. 8.3. Schematic diagram of the VWFA module of Mac-1 in the presence of Mn²⁺. Major conformational differences are shown in black (Mg²⁺) and dark gray (Mn²⁺) while the backbone is shown in gray. β strands are labeled A-F and α helices 1-7. (With permission from Lee J-O, Banckston LA, Arnaout MA, Liddington RC : Two conformations of the integrin A-domain (I-domain) : a pathway for activation? Structure 3 : 1333-1340, 1995. Copyright 1995, Current Biol Ltd).

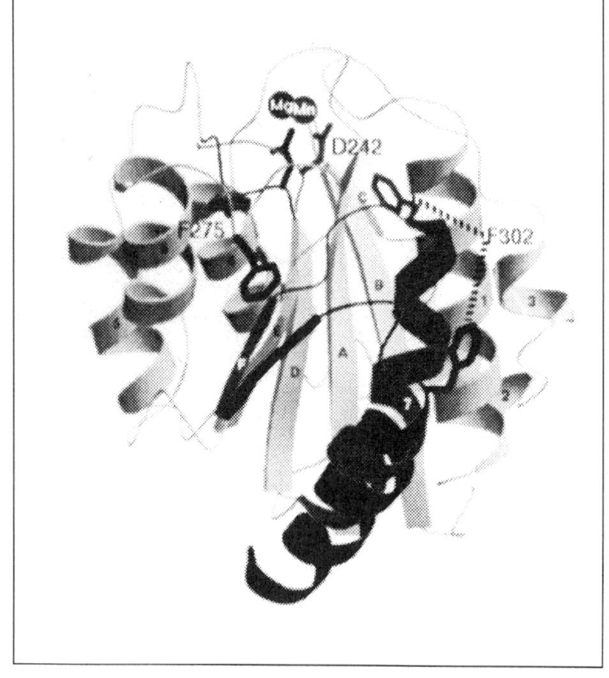

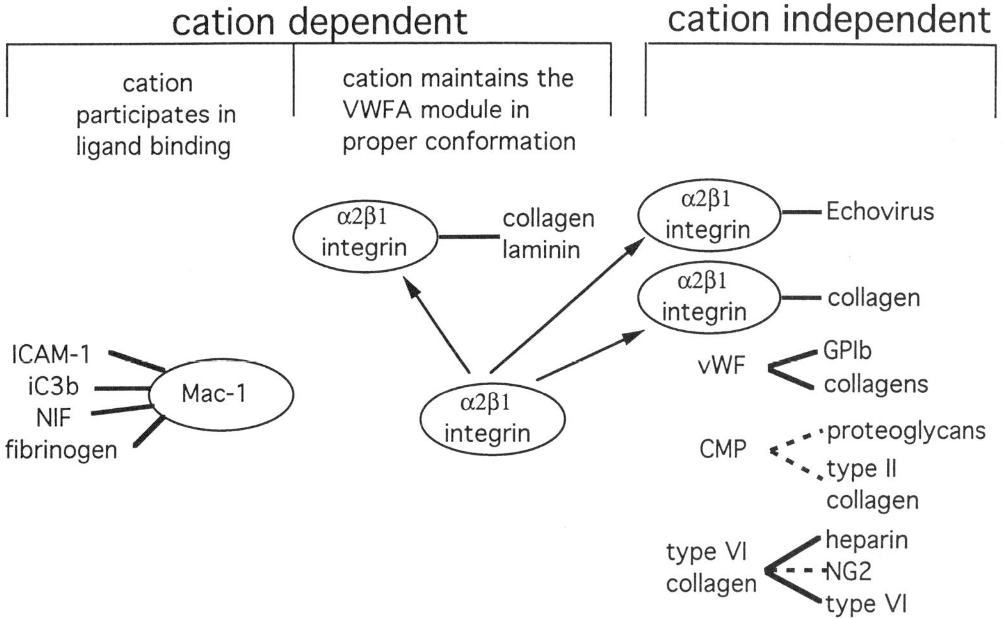

Fig. 8.4. Possible mechanisms of VWFA module-ligand interaction. Partners in which the recognition is mediated by the VWFA module are connected by a bold line and partners in which the interaction is not proven to be mediated by a VWFA module are connected by a dashed line.

Thus, it seems that the cation is not directly involved in ligand binding, as in the case of Mac-1, but contributes to the transition between the active and the inactive conformations of the module. The latter, once isolated from its context, assumes the active conformation able to constitutively bind collagens. It is worth mentioning that ligand recognition by β1 integrins is strictly dependent upon a native triple helical arrangement of the collagen molecules, although also in this case nonlinear acidic residues (Asp, Arg), spatially arranged in different collagen chains, are involved.[24] While the results of the functional role of the isolated modules seem consistent, in light of the above role of α2β1 there is a great need to quantify the binding potency of the isolated modules in comparison with the whole polypeptide chain.

The binding energy of the Mac-1 MIDAS motif for the cation is about one order of magnitude higher[13] than the energies of the non-VWFA containing integrins. The active and the inactive molecules also have about one order of magni-

tude different energies. Apart from the case of the Mac-1 VWFA, no values on cation binding affinities are yet available for the other modules. However, it could be predicted that, based on variations detected in the residues of the MIDAS consensus, differences will be found. Preliminary data on cation affinities of several modules of type VI collagen are in agreement with this hypothesis (Doliana R et al, unpublished).

The lack of cation dependency of some VWFA module-ligand interactions does not imply that the MIDAS residues are not involved in the interaction. In fact, a double mutation of the variant MIDAS motif of the vWF A1 module (D520A-R524A), abrogates the promotion of ristocetin induced binding to platelets.[25] These residues are not directly involved in the vWF-GPIb interaction, but could be part of the ristocetin binding site[26] around the crevice of the three-dimensional structure, and participate in the switch of the conformation of the A1 module toward an active state. Similarly, the segments of the vWFA A1 module affected by type 2B von Willebrand disease[27] that normally prevent vWF-GPIb interaction in the circulation, are distantly located from the GPIb as well as from the ristocetin binding sites if the coordinates of the crystal of the Mac-1 VWFA module are used to build a model of the vWFA A1 module.[25] Residues important in species-specific binding of LFA-1 to ICAM-1 and that define a ligand interface,[2] surround the Mg^{2+} binding site of the LFA-1 VWFA module. Conversely, two of the supposed GPIb binding sites of the vWF A1 module are distantly located from the MIDAS site. Therefore, the elucidation of the crystal structure of the Mac-1 VWFA module is proving beneficial to the localization of the sites involved in direct ligand binding versus those that, by affecting the conformation, play an indirect role.

The recognition of the primary ligand binding, the cooperative and the negative regulatory sites and their detailed positioning in the three-dimensional models of the VWFA modules is prompting rapid progress in the understanding of the structure-function relationships of the members of the Superfamily. The knowledge acquired could provide the basis for development of novel approaches aimed at the selective inhibition or potentiation of VWFA module dependent molecular interactions.

REFERENCES

1. Stanley P, Bates PA, Harvey J et al. Integrin LFA-1 α subunit contains an ICAM-1 binding site in domains V and VI. EMBO J 1994; 13:1790-1798.
2. Huang C, Springer TA. A binding interface on the I domain of Lymphocyte function-associated antigen-1 (LFA-1) required for specific interaction with intercellular adhesion molecule 1 (ICAM-1). J Biol Chem 1995; 270:19008-19016.
3. Diamond MS, Garcia-Aguilar J, Bickford JK et al. The I domain is a major recognition site on the leukocyte integrin Mac-1 (CD11b/CD18) for four distinct adhesion ligands. J Cell Biol 1993; 120:1031-1043.
4. Robson KJH, Frevert U, Reckmann I et al. Thrombospondin-related adhesive protein (TRAP) of *Plasmodium falciparum*: expression during sporozoite ontogeny and binding to human hepatocytes. EMBO J 1995; 14:3883-3894.
5. Muller HM, Reckmann I, Hollingdale MR et al. Thrombospondin related anonymous protein of *Plasmodium falciparum* binds specifically to sulfated glycoconjugates and to HepG2 hepatoma cell suggesting a role for this molecule in sporozoite invasion of hepatocytes. EMBO J 1993; 12:2881-2889.
6. Pryzdial ELG, Isenman DE. Alternative complement pathway activation fragment Ba binds to C3b. Evidence that the formation of the factor B-C3b complex involves two discrete points of contacts. J Biol Chem 1987; 262:1519-1525.
7. Kuo H-J, Keene D, Glanville RW. The macromolecular structure of type-VI collagen. Formation and stability of filaments. Eur J Biochem 1995; 232:364-372.
8. Ross JM, McIntire LV, Moake JL et al. Platelet adhesion and aggregation on human type VI collagen surfaces under physiological flow conditions. Blood 1995; 85:1826-1835.
9. Lee J-O, Rieu P, Arnaout AM et al. Crystal structure of the A domain from the α subunit of integrin CR3 (CD11b/CD18). Cell 1995; 80:631-638.
10. Lee J-O, Bankston LA, Arnaout MA et al. Two conformations of the integrin A-domain (I-domain): a pathway for activation? Structure 1995; 3:1333-1340.
11. Bork P, Rohde K. More von Willebrand factor type A domains? Sequence similarities with malaria thrombospondin-related anonymous protein, dihydropyridine-sensitive calcium channel and inter-α-trypsin inhibitor. Biochem J 1991; 279:908-910.
12. Edwards YJK, Perkins SJ. The protein fold of the von Willebrand factor type A domain is predicted to be similar to the open twisted β-sheet flanked by α-helices found in human ras-p21. FEBS Letters 1995; 358:283-286.
13. Michishita M, Videm V, Arnaout MA. A novel divalent cation-binding site in the A domain of the β2 integrin CR3 (CD11b/CD18) is essential for ligand binding. Cell 1993; 72:857-867.

14. Horiuchi T, Macon KJ, Engler JA et al. Site-directed mutagenesis of the region around Cys-241 of complement component C2: evidence for a C4b binding site. J Immunol 1991; 147:584-589.

15. Kamata T, Wright R, Takada Y. Critical Threonine and aspartic acid residues within the I domains of β2 integrins for interactions with intercellular adhesion molecule 1 (ICAM-1) and C3bi. J Biol Chem 1995; 270:12531-12535.

16. Altieri DC. Occupancy of CD11b/CD18 (Mac-1) divalent ion binding site(s) induces leukocyte adhesion. J Immunol 1991; 147:1891-1898.

17. Dransfield I, Cabanas C, Craig A et al. Divalent cation regulation of the function of the leukocyte integrin LFA-1. J Cell Biol 1992; 116:219-226.

18. Mohri H, Yoshioka A, Zimmerman TS et al. Isolation of the von Willebrand factor domain interacting with platelet glycoprotein Ib, heparin, and collagen, and characterization of its three distinct functional sites. J Biol Chem 1989; 264:17361-17367.

19. Pareti FI, Niiya K, McPherson JM et al. Isolation and characterization of two domains of human von Willebrand factor that interact with fibrillar collagen types I and III. J Biol Chem 1987; 262: 13835-13841.

20. Denis C, Baruch D, Kielty CM et al. Localization of von Willebrand factor binding domains to endothelial extracellular matrix and to type VI collagen. Arterioscler Thromb 1993; 13:396-406.

21. Kamata T, Puzon W, Takada Y. Identification of putative ligand binding sites within I domain of integrin α2β1 (VLA-2, CD49b/CD29). J Biol Chem 1994; 269:9659-9663.

22. Bergelson JM, Chan BMC, Finberg RW et al. The integrin VLA-2 binds Echovirus 1 and extracellular matrix ligands by different mechanisms. J Clin Invest 1993; 92:232-239.

23. Kamata T, Takada Y. Direct binding of collagen to the I domain of integrin α2β1 (VLA-2, CD49b/CD29) in a divalent cation-independent manner. J Biol Chem 1994; 269:26006-26010.

24. Kühn K, Eble J. The structural basis of integrin-ligand interactions. Trends Cell Biol1994; 4:256-261.

25. Matsushita T, Sadler JE. Identification of amino acid residues essential for von Willebrand factor binding to platelet glycoprotein Ib. J Biol Chem 1995; 270: 13406-13414.

26. Berndt MC, Ward CM, Booth WJ et al. Identification of aspartic acid 514 through glutamic acid 542 as a glycoprotein Ib-IX complex receptor recognition sequence in von Willebrand factor-Mechanism of modulation of von Willebrand factor by ristocetin and botrocetin. Biochemistry 1992; 31: 11144-11151.

27. Sadler JE. A revised classification of von Willebrand disease. Thromb Haemost 1994; 71:520-525.